£5.99

This book is due for return on or before the last date shown below.

ADVANCES IN

Surgery

Editor-in-Chief
John L. Cameron, MD

ELSEVIER

PHILADELPHIA   LONDON   TORONTO   MONTREAL   SYDNEY   TOKYO

VOLUME 45

VOLUME 43

Vice President, Continuity Publishing: Kimberly Murphy
Editor: Jessica McCool

Printed and bound by CPI Group (UK) Ltd, Croydon, CR0 4YY
Transferred to Digital Print 2012

Editorial Office:
Elsevier
1600 John F. Kennedy Blvd,
Suite 1800
Philadelphia, PA 19103-2899

International Standard Serial Number: 0065-3411
International Standard Book Number: 978-0-323-08872-5

Editor-in-Chief

JOHN L. CAMERON, MD, The Alfred Blalock Distinguished Service Professor, Department of Surgery, Johns Hopkins University, Baltimore, Maryland

Associate Editors

B. MARK EVERS, MD, Director, Markey Cancer Center; Professor and Vice-Chair for Research, Department of Surgery, Markey Cancer Foundation Endowed Chair, Physician-in-Chief Oncology Service Line, University of Kentucky, Lexington, Kentucky

YUMAN FONG, MD, Murray F. Brennan Chair in Surgery, Memorial Sloan Kettering Cancer Center; Professor of Surgery, Weill Cornell Medical Center, New York, New York

DAVID HERNDON, MD, Professor of Surgery and Pediatrics, Jesse H. Jones Distinguished Chair in Burn Surgery, University of Texas Medical Branch; Chief of Staff and Director of Research, Shriners Hospitals for Children, Galveston, Texas

KEITH D. LILLEMOE, MD, Surgeon-in-Chief and Chief, Department of Surgery, Massachusetts General Hospital; W. Gerald Austen Professor, Harvard Medical School, Boston, Massachusetts

JOHN A. MANNICK, MD, Moseley Distinguished Professor Emeritus of Surgery, Harvard Medical School; Surgeon-in-Chief Emeritus, Brigham and Women's Hospital, Boston, Massachusetts

CHARLES J. YEO, MD, Samuel D. Gross Professor and Chair of Surgery, Jefferson Medical College of Thomas Jefferson University and Thomas Jefferson University Hospital, Philadelphia, Pennsylvania

CONTRIBUTORS

WADDAH B. AL-REFAIE, MD, FACS, Associate Professor of Surgery and Co-Director of the Minnesota Surgical Outcomes Research Center, Department of Surgery, Surgical Outcomes Research Center, University of Minnesota and Minneapolis VAMC, Minneapolis, Minnesota

JOSEPH L. BOBADILLA, MD, Department of Surgery, University of Wisconsin–Madison, Madison, Wisconsin

EILEEN M. BULGER, MD, Professor of Surgery, Department of Surgery, Harborview Medical Center, University of Washington, Seattle, Washington

EVIE H. CARCHMAN, MD, Resident in General Surgery, Department of Surgery, University of Pittsburgh, Pittsburgh, Pennsylvania

HERBERT CHEN, MD, FACS, Professor and Chairman, Division of General Surgery, Department of Surgery; Layton F. Rikkers Chair in Surgical Leadership, University of Wisconsin, Madison, Wisconsin

MARTIN A. CROCE, MD, Department of Surgery, University of Tennessee Health Science Center, Memphis, Tennessee

BARISH H. EDIL, MD, Assistant Professor of Surgery and Oncology, Department of Surgery, The Johns Hopkins Hospital, Baltimore, Maryland

TREVOR A. ELLISON, MD, MBA, Halsted Surgery Resident, Department of Surgery, The Johns Hopkins Hospital, Baltimore, Maryland

DAVID R. FARLEY, MD, Department of Surgery, College of Medicine, Mayo Clinic, Rochester, Minnesota

JOSE G. GUILLEM, MD, MPH, Professor of Surgery, Department of Surgery, Memorial Sloan-Kettering Cancer Center, New York, New York

ROBERTO HERNANDEZ-IRIZARRY, BS, Department of Surgery, College of Medicine, Mayo Clinic, Rochester, Minnesota

JOHNNY C. HONG, MD, FACS, Associate Professor of Surgery, Director, Multi-Organ Transplant and Hepatobiliary Surgery Fellowship Training Program; Director, Living Donor Liver Transplant Program; Director, Liver Transplantation Service; Division of Liver and Pancreas Transplantation, Department of Surgery, David Geffen School of Medicine at University of California, Los Angeles, Los Angeles, California

DAVID B. HOYT, MD, Executive Director, American College of Surgeons, Chicago, Illinois

MATTHEW M. HUTTER, MD, MPH, Director, The Codman Center for Clinical Effectiveness in Surgery; Division of General and Gastrointestinal Surgery, Department of Surgery, Massachusetts General Hospital, Boston, Massachusetts

TIMOTHY D. JACKSON, MD, MPH, The Codman Center for Clinical Effectiveness in Surgery, Massachusetts General Hospital, Boston, Massachusetts; Assistant Professor of Surgery, Department of Surgery, University of Toronto, Toronto, Ontario, Canada

K. CRAIG KENT, MD, Chairman, Department of Surgery, University of Wisconsin–Madison, Madison, Wisconsin

JOHN W. KUNSTMAN, MD, Resident in General Surgery, Yale University School of Medicine, New Haven, Connecticut

HAROLD L. LAZAR, MD, Professor of Cardiothoracic Surgery, Director, Cardiothoracic Research, Boston University School of Medicine; Attending Cardiothoracic Surgeon, Boston Medical Center, Boston, Massachusetts

THOMAS J. LEE, MD, Division of Surgical Oncology, University of Louisville School of Medicine, Louisville, Kentucky

RICARDO LLOYD, MD, PhD, Professor, Department of Pathology, University of Wisconsin, Madison, Wisconsin

ROBERT C.G. MARTIN II, MD, PhD, FACS, Sam and Lolita Weakley Professor, Division Director, Division of Surgical Oncology, University of Louisville School of Medicine, Louisville, Kentucky

SEAN T. MARTIN, MD, FRCSI, Associate Staff Surgeon, Department of Colorectal Surgery, Digestive Disease Institute, The Cleveland Clinic, Cleveland, Ohio

IBRAHIM NASSOUR, MD, Research Fellow, Department of Surgery, University of Pittsburgh, Pittsburgh, Pennsylvania

NANCY A. PARKS, MD, Department of Surgery, University of Tennessee Health Science Center, Memphis, Tennessee

ERIN E. SALO-MULLEN, MS, CGC, Senior Genetic Counselor, Department of Medicine, Memorial Sloan-Kettering Cancer Center, New York, New York

THOMAS M. SCALEA, MD, Francis X. Kelly Professor of Trauma Surgery, University of Maryland School of Medicine; Physician in Chief, R Adams Cowley Shock Trauma Center, Baltimore, Maryland

RICHARD L. SIMMONS, MD, Professor of Surgery, Chairman Emeritus, Department of Surgery, University of Pittsburgh, Pittsburgh, Pennsylvania

C. DANIEL SMITH, MD, FACS, Professor and Chair, Department of Surgery; Surgeon-in-Chief, Mayo Clinic, Jacksonville, Florida

DEBORAH M. STEIN, MD, MPH, FACS, FCCM, Associate Professor, Department of Surgery, University of Maryland School of Medicine; Chief of Critical Care, R Adams Cowley Shock Trauma Center, Baltimore, Maryland

ROBERT UDELSMAN, MD, MBA, FACS, FACE, Surgeon-in-Chief, Yale-New Haven Hospital; Carmalt Professor of Surgery and Oncology, Chairman of Surgery, Yale University School of Medicine, New Haven, Connecticut

SELWYN M. VICKERS, MD, FACS, Jay Phillips Professor of Surgery and Chairman of Surgery, Department of Surgery, Surgical Outcomes Research Center, University of Minnesota and Minneapolis VAMC, Minneapolis, Minnesota

JON D. VOGEL, MD, FACS, FASCRS, Department of Colorectal Surgery, Digestive Disease Institute, The Cleveland Clinic, Cleveland, Ohio

RICHELLE T. WILLIAMS, MD, Department of Surgery, University of Chicago; Clinical Scholar, Cancer Programs, American College of Surgeons, Chicago, Illinois

DAVID J. WINCHESTER, MD, Clinical Professor of Surgery, Department of Surgery, University of Chicago, Pritzker School of Medicine; Chief, Division of Surgical Oncology, NorthShore University HealthSystem, Evanston Hospital, Evanston, Illinois

DAVID P. WINCHESTER, MD, Medical Director, Cancer Programs, American College of Surgeons; Clinical Professor of Surgery, Department of Surgery, University of Chicago, Pritzker School of Medicine, NorthShore University HealthSystem, Evanston Hospital, Evanston, Illinois

KATHARINE YAO, MD, Clinical Associate Professor of Surgery, Department of Surgery, University of Chicago, Pritzker School of Medicine, NorthShore University HealthSystem, Evanston Hospital, Evanston, Illinois

XIAO-MIN YU, MD, PhD, Post-Doctoral Research Fellow, Department of Surgery, University of Wisconsin, Madison, Wisconsin

ALI ZARRINPAR, MD, PhD, Clinical Instructor of Surgery, Division of Liver and Pancreas Transplantation, Department of Surgery, David Geffen School of Medicine at University of California, Los Angeles, Los Angeles, California

BENJAMIN ZENDEJAS, MD, MSc, Department of Surgery, College of Medicine, Mayo Clinic, Rochester, Minnesota

BRIAN S. ZUCKERBRAUN, MD, Associate Professor of Surgery, Department of Surgery, University of Pittsburgh; VA Pittsburgh Healthcare System, Pittsburgh, Pennsylvania

Zero Surgical Site Infections: Is It Possible?
C. Daniel Smith

Does Simulation Training Improve Outcomes in Laparoscopic Procedures?
Benjamin Zendejas, Roberto Hernandez-Irizarry, and
David R. Farley

Hypertonic Resuscitation After Severe Injury: Is it of Benefit?
Eileen M. Bulger and David B. Hoyt

What is the Prognosis After Retransplantation of the Liver?

Ali Zarrinpar and Johnny C. Hong

Screening for Abdominal Aortic Aneurysms

Joseph L. Bobadilla and K. Craig Kent

Novel Management Strategies in the Treatment of Severe *Clostridium difficile* Infection

Ibrahim Nassour, Evie H. Carchman, Richard L. Simmons, and Brian S. Zuckerbraun

Current Treatment of Papillary Thyroid Microcarcinoma
Xiao-Min Yu, Ricardo Lloyd, and Herbert Chen

Use of Computed Tomography in the Emergency Room to Evaluate Blunt Cerebrovascular Injury
Nancy A. Parks and Martin A. Croce

How Important is Glycemic Control During Coronary Artery Bypass?
Harold L. Lazar

Capillary Leak Syndrome in Trauma: What is it and What are the Consequences?
Deborah M. Stein and Thomas M. Scalea

Morbidity and Effectiveness of Laparoscopic Sleeve Gastrectomy, Adjustable Gastric Band, and Gastric Bypass for Morbid Obesity
Timothy D. Jackson and Matthew M. Hutter

Are Cancer Trials Valid and Useful for the General Surgeon and Surgical Oncologist?
Waddah B. Al-Refaie and Selwyn M. Vickers

The Current Management of Pancreatic Neuroendocrine Tumors
Trevor A. Ellison and Barish H. Edil

Who Should Have or Not Have an Axillary Node Dissection with Breast Cancer?

Richelle T. Williams, MD[a,b], David P. Winchester, MD[b,c], Katharine Yao, MD[c], David J. Winchester, MD[c,*]

[a]Department of Surgery, University of Chicago, 5841 South Maryland Avenue, Chicago, IL 60637, USA; [b]Cancer Programs, American College of Surgeons, 633 North St Clair Street, Chicago, IL 60611, USA; [c]Department of Surgery, University of Chicago, Pritzker School of Medicine, NorthShore University HealthSystem, Evanston Hospital, 2650 Ridge Avenue, Walgreen Building, Suite 2507, Evanston, IL 60201, USA

Keywords
• Breast cancer • Axillary lymph node dissection • Sentinel lymph node biopsy

Key Points
• Axillary recurrence rates have fallen dramatically.
• Low axillary recurrence rates relate to improved detection, earlier stage disease, frequent utilization of adjuvant therapy, and possibly targeted lymph node removal.
• Axillary dissection should be reserved for therapeutic removal of clinically evident disease.

THE EVOLUTION OF AXILLARY SURGERY FOR BREAST CANCER

The treatment of breast cancer has evolved from the aggressive approach of radical mastectomy to less invasive breast conservation therapy (BCT). In concert with this evolution, there have been significant changes in the management of the axilla. Radical mastectomy was popularized by William Halsted in the late 1800s, and was the standard of care for the treatment of breast cancer from the 1900s to the early 1970s [1,2]. With this procedure, the breast, pectoral muscles, draining lymphatics, and axillary nodes were removed en bloc (Fig. 1). This strategy was in keeping with the prevailing dogma of the nineteenth century (supported by work from von Volkmann, Moore, Banks, and others) that complete removal of the breast along with the axillary nodes, even when not clinically involved, was the treatment of choice

Disclosure: The authors have no financial relationships to disclose.

*Corresponding author. E-mail address: djwinchester@northshore.org

0065-3411/12/$ – see front matter
doi:10.1016/j.yasu.2012.04.001

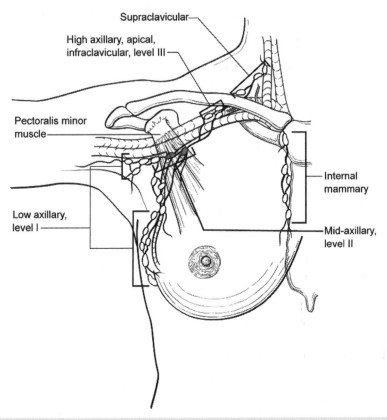

Fig. 1. Regional lymph nodes of the breast. (*From* Edge SB, Byrd DR, Compton CC, et al, editors. AJCC cancer staging manual. 7th edition. New York: Springer-Verlag; 2010; with permission of the American Joint Committee on Cancer, Chicago, IL.)

for breast cancer [1–4]. Specifically, Halsted's theory of centrifugal spread of breast cancer via the lymphatics and deep fascial planes in continuity with the primary tumor justified en bloc removal as the only chance for cure in patients with this disease [5]. Radical mastectomy decreased locoregional recurrence rates from 60% to 80% to 10% to 15% (31.9% in Halsted's initial experience) and resulted in approximately 50% to 60% overall 5-year survival [2,5,6]. However, the procedure was extremely morbid, producing significant disability of the ipsilateral arm as well as chest wall deformity. First described by Patey and Dyson in 1948, the modified radical mastectomy (MRM) included removal of the breast and axillary nodes but spared the pectoralis major muscle [7]. When randomized clinical trials showed no difference in survival for patients treated with MRM, it replaced the Halsted mastectomy as the standard of care [8–11].

The treatment paradigm continued to evolve with the concept of removing only nodes that were clinically evident, particularly as procedures that decoupled the surgical treatment of the axilla and the primary tumor began to emerge. George

Crile, one of the early advocates of breast conservation, championed this approach in the 1960s. Drawing on experiences with other tumors, such as melanoma, as well as observations of the natural history of nodal disease in patients who for various reasons did not undergo an initial node dissection, Crile and others began to selectively use axillary dissection. Reports comparing these cohorts of patients with those treated by radical mastectomy suggested no difference in survival [11–14]. In addition, there was evidence that radiation might represent a reasonable alternative to surgery in the treatment of the axilla [2]. This was the milieu when the landmark National Surgical Adjuvant Breast and Bowel Project (NSABP) B-04 trial by Fisher and colleagues [11] began in 1971. NSABP B-04 found no survival advantage for patients treated with radical versus simple mastectomy, which refuted the Halstedian view of an anatomic, orderly progression of disease in favor of tumor biology defined at the time of diagnosis [2,11]. These results laid the groundwork for the modern era of BCT and axillary surgery utilizing sentinel node biopsy.

Management of the axilla remains an evolving focus of investigation, but is currently dictated by several factors, including the patient's age, comorbid conditions, life expectancy, presenting stage, sentinel lymph node status, burden of axillary disease, receptor profile, and local therapy. These factors are important in selecting one of the 4 surgical management options for the axilla that consist of: (1) observation, (2) sentinel node biopsy alone, (3) sentinel node biopsy followed by axillary dissection, or (4) axillary dissection. During this time of transition, clinical trials have been conducted in multiple areas, creating advances simultaneously in early detection, diagnostic imaging, molecular profiling, surgical techniques, endocrine therapy, cytotoxic chemotherapy, targeted therapy, and radiation therapy. Improved outcomes with regard to locoregional control most likely relate to multiple influences, leading to an overall diminished impact of a single treatment modality (ie, axillary dissection).

SURGICAL APPROACHES FOR THE CLINICALLY POSITIVE AXILLA

There is little controversy regarding the management of the clinically positive axilla, defined as abnormal nodes detected on physical examination or imaging studies. It is widely accepted that patients with resectable disease should undergo tissue sampling with fine needle aspiration (FNA) or core needle biopsy, followed by axillary lymph node dissection (ALND). However, the decision to resect axillary disease also remains contingent on the extent and status of the primary tumor as well as distant disease. The timing of this intervention has also evolved, in part because of the findings of B-04, showing that initial or delayed ALND does not affect survival [10,11]. More importantly, significant advances in cytotoxic chemotherapy, endocrine therapy, and targeted therapy may lead to either a partial or complete response to axillary disease, favoring a neoadjuvant approach, followed by resection. Although it remains the standard of care to resect subclinical axillary disease after neoadjuvant therapy [15], we are moving closer to observation of this group of patients based on increasing rates of a complete pathologic response or considering sentinel node biopsy as a selection criterion to complete an axillary dissection.

SURGICAL APPROACHES FOR THE CLINICALLY NEGATIVE AXILLA

Of the 4 surgical options listed earlier, initial ALND is no longer considered appropriate except in selected circumstances. These include inflammatory breast cancer, in which the false-negative rate of sentinel node biopsy is increased, and unsuccessful lymphatic mapping [15–17]. Contraindications and limitations of sentinel node biopsy are discussed in further detail later.

Observation is an appropriate option for patients with a low probability of developing overt disease, particularly in the setting of competing causes of mortality. This approach is supported by randomized clinical data. In NSABP B-04, patients with clinically negative axillae were randomly assigned to radical mastectomy, simple mastectomy with regional radiation, or simple mastectomy alone. Those patients treated with radical mastectomy had a 40% incidence of pathologically positive nodes, whereas those patients treated with observation of the axilla had an 18.6% incidence of subsequent overt axillary disease [10,11]. A delayed axillary recurrence was not considered as an event in this treatment arm unless the regional disease was unresectable or subsequently recurred again in the axilla. There was no difference in regional recurrence or overall survival between the 3 treatment arms. This study suggests that less than half of all axillary nodal disease becomes clinically evident in the absence of any systemic adjuvant therapy, which was not routinely administered in this trial. Although not considered definitive evidence of equivalence with ALND, the 25-year update of this study has continued to show no difference in overall or relapse-free survival [10].

In a more recent trial comparing the outcome of 435 patients with tumors less than 1.2 cm treated with breast conservation surgery then randomized to axillary radiation or observation, there was no significant difference in the rate of axillary recurrence (1.5% without axillary treatment, 0.5% for those having axillary radiation) after a median follow-up of 63 months [18,19]. Eighty percent of patients received some form of systemic treatment [18,19]. This low rate of axillary recurrence is most likely related to multiple factors, including more favorable tumor biology and the frequent use of adjuvant therapy.

SENTINEL LYMPH NODE BIOPSY

Sentinel lymph node biopsy (SLNB) was first introduced by Cabanas in 1977 for penile cancer [20]. The technique was subsequently adopted for breast cancer by Giuliano and colleagues and Krag and colleagues in the 1990s [21,22]. The basic premise of SLNB is that the first draining node(s) in a lymph node basin reliably predict(s) the status of the remaining nodes. Using blue dye or radioisotope as the mapping agent, the sentinel nodes(s) can be identified and removed. If these nodes are negative for tumor, no further dissection of the axilla is required. The advantages of this approach in the assessment of the axilla are readily apparent. These include less invasive surgical staging of the axilla with diminished morbidity compared with ALND and identifying a subset of patients who may derive benefit from a completion ALND.

Safety and outcomes

SLNB in breast cancer is now a well-established technique, which has been validated in numerous studies, including multiple randomized controlled trials [23–30]. These studies have shown successful identification of the sentinel node in as many as 98% of patients using radioisotope and/or blue dye. The frequency of unsuccessful sentinel node mapping has been shown to be associated with several patient, provider, and tumor factors. Obesity, increasing age, upper outer quadrant tumors, low surgeon SLNB procedure volume, and increased lymphatic/nodal tumor burden all decrease the likelihood of successful mapping [30–32].

The overall accuracy of SLNB is 97% to 98%, with a false-negative rate from 5.5% to 9.8%. SLNB has been shown to be safe, with an incidence of serious allergy (to isosulfan blue) of less than 1% [24,25], 1.25% incidence of skin necrosis (with methylene blue) [33], an axillary recurrence rate less than 1%, and no difference in survival compared with patients treated with ALND [23–25,28–30]. Several large studies have reported a significant decrease in pain, paresthesias, lymphedema, and arm immobility with SLNB compared with ALND. Table 1 summarizes the main findings from several prospective randomized studies examining SLNB.

Indications, contraindications, and limitations

Currently, SLNB represents the standard of care in the assessment of the axilla in patients with clinically node-negative, T1-T3 breast tumors [15,34]. Beyond these general indications for SLNB, there are several clinical situations that warrant special consideration. These include inflammatory breast cancer, locally advanced breast cancer, neoadjuvant chemotherapy, pregnancy, ductal

Table 1
Accuracy and outcomes of SLNB compared with ALND

Study [Ref.] (Number of patients)	FN (%)	Accuracy (%)	AR (%)	Survival (%)	LE	Paresthesias	ROM
Milan Trial [23] (516)	8.8	96.9	0.4→	→	↓	↓	↑
NSABP B32 [24–26] (5611)	9.8	97.1	0.7→	→	↓	↓	↑
ALMANAC [28,31] (1031)	6.7	97.6	0.2→		↓	↓	↑
RACS SNAC [29] (1088)	5.5		0.3→		↓		
ACOSOG Z0010 [30] (5327)			0.3		↓	↓	

→, unchanged relative to ALND; ↓, decreased relative to ALND; ↑, increased relative to ALND.
   Abbreviations: ACOSOG, American College of Surgeons Oncology Group; ALMANAC, Axillary Lymphatic Mapping Against Nodal Axillary Clearance; AR, axillary recurrence; FN, false-negative; LE, lymphedema; RACS SNAC, Royal Australasian College of Surgeons Sentinel Node biopsy versus Axillary Clearance; ROM, range of motion (arm).

carcinoma in situ (DCIS), male breast cancer, patients with a previous history of breast or axillary surgery, and multicentric disease.

Inflammatory and locally advanced breast cancer
Inflammatory breast cancer is a relative contraindication to SLNB. Subdermal lymphatic invasion may inhibit migration of lymphatic mapping substrate, decreasing the accuracy in a patient population that has a 55% to 85% incidence of clinically node-positive disease [35]. In their study examining SLNB after neoadjuvant chemotherapy in inflammatory breast cancer, Hidar and colleagues [16] found an identification rate of 80% and a false-negative rate of 18%. Similarly, Stearns and colleagues [17] in their study of SLNB in locally advanced and inflammatory breast cancers reported an identification rate of 75% with a false-negative rate of 25% in the inflammatory breast cancer subgroup. The data are limited, but given the higher false-negative and lower identification rates, consensus guidelines do not recommend SLNB in this subgroup of patients [15,34–36]. This subset of patients is also at high risk for distant disease and breast cancer mortality. The use of ALND in this group of patients should be reserved for patients showing a complete or significant partial response to neoadjuvant therapy in the absence of distant disease. In addition, most patients presenting with inflammatory breast cancer are not offered surgery as the initial treatment modality. Restaging after systemic therapy should be strongly considered to determine the benefit of any locoregional therapy, including a possible ALND.

The data regarding SLNB in locally advanced breast cancer (T4a-c or N2-3M0 disease) are mixed. Because most of these patients are initially node-positive, many publications focus on the role of SLNB after neoadjuvant systemic therapy (see next section). The accuracy of SLNB for T4 tumors is uncertain, and consensus recommendations do not support the routine use of SLNB in these patients [34,37]. As is the case with patients presenting with inflammatory breast cancer, the initial treatment modality for this patient population should be systemic therapy, followed by restaging. Surgical interventions may offer locoregional control, particularly for those patients showing a complete or near-complete response rate. Aggressive surgical intervention including ALND should be recommended for patients with reasonable life expectancy and long-term disease control.

Neoadjuvant therapy
Neoadjuvant chemotherapy or endocrine therapy is the initial treatment modality for most patients with inflammatory breast cancer, locally advanced breast cancer, or patients not meeting criteria for breast conservation. Debates regarding SLNB and neoadjuvant systemic therapy have been centered on 2 issues: (1) the optimal timing of SLNB (ie, before or after chemotherapy) in patients with clinically negative axillae and (2) whether or not SLNB is accurate in clinically node-positive patients who become clinically node-negative after treatment.

With respect to timing, some have reported a higher false-negative rate after neoadjuvant chemotherapy (on the order of 10%–15%), whereas others report results similar to those with initial SLNB [16,17,34–36,38]. Higher false-negative rates are postulated to be caused by the unpredictable effects of neoadjuvant chemotherapy on lymphatic pathways or by the initial extent of disease, encompassing a broader network of draining lymphatics not accurately identified at the time of lymphatic mapping. A total of 428 patients from the NSABP B-27 trial underwent SLNB and completion ALND after receiving neoadjuvant chemotherapy. The SLNB false-negative rate was 11%, with successful sentinel node identification in 85% of patients and accuracy of 95.6%. The investigators concluded that SLNB was reasonable in this patient population [38]. The 2005 American Society of Clinical Oncology (ASCO) guidelines concluded that there were insufficient data to suggest appropriate timing of SLNB, whereas current National Comprehensive Cancer Network guidelines recommend SLNB before chemotherapy [15,34]. An international consensus panel published guidelines in 2010 stating that SLNB either before or after neoadjuvant therapy was acceptable, but that further study is needed [37].

For clinically node-positive patients rendered node-negative after neoadjuvant therapy, data remain inconsistent [35,36,38]. The American College of Surgeons Oncology Group (ACOSOG) Z1071 trial, designed to address the neoadjuvant therapy setting, has met accrual and results are pending [39]. Currently, axillary dissection remains the standard in this circumstance.

Pregnancy
SLNB was previously contraindicated in pregnant or breast-feeding patients, but recent studies have determined that sentinel node biopsy using radiolabeled sulfur colloid is safe and accurate in this patient population, with fetal radioactivity exposure falling well below recommended thresholds. However, isosulfan blue and methylene blue remain contraindicated during pregnancy and should not be used because of risks of anaphylaxis and teratogenicity, respectively [40,41].

DCIS
Routine axillary staging is not required for pure DCIS unless a total mastectomy or an excision that may compromise future performance of SLNB is planned [15]. Some advocate SLNB with high-grade, high-volume disease or microinvasion seen on core biopsy. If metastatic disease is found on SLNB in what was presumed to be pure DCIS, the disease is upstaged to reflect the nodal involvement and treated accordingly. It is estimated that 10% to 20% of patients diagnosed with DCIS are found to have occult invasive disease [34].

Male breast cancer
Male breast cancer is rare, accounting for less than 1% of all breast cancer diagnoses. Because of this rarity, data regarding SLNB accuracy are limited. Multiple small single institutional studies have reported high success rates for sentinel node identification [42–48]. Controversy continues to exist for the positive sentinel node because most men with breast cancer are treated with mastectomy, not BCT, and

do not receive chest wall or breast irradiation, postulated to be a contributing factor for the low recurrence rates noted in the ACOSOG Z011 trial [49,50].

Previous breast or axillary surgery
The effect of previous breast or axillary surgery on the accuracy of SLNB is unclear. The effect is likely variable and depends on the elapsed time, extent, and location of the previous surgical procedure. SLNB is feasible after diagnostic or excisional breast biopsies, but it has not been well studied in the setting of procedures such as augmentation or reduction mammoplasty. ASCO guidelines cite insufficient data to make any recommendations for or against SLNB in these patients, but suggest lymphoscintigraphy be performed [34].

In addition, ASCO guidelines recommend against SLNB in women with previous axillary surgery because of higher failure rates, but several reports note successful SLNB with recurrent breast cancer [51,52]. Attempted SLNB in this patient population does not increase morbidity and may identify nodal disease in otherwise unsuspected nodal basins as a consequence of previous surgical interventions.

Multicentric disease
SLNB has been successfully used in patients with multicentric disease, with similar false-negative rates as in patients with unicentric disease [53–55]. However, there may be a higher likelihood of additional axillary disease on completion ALND with multicentric disease compared with unicentric disease. In a study of 142 patients with multicentric cancer, 61% of patients with multicentric disease had positive nonsentinel nodes after completion ALND compared with 38% of patients with unicentric disease [56], suggesting a greater burden of disease may be present after SLNB, potentially increasing the benefit of a completion ALND.

THE POSITIVE SENTINEL NODE
After the widespread adoption of SLNB, most reports showed that a substantial percentage of patients with positive sentinel nodes were found to have no further axillary involvement on completion ALND. Adding to the controversy, increasingly sensitive techniques for detecting tumor cells, including finer sections through each node during pathologic evaluation, immunohistochemistry (IHC), and reverse transcriptase-polymerase chain reaction (RT-PCR), led to the identification of sentinel nodes with perhaps clinically insignificant disease, consisting of micrometastatic disease (≤ 2 mm and >0.2 mm or more than 200 cells) or isolated tumor cells (ITCs, ≤ 0.2 mm). For clarity in the remaining discussion, a positive sentinel node refers only to macrometastatic or micrometastatic disease. In keeping with American Joint Committee on Cancer (AJCC) seventh edition staging, ITCs will be classified as pN0(i+) and pN0(mol+) if they were detected by hematoxylin and eosin (H&E) or IHC and RT-PCR respectively (Table 2) [57].

Table 2
AJCC 7th edition TNM staging with pathologic nodal categories defined

Stage grouping	T	N	M
Stage 0	Tis	N0	M0
Stage IA	T1[a]	N0	M0
Stage IB	T0	N1mi	M0
	T1[a]	N1mi	M0
Stage IIA	T0	N1[b]	M0
	T1[a]	N1[b]	M0
	T2	N0	M0
Stage IIB	T2	N1	M0
	T3	N0	M0
Stage IIIA	T0	N2	M0
	T1[a]	N2	M0
	T2	N2	M0
	T3	N1	M0
	T3	N2	M0
Stage IIIB	T4	N0	M0
	T4	N1	M0
	T4	N2	M0
Stage IIIC	Any T	N3	M0
Stage IV	Any T	Any N	M1

Pathologic regional nodes (pN)

pNX[c]	Regional lymph nodes cannot be assessed (eg, previously removed, or not removed for pathologic study)
pN0	No regional lymph node metastasis identified histologically
pN0(i-)	No regional lymph node metastases histologically, negative IHC
pN0(i+)	Malignant cells in regional lymph node(s) no greater than 0.2 mm (detected by H&E or IHC including ITC)
pN0(mol-)	No regional lymph node metastases histologically, negative molecular findings (RT-PCR)
pN0(mol+)	Positive molecular findings (RT-PCR), but no regional lymph node metastases detected by histology or IHC
pN1	Micrometastases; or metastases in 1–3 axillary lymph nodes; and/or in internal mammary nodes with metastases detected by SLNB but not clinically detected[d]
pN1mi	Micrometastases (>0.2 mm and/or more than 200 cells, but none greater than >2.0 mm)
pN1a	Metastases in 1–3 axillary lymph nodes, at least 1 metastasis greater than 2.0 mm
pN1b	Metastases in internal mammary nodes with micrometastases or macrometastases detected by SLNB but not clinically detected[d]
pN1c	Metastases in 1–3 axillary lymph nodes and in internal mammary lymph nodes with micrometastases or macrometastases detected by SLNB but not clinically detected[d]
pN2	Metastases in 4–9 axillary lymph nodes; or in clinically detected[e] internal mammary lymph nodes in the absence of axillary lymph node metastases

(continued on next page)

Table 2
(continued)

Stage grouping	T	N	M
	pN2a	Metastases in 4–9 axillary lymph nodes (at least 1 tumor deposit >2.0 mm)	
	pN2b	Metastases in clinically detected[e] internal mammary lymph nodes in the absence of axillary lymph node metastases	
pN3		Metastases in 10 or more axillary lymph nodes; or in infraclavicular (level III axillary) lymph nodes; or in clinically detected[e] ipsilateral internal mammary lymph nodes in the presence of 1 or more positive level I, II axillary lymph nodes; or in more than 3 axillary lymph nodes and in internal mammary lymph nodes with micrometastases or macrometastases detected by SLNB but not clinically detected[d]; or in ipsilateral supraclavicular lymph nodes	
	pN3a	Metastases in 10 or more axillary lymph nodes (at least 1 tumor deposit >2.0 mm); or metastases to the infraclavicular (level III axillary lymph) nodes	
	pN3b	Metastases in clinically detected[e] ipsilateral internal mammary lymph nodes in the presence of 1 or more positive axillary lymph nodes; or in more than 3 axillary lymph nodes and in internal mammary lymph nodes with micrometastases or macrometastases detected by SLNB but not clinically detected[d]	
	pN3c	Metastases in ipsilateral supraclavicular lymph nodes	

ITC clusters are defined as small clusters of cells not greater than 0.2 mm, or single tumor cells, or a cluster of fewer than 200 cells in a single histologic cross-section. ITCs may be detected by routine histology or by immunohistochemical methods. Nodes containing only ITCs are excluded from the total positive node count for purposes of N classification but should be included in the total number of nodes evaluated.

[a] T1 includes T1mi.

[b] T0 and T1 tumors with nodal micrometastases only are excluded from stage IIA and are classified stage IB.

[c] Classification is based on ALND with or without SLNB. Classification based solely on SLNB without subsequent ALND is designated (sn) for sentinel node, for example, pN0(sn).

[d] Not clinically detected is defined as not detected by imaging studies (excluding lymphoscintigraphy) or not detected by clinical examination.

[e] Clinically detected is defined as detected by imaging studies (excluding lymphoscintigraphy) or by clinical examination and having characteristics highly suspicious for malignancy or a presumed pathologic macrometastasis based on FNA biopsy with cytologic examination. Pathologic classification (pN) is used for excision or SLNB only in conjunction with a pathologic T assignment.

From Edge SB, Byrd DR, Compton CC, et al, editors. AJCC cancer staging manual. 7th edition. New York: Springer-Verlag; 2010; with permission of the American Joint Committee on Cancer, Chicago, IL.

Although studies have shown the prognostic significance of micrometastatic disease compared with those deemed negative with serial sections, the appropriate management of the axilla remains unclear [58,59]. When the sentinel node contains macrometastatic disease, 52% of patients do not have additional disease recognized with ALND. This number increases to 85% in the setting of micrometastatic disease [23,60]. These observations have sparked considerable interest in omitting ALND in this subgroup of patients [61]. In an attempt to assess the likelihood of residual axillary disease after SLNB, a proliferation of predictive models has emerged [62,63]. These models perform fairly well in their predictions; however, they are limited by lack of long-term follow-up and do not address the biologic significance of residual disease.

Several randomized trials were launched to address these questions. The ACOSOG Z0011 trial opened in 1999 with a plan to randomize 1900 BCT patients with 1 or 2 positive sentinel nodes to observation versus completion ALND [50]. The International Breast Cancer Study Group (IBCSG) trial 23-01 began in 2001 and aimed to recruit 1960 patients with micrometastases in 1 sentinel node only to either undergo completion ALND or no further axillary treatment [64]. Both studies failed to meet their targeted accrual and were closed early, in part because of low event rate. Poor accrual was believed to be caused by reluctance to randomize sentinel node-positive patients to no ALND in the early 2000s when these trials were open [65]. However, in the interim, there has been mounting observational data reporting equivalent outcomes for patients observed after a positive SLNB compared with ALND counterparts [61,66–69]. By 2009, a survey indicated that only 23% of surgeons and medical oncologists would always perform ALND for patients with micro-metastatic disease, contrary to published guidelines [70]. A study from the National Cancer Data Base (NCDB) confirmed this change in practice patterns, with a significant increase (24.7% in 1998 to 45.3% in 2005) in the percentage of patients with micrometastatic sentinel node disease who received no further axillary surgery [61].

ALND VERSUS SLNB ONLY: THE EVIDENCE

Potential benefits of axillary clearance in the treatment of sentinel node-positive breast cancer are 3-fold: (1) decreased locoregional recurrence, (2) a possible survival benefit, and (3) additional staging information that may influence adjuvant therapy. We examine each of these in turn with respect to the current evidence.

Recurrence

As mentioned in the previous section, there have been numerous observational studies examining outcomes in patients treated with SLNB only for positive sentinel nodes. These studies were frequently single-institution reports of patients with only 1 or 2 positive nodes who for various reasons (eg, patient refusal or co-morbid disease) did not undergo completion ALND. Although these studies may be limited by selection bias, the striking and consistent finding among them is the low axillary recurrence rates, often less than 1% [66–69]. These rates are lower than the expected values extrapolated from historical data of patients whose axillae were observed (18.6% in NSABP B-04) and multiple factors are likely at play. First, with improved screening, breast cancer is now diagnosed earlier, leading to a lower axillary disease burden. As noted earlier, sentinel nodes are frequently the only involved nodes, raising the possibility that SLNB confers a therapeutic benefit. Also, unlike patients treated in NSABP B-04, most patients are now treated with breast conservation surgery and whole breast radiation, which may reduce regional recurrence rates with inclusion of the lower axilla within the radiation field (see Fig. 1) [50]. Most patients currently receive adjuvant systemic therapy, which may contribute to lower rates of axillary recurrence [71].

ACOSOG Z0011 randomized 891 women with tumors 5 cm or less treated with BCT and whole breast radiation to ALND versus no further surgery after a positive SLNB and found no difference in locoregional control. Regional recurrence in the SLNB only group was 0.9%, which is similar to the rates that were observed in observational studies, whereas the ALND group had a rate of 0.5% [50]. These results indicate that SLNB only is as effective as ALND in achieving locoregional control in this subgroup of patients within the current treatment paradigm of early detection and multimodal therapy.

Survival
The IBCSG 23-01 trial included 931 patients with tumors 5 cm or less with 1 or more micrometastatic sentinel nodes, randomly assigned to either completion ALND or SLNB only [72]. There was no difference in 5-year disease-free or overall survival between the groups. Similarly, ACOSOG Z0011 found no significant difference in 5-year disease-free or overall survival between patients in the axillary dissection versus no dissection groups [49]. These findings are consistent with the survival results of NSABP B-04 [10,11].

Staging
Having already outlined the excellent staging results achieved with SLNB, the 1 remaining potential advantage of ALND is to provide additional prognostic information, which may alter the patient's adjuvant therapy. Historically, the extent of nodal involvement was one of the main determinants of adjuvant chemotherapy or radiation therapy use. However, as our knowledge about molecular markers of the primary tumor (eg, hormone receptor status, HER2 status, 21-gene assay) and their prognostic implications have increased, there has been less and less emphasis placed on determining the extent of nodal metastases. In the AMAROS (After Mapping of the Axilla: Radiotherapy or Surgery) trial, patients with a positive SLNB were randomized to ALND or axillary radiation. Patients in both study arms received adjuvant chemotherapy and hormone therapy at the same rates; thus further knowledge of the axillary status beyond SLNB did not influence systemic adjuvant therapy recommendations [73]. Postmastectomy chest wall radiation or more extensive radiation fields for patients with BCT are currently dictated by the extent of lymph node disease. SLNB surgery alone for node-positive disease may lead to either overuse or under use of radiation therapy in this subset of patients. This may remain a valid argument to consider an ALND until other markers of regional recurrence risk emerge.

Implications and limitations
Overall, the best evidence shows no recurrence, survival, or significant staging advantage of completion ALND over SLNB only in patients with early-stage cancers and 1 or 2 positive sentinel nodes. Given the significant morbidity difference between these procedures, SLNB represents the preferred procedure

in this patient subset. However, some restraint is necessary in these conclusions because of the limitations of the various studies. Both randomized controlled trials directly exploring ALND versus SLNB only in the setting of a positive node closed early because of poor accrual, with less than half the intended number of patients. In addition, both have relatively short follow-up (5 years for IBCSG and 6.3 years for Z0011) and many patients had a low axillary tumor burden with micrometastatic nodal disease (98% of patients in IBCSG trial 23-01 and 41% of patients in Z0011) [49,50,72]. These factors may obscure a small difference between the treatment groups if one does exist. The narrow inclusion criteria of ACOSOG Z0011 limit the extrapolation of the data to other patient subgroups (mastectomy, neoadjuvant chemotherapy; patients with 3 or more involved sentinel nodes, inflammatory breast cancer, locally advanced breast cancer, multicentric disease; patients with prepectoral breast implants or a history of ipsilateral axillary surgery; male breast cancer or pregnant patients) [50]. A major question going forward is whether ALND can be safely omitted in these patient populations. The early results presented from IBCSG 23-01, which included mastectomy patients in its cohort, suggest that observation of the positive sentinel node in mastectomy patients may be appropriate [72]. Nonrandomized data from the NCDB and SEER (Surveillance, Epidemiology and End Results) have been analyzed to address this question as well. In both data sets, women treated with mastectomy had equivalent rates of axillary recurrence (1%) and survival irrespective of observation or ALND after removal of a positive sentinel lymph node [61,74]. It is a safe assumption that if there is an added benefit for a completion ALND in patients undergoing mastectomy, it is low. Debate continues as to the necessity and feasibility of creating additional randomized controlled trials to confirm equivalent or small regional recurrence rates for other clinical scenarios, such as mastectomy, with the current level of knowledge and the accrual challenges observed in the ACOSOG Z011 and IBCSG 23-01 trials.

Other clinical trials have indirectly supported more conservative management for patients with limited axillary disease. In the CALGB 9343 trial, women aged 70 years and older treated with BCT plus tamoxifen were randomized to breast radiation or no further treatment. Sixty-three percent and 64% of the patients in the respective treatment arms did not undergo ALND. The rate of axillary recurrence in both arms was less than 1% and the overall survival was equivalent [75]. These observations suggest that the regional recurrence risk is low with or without the use of radiation therapy. In a prospective study by Martelli and colleagues [76], 354 elderly women were treated with BCT and tamoxifen and no axillary surgery. The 15-year cumulative incidence for axillary disease was 4.2% (95% confidence interval [CI], 2.6%–7%), and the corresponding incidence for women with pT1 tumors was 4.0% (95% CI, 2.3%–7.2%). IBCSG 10-93 was a randomized controlled trial that included patients 60 years of age and older. Four hundred and seventy-three patients were randomized to either breast surgery with axillary dissection or breast surgery alone. In each of the 2 treatment arms, 45% and

Table 3
Who should have or not have an axillary dissection in breast cancer

ALND	No ALND
cN1-N2, FNA or core biopsy confirmed	DCIS, wide excision, no invasion
Initially cN1-N2 or positive SN treated with neoadjuvant therapy	Negative SN with:
	Extensive DCIS, total mastectomy
Inflammatory breast cancer (if patient becomes resectable)	DCIS with microinvasion, excision or total mastectomy
3 or more involved sentinel nodes, BCS	Paget disease with invasive cancer
Positive SN with:	Clinical stage I, II (all with cN0 disease)
Multicentric disease[a]	pN0(i+) or pN0(mol+) sentinel
Male breast cancer[a]	nodes only
Pregnant patient[a]	Initially cN0 and negative SN before or
Plan for PBI after BCS[a]	after neoadjuvant therapy
Mastectomy[a]	
Failure to map SN	pN1 disease established by SLNB in elderly patients or in patients with extensive comorbidities
	1 or 2 positive sentinel nodes with:
	T1 or T2 unilateral, unicentric primary tumor, BCS, plan for WBI, and no neoadjuvant therapy

Abbreviations: BCS, breast-conserving surgery; PBI, partial breast irradiation; SN, sentinel node; WBI, whole breast irradiation.
[a]Consider other clinical factors to support SLNB alone.

44% of the women of each respective arm were treated with mastectomy; overall, only 22 and 23%, respectively, of each treatment arm received breast radiation. With a median follow-up of 6.6 years, the axillary recurrence rates for the 2 treatment arms was similar (2.5% vs 1.0%), suggesting that the surgical treatment (mastectomy or BCT) or inclusion of radiation therapy are not important factors in accounting for low rates of axillary recurrence [77].

Taking a more global view, given the lack of evidence of a significant survival advantage with ALND, the decision to perform ALND should also consider patient and tumor factors. For patients with favorable tumors, significant comorbidity, ages 70 years and older, or those for whom the selection of adjuvant systemic therapy is unlikely to be affected by more aggressive lymph node surgery, observation should be preferentially considered over ALND [15]. With these considerations, the current best answers to the question posed by title of this article, "Who should have or not have an axillary node dissection with breast cancer?", are summarized in Table 3.

SUMMARY

There have been dramatic changes in the approach to the axilla in women with breast cancer over the last 100 years, reflecting the evolution in our understanding of the underlying tumor biology, reduced disease burden because of early detection, and advances in all breast cancer treatment modalities.

The approach to the axilla needs to be individualized, much like the extent of surgery for the primary tumor. Axillary dissection remains an important intervention for patients with more locally advanced disease. However, in patients with early-stage breast cancer, in whom regional recurrence is extremely low, the added benefit of an ALND has yet to be confirmed.

References

[1] Halsted WS. The results of operations for the cure of cancer of the breast performed at the Johns Hopkins Hospital from June, 1889 to January 1894. Ann Surg 1894;20(5):497–555.

[2] Fisher B. The surgical dilemma in the primary therapy of invasive breast cancer: a critical appraisal. Curr Probl Surg 1970;October:3–53.

[3] Moore CH. On the influence of inadequate operations on the theory of cancer. Med Chir Trans 1867;50:245–80.

[4] Banks WM. On free removal of mammary cancer, with extirpation of the axillary glands as a necessary accompaniment. Br Med J 1882;2(1145):1138–41.

[5] Halsted WS. I. The results of radical operations for the cure of carcinoma of the breast. Ann Surg 1907;46(1):1–19.

[6] Lewis D, Rienhoff WF. Results of operations at the Johns Hopkins Hospital for Cancer of the Breast: performed at the Johns Hopkins Hospital from 1889 to 1931. Ann Surg 1932;95(3): 336–400.

[7] Patey DH, Dyson WH. The prognosis of carcinoma of the breast in relation to the type of operation performed. Br J Cancer 1948;2(1):7–13.

[8] Davidson AT Sr. Modified radical mastectomy: treatment of choice in carcinoma of breast. J Natl Med Assoc 1976;68(1):16–9.

[9] Crile G Jr. Primary treatment of breast cancer. Bull N Y Acad Med 1979;55(5):492–7.

[10] Fisher B, Jeong JH, Anderson S, et al. Twenty-five-year follow-up of a randomized trial comparing radical mastectomy, total mastectomy, and total mastectomy followed by irradiation. N Engl J Med 2002;347(8):567–75.

[11] Fisher B, Montague E, Redmond C, et al. Comparison of radical mastectomy with alternative treatments for primary breast cancer. A first report of results from a prospective randomized clinical trial. Cancer 1977;39(Suppl 6):2827–39.

[12] Crile G. Simplified treatment of cancer of the breast: early results of a clinical study. Ann Surg 1961;153(5):745–58.

[13] Crile G Jr. Metastases from involved lymph nodes after removal of various primary tumors: evaluation of radical and of simple mastectomy for cancers of the breast. Ann Surg 1966;163(2):267–71.

[14] Crile G Jr. Results of conservative treatment of breast cancer at ten and 15 years. Ann Surg 1975;181(1):26–30.

[15] National Comprehensive Cancer Network practice guidelines in oncology–V.1.2012. Available at: http://www.nccn.org/professionals/physician_gls/PDF/breast.pdf. Accessed February 1, 2012.

[16] Hidar S, Bibi M, Gharbi O, et al. Sentinel lymph node biopsy after neoadjuvant chemotherapy in inflammatory breast cancer. Int J Surg 2009;7(3):272–5.

[17] Stearns V, Ewing CA, Slack R, et al. Sentinel lymphadenectomy after neoadjuvant chemotherapy for breast cancer may reliably represent the axilla except for inflammatory breast cancer. Ann Surg Oncol 2002;9(3):235–42.

[18] Veronesi U, Orecchia R, Zurrida S, et al. Avoiding axillary dissection in breast cancer surgery: a randomized trial to assess the role of axillary radiotherapy. Ann Oncol 2005;16(3):383–8.

[19] Zurrida S, Orecchia R, Galimberti V, et al. Axillary radiotherapy instead of axillary dissection: a randomized trial. Italian Oncological Senology Group. Ann Surg Oncol 2002;9(2): 156–60.

[20] Cabanas RM. An approach for the treatment of penile carcinoma. Cancer 1977;39(2): 456–66.

[21] Krag DN, Weaver DL, Alex JC, et al. Surgical resection and radiolocalization of the sentinel lymph node in breast cancer using a gamma probe. Surg Oncol 1993;2(6):335–9 [discussion: 340].

[22] Giuliano AE, Kirgan DM, Guenther JM, et al. Lymphatic mapping and sentinel lymphadenectomy for breast cancer. Ann Surg 1994;220(3):391–8 [discussion: 398–401].

[23] Veronesi U, Paganelli G, Viale G, et al. A randomized comparison of sentinel-node biopsy with routine axillary dissection in breast cancer. N Engl J Med 2003;349(6): 546–53.

[24] Krag DN, Anderson SJ, Julian TB, et al. Technical outcomes of sentinel-lymph-node resection and conventional axillary-lymph-node dissection in patients with clinically node-negative breast cancer: results from the NSABP B-32 randomised phase III trial. Lancet Oncol 2007;8(10):881–8.

[25] Krag DN, Anderson SJ, Julian TB, et al. Sentinel-lymph-node resection compared with conventional axillary-lymph-node dissection in clinically node-negative patients with breast cancer: overall survival findings from the NSABP B-32 randomised phase 3 trial. Lancet Oncol 2010;11(10):927–33.

[26] Ashikaga T, Krag DN, Land SR, et al. Morbidity results from the NSABP B-32 trial comparing sentinel lymph node dissection versus axillary dissection. J Surg Oncol 2010;102(2): 111–8.

[27] Krag D, Weaver D, Ashikaga T, et al. The sentinel node in breast cancer—a multicenter validation study. N Engl J Med 1998;339(14):941–6.

[28] Mansel RE, Fallowfield L, Kissin M, et al. Randomized multicenter trial of sentinel node biopsy versus standard axillary treatment in operable breast cancer: the ALMANAC Trial. J Natl Cancer Inst 2006;98(9):599–609.

[29] Gill G. Sentinel-lymph-node-based management or routine axillary clearance? One-year outcomes of sentinel node biopsy versus axillary clearance (SNAC): a randomized controlled surgical trial. Ann Surg Oncol 2009;16(2):266–75.

[30] Posther KE, McCall LM, Blumencranz PW, et al. Sentinel node skills verification and surgeon performance: data from a multicenter clinical trial for early-stage breast cancer. Ann Surg 2005;242(4):593–9 [discussion: 599–602].

[31] Goyal A, Newcombe RG, Chhabra A, et al. Factors affecting failed localisation and false-negative rates of sentinel node biopsy in breast cancer—results of the ALMANAC validation phase. Breast Cancer Res Treat 2006;99(2):203–8.

[32] Sener SF, Winchester DJ, Brinkmann E, et al. Failure of sentinel lymph node mapping in patients with breast cancer. J Am Coll Surg 2004;198(5):732–6.

[33] Zakaria S, Hoskin TL, Degnim AC. Safety and technical success of methylene blue dye for lymphatic mapping in breast cancer. Am J Surg 2008;196(2):228–33.

[34] Lyman GH, Giuliano AE, Somerfield MR, et al. American Society of Clinical Oncology guideline recommendations for sentinel lymph node biopsy in early-stage breast cancer. J Clin Oncol 2005;23(30):7703–20.

[35] Singletary SE. Surgical management of inflammatory breast cancer. Semin Oncol 2008;35(1):72–7.

[36] Chung A, Giuliano A. Axillary staging in the neoadjuvant setting. Ann Surg Oncol 2010;17(9):2401–10.

[37] Kaufmann M, Morrow M, von Minckwitz G, et al. Locoregional treatment of primary breast cancer: consensus recommendations from an International Expert Panel. Cancer 2010;116(5):1184–91.

[38] Mamounas EP, Brown A, Anderson S, et al. Sentinel node biopsy after neoadjuvant chemotherapy in breast cancer: results from National Surgical Adjuvant Breast and Bowel Project Protocol B-27. J Clin Oncol 2005;23(12):2694–702.

[39] National Institutes of Health, ClinicalTrials.gov, ACOSOG Z1071. Available at: http://clinicaltrials.gov/ct2/show/NCT00881361?term=acosog+z1071&rank=1. Accessed February 1, 2012.

[40] Gentilini O, Cremonesi M, Toesca A, et al. Sentinel lymph node biopsy in pregnant patients with breast cancer. Eur J Nucl Med Mol Imaging 2010;37(1):78–83.
[41] Guidroz JA, Scott-Conner CE, Weigel RJ. Management of pregnant women with breast cancer. J Surg Oncol 2011;103(4):337–40.
[42] De Cicco C, Baio SM, Veronesi P, et al. Sentinel node biopsy in male breast cancer. Nucl Med Commun 2004;25(2):139–43.
[43] Goyal A, Horgan K, Kissin M, et al. Sentinel lymph node biopsy in male breast cancer patients. Eur J Surg Oncol 2004;30(5):480–3.
[44] Cimmino VM, Degnim AC, Sabel MS, et al. Efficacy of sentinel lymph node biopsy in male breast cancer. J Surg Oncol 2004;86(2):74–7.
[45] Flynn LW, Park J, Patil SM, et al. Sentinel lymph node biopsy is successful and accurate in male breast carcinoma. J Am Coll Surg 2008;206(4):616–21.
[46] Hill AD, Borgen PI, Cody HS 3rd. Sentinel node biopsy in male breast cancer. Eur J Surg Oncol 1999;25(4):442–3.
[47] Port ER, Fey JV, Cody HS 3rd, et al. Sentinel lymph node biopsy in patients with male breast carcinoma. Cancer 2001;91(2):319–23.
[48] Boughey JC, Bedrosian I, Meric-Bernstam F, et al. Comparative analysis of sentinel lymph node operation in male and female breast cancer patients. J Am Coll Surg 2006;203(4):475–80.
[49] Giuliano AE, Hunt KK, Ballman KV, et al. Axillary dissection vs no axillary dissection in women with invasive breast cancer and sentinel node metastasis: a randomized clinical trial. JAMA 2011;305(6):569–75.
[50] Giuliano AE, McCall L, Beitsch P, et al. Locoregional recurrence after sentinel lymph node dissection with or without axillary dissection in patients with sentinel lymph node metastases: the American College of Surgeons Oncology Group Z0011 randomized trial. Ann Surg 2010;252(3):426–32 [discussion: 432–3].
[51] Intra M, Trifiro G, Viale G, et al. Second biopsy of axillary sentinel lymph node for reappearing breast cancer after previous sentinel lymph node biopsy. Ann Surg Oncol 2005;12(11):895–9.
[52] Newman EA, Cimmino VM, Sabel MS, et al. Lymphatic mapping and sentinel lymph node biopsy for patients with local recurrence after breast-conservation therapy. Ann Surg Oncol 2006;13(1):52–7.
[53] Tousimis E, Van Zee KJ, Fey JV, et al. The accuracy of sentinel lymph node biopsy in multicentric and multifocal invasive breast cancers. J Am Coll Surg 2003;197(4):529–35.
[54] Kumar R, Potenta S, Alavi A. Sentinel lymph node biopsy in multifocal and multicentric breast cancer. J Am Coll Surg 2004;198(4):674–6.
[55] Goyal A, Newcombe RG, Mansel RE, et al. Sentinel lymph node biopsy in patients with multifocal breast cancer. Eur J Surg Oncol 2004;30(5):475–9.
[56] Knauer M, Konstantiniuk P, Haid A, et al. Multicentric breast cancer: a new indication for sentinel node biopsy—a multi-institutional validation study. J Clin Oncol 2006;24(21):3374–80.
[57] Edge SB, Byrd DR, Compton CC, et al, editors. AJCC cancer staging manual. 7th edition. New York: Springer-Verlag; 2010.
[58] Tan LK, Giri D, Hummer AJ, et al. Occult axillary node metastases in breast cancer are prognostically significant: results in 368 node-negative patients with 20-year follow-up. J Clin Oncol 2008;26(11):1803–9.
[59] Clare SE, Sener SF, Wilkens W, et al. Prognostic significance of occult lymph node metastases in node-negative breast cancer. Ann Surg Oncol 1997;4(6):447–51.
[60] Goyal A, Douglas-Jones A, Newcombe RG, et al. Predictors of non-sentinel lymph node metastasis in breast cancer patients. Eur J Cancer 2004;40(11):1731–7.
[61] Bilimoria KY, Bentrem DJ, Hansen NM, et al. Comparison of sentinel lymph node biopsy alone and completion axillary lymph node dissection for node-positive breast cancer. J Clin Oncol 2009;27(18):2946–53.

[62] Van Zee KJ, Manasseh DM, Bevilacqua JL, et al. A nomogram for predicting the likelihood of additional nodal metastases in breast cancer patients with a positive sentinel node biopsy. Ann Surg Oncol 2003;10(10):1140–51.

[63] Katz A, Smith BL, Golshan M, et al. Nomogram for the prediction of having four or more involved nodes for sentinel lymph node-positive breast cancer. J Clin Oncol 2008;26(13):2093–8.

[64] Mansel RE, Goyal A. European studies on breast lymphatic mapping. Semin Oncol 2004;31(3):304–10.

[65] Morrow M. Patterns of care with a positive sentinel node: echoes of an opportunity missed. Ann Surg Oncol 2009;16(9):2429–30.

[66] Naik AM, Fey J, Gemignani M, et al. The risk of axillary relapse after sentinel lymph node biopsy for breast cancer is comparable with that of axillary lymph node dissection: a follow-up study of 4008 procedures. Ann Surg 2004;240(3):462–8 [discussion: 468–71].

[67] Jeruss JS, Winchester DJ, Sener SF, et al. Axillary recurrence after sentinel node biopsy. Ann Surg Oncol 2005;12(1):34–40.

[68] Fant JS, Grant MD, Knox SM, et al. Preliminary outcome analysis in patients with breast cancer and a positive sentinel lymph node who declined axillary dissection. Ann Surg Oncol 2003;10(2):126–30.

[69] Guenther JM, Hansen NM, DiFronzo LA, et al. Axillary dissection is not required for all patients with breast cancer and positive sentinel nodes. Arch Surg 2003;138(1):52–6.

[70] Wasif N, Ye X, Giuliano AE. Survey of ASCO members on management of sentinel node micrometastases in breast cancer: variation in treatment recommendations according to specialty. Ann Surg Oncol 2009;16(9):2442–9.

[71] Buchholz TA, Tucker SL, Erwin J, et al. Impact of systemic treatment on local control for patients with lymph node-negative breast cancer treated with breast-conservation therapy. J Clin Oncol 2001;19(8):2240–6.

[72] San Antonio Breast Cancer Symposium 2011. Abstract [S3–1]. Galimberti V, Cole BF, Zurrida S, et al. Update of International Breast Cancer Study Group Trial 23-01 to compare axillary dissection versus no axillary dissection in patients with clinically node negative breast cancer and micrometastases in the sentinel node. Available at: http://www.abstracts2view.com/sabcs11/view.php?nu=SABCS11L_150. Accessed February 1, 2012.

[73] Straver ME, Meijnen P, van Tienhoven G, et al. Role of axillary clearance after a tumor-positive sentinel node in the administration of adjuvant therapy in early breast cancer. J Clin Oncol 2010;28(5):731–7.

[74] Yi M, Giordano SH, Meric-Bernstam F, et al. Trends in and outcomes from sentinel lymph node biopsy (SLNB) alone vs. SLNB with axillary lymph node dissection for node-positive breast cancer patients: experience from the SEER database. Ann Surg Oncol 2010;17(Suppl 3):343–51.

[75] Hughes KS, Schnaper LA, Berry D, et al. Lumpectomy plus tamoxifen with or without irradiation in women 70 years of age or older with early breast cancer. N Engl J Med 2004;351(10):971–7.

[76] Martelli G, Miceli R, Costa A, et al. Elderly breast cancer patients treated by conservative surgery alone plus adjuvant tamoxifen: fifteen-year results of a prospective study. Cancer 2008;112(3):481–8.

[77] Rudenstam CM, Zahrieh D, Forbes JF, et al. Randomized trial comparing axillary clearance versus no axillary clearance in older patients with breast cancer: first results of International Breast Cancer Study Group Trial 10-93. J Clin Oncol 2006;24(3):337–44.

Intestinal Stomas
Indications, Management, and Complications

Sean T. Martin, MD, FRCSI*, Jon D. Vogel, MD

Department of Colorectal Surgery, Digestive Disease Institute, The Cleveland Clinic, 9500 Euclid Avenue, Cleveland, OH 44195, USA

Keywords
- Stomas • Ileostomy • Colostomy • Indications • Construction • Management
- Complications

Key Points
- An ostomy may be temporary or permanent.
- Prudent utilization of an ostomy at time of surgery may prevent adverse sequelae in the acute or elective setting.
- Appropriate marking of an ostomy site by enterostomal therapy is crucial for construction of a well-functioning ostomy.
- Appropriate use of ostomy appliances and management of complications by skilled enterostomal therapists maximize patient satisfaction and QoL.

INTRODUCTION

The word ostomy, derived from the Latin word *ostium*, means mouth or opening. Surgical creation and subsequent management of the patient with an ostomy encompass an important aspect of the colorectal surgeon's workload. The first recorded surgical ileostomy was created in 1879 by a German surgeon, Baum, to divert an obstructing carcinoma of the right colon. Originally, the ileostomy was created flush with the skin, with severe excoriation of the peristomal skin inevitable. This strategy, allied to the lack of good available pouching systems, resulted in the failure of the ileostomy to gain popularity. As a result of high morbidity (and mortality), an ileostomy was created as a last resort for severe colitis or mechanical obstruction. In 1912, John Y. Brown, a St Louis surgeon, reported a major advance in ileostomy management with the creation of a spouted ostomy; the spouted ileostomy was created from several centimeters of terminal ileum delivered through the lower aspect of a midline laparotomy incision, which was held in place by a surgical clamp. The stoma emptied through a catheter, which was sutured

*Corresponding author. *E-mail address:* MARTINS7@ccf.org

0065-3411/12/$ – see front matter
doi:10.1016/j.yasu.2012.04.005

in place and subsequently removed. The distal portion of the ostomy sloughed off when ischemic and the remaining ileostomy self-matured. The ensuing mucosal eversion produced severe associated peristomal skin inflammation and recurrent partial small bowel obstruction but did produce a more pouchable ileostomy [1,2]. In 1942, George Crile of the Cleveland Clinic described the mucosal grafted ileostomy to circumvent ileostomy dysfunction. The entity of ileostomy dysfunction was described by Crile and Rupert Turnbull as an ileal serositis, which resulted from the caustic nature of the small bowel effluent coming into contact with the serosal surface of the ileostomy. As a result, serosal edema led to ileostomy obstruction. The mucosal grafted ileostomy involved stripping the serosa and muscle from the terminal 3 to 4 cm of the ileostomy, inverting and suturing the redundant mucosa to the skin edges. Unaware of these advances in ileostomy creation, Dr Bryan Brooke of the University of Birmingham, England, described a spouted ileostomy by full-thickness eversion of the protruding distal ileum. This description, accompanied by a single illustration, revolutionized ileostomy surgery and remains the gold-standard, budded ileostomy that remains in vogue in colorectal surgery [3].

INDICATIONS FOR ILEOSTOMY CREATION

Typically, an ileostomy is created to protect a distal anastomosis, relieve a distal obstruction, or to divert stool from pelvic or perianal/perineal sepsis (Table 1). An ileostomy may be temporary or permanent. A temporary ileostomy is created to divert the fecal stream from a distal anastomosis at high risk of anastomotic leak (extraperitoneal colorectal or coloanal anastomosis postneoadjuvant chemoradiotherapy), severe perianal sepsis in complex Crohn disease or after traumatic rectal injury. A permanent ileostomy is used if a restorative procedure is not possible (eg, total proctocolectomy for Crohn disease or a patient with familial adenomatous polyposis [FAP] and low rectal cancer not suitable for a sphincter-preserving procedure). It is helpful when patients

Table 1
Indications for ileostomy

Defunctioning loop ileostomy	End or loop-end ileostomy
Low rectal/coloanal anastomosis	Total abdominal colectomy for medically refractory
Treatment of anastomotic leak	mucosal ulcerative colitis
Relieve distal obstruction–diverticular/	Familial adenomatous polyposis/hereditary
malignant/radiation stricture	nonpolyposis colon cancer with low rectal
Severe Crohn perianal sepsis	cancer total proctocolectomy for Crohn
Rectal trauma/sphincter injury	proctocolitis
Fournier gangrene	
Perineal necrotizing fasciitis	
Complex rectovaginal/rectourethral	
or ileal pouch-vaginal fistulae	
Fecal incontinence	
Fulminant toxic colitis	

are seen by an enterostomal therapist before surgery to mark the most appropriate site for an ileostomy, if one is required. This strategy minimizes potential skin and appliance problems. An appropriate site is marked on the patient's abdominal wall, which is visible in the erect, supine, and seated position. It is essential to avoid any scars, bony prominences, interference with belts or clothing, and classically it should be at the apex of any fat pads. An ileostomy is usually created within the rectus sheath, in the infraumbilical fat pad. In obese patients, visibility is often best by situating the ostomy above the umbilicus. It is worth paying attention to preoperative marking of the ileostomy site because a poorly constructed ileostomy can cause skin excoriation and difficulty with appliance application, and may significantly affect patient quality of life (QoL).

ILEOSTOMY PHYSIOLOGY

Ileostomy output is directly related to how distal the ostomy is located. The more proximal the ostomy, the less surface area that is available for water and electrolyte absorption [4,5]. After ileostomy creation, the output is initially bilious in color and watery. With resumption of diet, the ostomy output thickens. Typically, the consistency of the output is soft but can be affected by food and fluid intake, medications, active Crohn disease, adhesions, and radiation therapy. In patients in whom a substantial length of small bowel has been resected, output can be watery and patients may be prone to dehydration. Occasionally, short bowel syndrome may ensue, requiring input from an intestinal rehabilitation team and total parenteral nutrition (TPN) may be required. Patients with an ileostomy can often recognize undigested foodstuffs in the ileostomy output. Classically, corn, other vegetables, nuts, and certain pills may be secreted wholly undigested.

Ileostomy output ranges from 500 to 700 mL per day. In the fasting state, this amount may be reduced by half. A normally functioning, healthy ileostomy may have an output of 1000 to 1500 mL. An output more than 1500 mL is considered excessive and may provoke dehydration [6,7]. Reduced oral fluid intake may reduce ileostomy output and make it thicker. Increased fluid intake and high fat content foods increase output and fluidity. There are few dietary restrictions on a patient with an ileostomy [8,9]; in the first few months after surgery, patients are advised to consume a low-fiber diet because small bowel edema after surgery makes absorption of fiber difficult. An ileostomy periodically empties throughout the day, with output increased after eating and drinking. Small bowel transit is delayed after proctocolectomy; the pathophysiology underpinning this is poorly understood, but it likely occurs secondary to mucosal hypertrophy, which compensates for decreased absorptive capacity. Transit time may be further retarded by drugs such as diphenoxylate-atropine (Lomotil), loperamide (Imodium), codeine, or tincture of opium, which act on intestinal mucosal opioid receptors to decrease activity of the myenteric plexus, resulting in relaxation of smooth muscle in the small bowel wall. This situation increases the amount of time substances stay in the intestine, allowing for more water to be absorbed [10,11]. An ileostomy should not interfere with the patient's nutrition because the colon and rectum have little or no absorptive capacity. If the distal ileum remains intact, nutrition status is largely unaffected. However, if a meter or two of the terminal ileum is resected fat, fat-soluble vitamins and bile acids are not resorbed. As a result, vitamin B_{12} deficiency can occur, producing a macrocytic or pernicious anemia [12]. Such patients require monthly adjunctive intramuscular B_{12} therapy. Similarly, failure to absorb bile salts can predispose to cholelithiasis, depending on the extent of small bowel disease (Crohn) or extent of resection [12]. Cholestyramine (Questran), a bile salt binding resin, may be useful in this situation. Urolithiasis may also be observed after ileostomy formation as a consequence of chronic dehydration and the urine being more acidic. This situation can be circumvented by counseling the patient on appropriate fluid intake and adding 4 g of sodium bicarbonate to the diet to alkalinize the urine [13,14].

ENTEROSTOMAL THERAPY

The concept of enterostomal therapy originated from the Cleveland Clinic in the late 1950s. Norma Gill, the first enterostomal therapist, underwent a colectomy and end ileostomy by Dr Rupert Turnbull at the Cleveland Clinic for refractory colitis. Subsequently, she developed an interest in ostomy management and in 1958 was appointed by Turnbull to care for patients with an ostomy. As the popularity of ileostomy surgery increased, and with it, the need for specially trained enterostomal therapists, the first school of enterostomal therapy was opened at the Cleveland Clinic in 1961. The United Ostomy Association was born in 1968 and Norma Gill was its first secretary. Today, enterostomal therapists play a crucial role in the preoperative assessment of, and postoperative management of, patients with an ileostomy. Colorectal surgeons should also be familiar with the preoperative assessment for ileostomy because in the emergent setting, enterostomal therapists may be unavailable for ostomy marking. A well-placed ileostomy is associated with better functional outcomes, less morbidity, and improved patient QoL [15–17].

END ILEOSTOMY

Indications for end ileostomy are listed in Table 1. When preparing the end of the ileum for creation of the ileostomy, it is important to be able to bring the well-vascularized ileum through the abdominal wall without tension. The opening in the peritoneum and fascia must be sufficient to allow the small bowel to be delivered through the abdominal wall. Otherwise, a small peritoneal or fascial opening can obstruct the small bowel lumen and potentially strangulate the blood supply to the end of the ileum, causing stoma ischemia and, occasionally, necrosis. Before closing the abdominal incision, the stoma aperture is created at the premarked skin site. A Kocher clamp is placed on the fascia of the abdominal wall and another placed on the skin to keep all of the abdominal wall components in-line, preventing angulation of the bowel as it passes through the abdominal wall. The operating surgeon places traction on the clamps, gently drawing them medially. A folded sponge is then placed beneath the ileostomy site in the abdomen and the abdominal wall is tented up from within. A disk of skin is then excised from the ileostomy site. Typically, we do not excise much subcuticular fat because it provides support for the ileostomy. The first assistant retracts the skin and subcuticular fat with right angle retractors as the surgeon uses electrocautery to expose the fascia. While maintaining upward tension on the abdominal wall using the left hand, the surgeon incises the fascia in a longitudinal manner. On exposure of the underlying rectus muscle, a straight scissors or Kelly clamp is used to split the muscle, taking care to avoid the inferior epigastric vessels. The assistant then repositions the right angle retractors to expose the parietal peritoneum. Using the electrocautery, the surgeon opens the peritoneum on to the sponge held within the abdomen. A large Kelly or Babcock clamp is placed through the aperture from the skin into the abdominal cavity, the abdominal wall is leveled anteriorly using the clamp, and the internal (peritoneal) opening is visualized. If the opening is deemed too small, it can be incised from within the abdomen using electrocautery. The ileal mesentery is rechecked to ensure good blood supply to the terminal ileum. A Babcock grasper is then passed through the skin aperture, and the ileostomy is grasped and delivered on to the surface of the skin. This procedure is facilitated by gently delivering the ileum through the abdominal wall opening from within the abdomen. Next, it is critical to check the orientation of the ileal mesentery by following the cut end down to its origin from the third part of the duodenum. The ileal mesentery abutting the abdominal wall is then sutured to the parietal peritoneum to prevent volvulus around the ileostomy. Typically, 4 to 5 cm of ileum should protrude above the level of the skin on the abdominal wall to ensure an appropriately spouted end ileostomy. We secure the ileostomy in its position by applying a Babcock grasper to the end of the ileum and securing it in place with a towel clamp. Before proceeding to close the abdomen, we once again check the orientation of the ileostomy and ensure an appropriate blood supply.

The ileostomy is then matured using 4 or 5 everting full-thickness absorbable sutures to the subcuticular portion of the skin. These sutures are tagged and tied in turn. It is important that the sutures do not pass through the skin because this may result in mucosal islands forming adjacent to the ostomy, which can weep and cause peristomal skin irritation. We often take a serosal bite on the ileostomy at skin level to facilitate ostomy eversion, but may avoid this when there is concern that it will predispose to fistula formation between the ileostomy and the skin, such as in patients with ileal Crohn disease. The ostomy is matured with a 2-cm to 3-cm spout by placing traction on the tagged sutures and everting the serosal surface of the ileum. The sutures are tied perpendicular to the small bowel wall. If additional sutures are required to bury redundant fat, they can easily be placed between the ostomy and the subcuticular portion of the skin (Fig. 1). The stoma appliance is then placed after the abdominal wound has been dressed. The faceplate is cut approximately 7 to 8 mm larger than the diameter of the ostomy to allow for ostomy edema, which is inevitable.

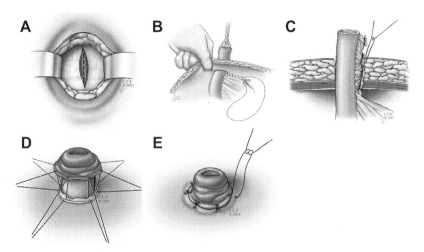

Fig. 1. (A–E) Creating an end ileostomy. The peritoneum is incised longitudinally, the ileum delivered through the interior abdominal wall and sutured in place with everting sutures. (*Reprinted* with permission, Cleveland Clinic Center for Medical Art & Photography © 2009–2012. All Rights Reserved.)

Occasionally, it may be difficult to construct an end ileostomy in an obese patient because of the depth of the abdominal pannus. In such circumstances, it is prudent to construct a loop end ileostomy (Fig. 2). This technique, first described by Unti and colleagues [18], allows construction of an ostomy, minimizing undue tension and preventing shearing of the small bowel mesentery. The loop end ileostomy may be constructed by first closing the end of the

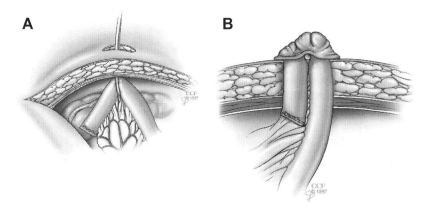

Fig. 2. (A, B) The loop-end ileostomy. A loop of small bowel is delivered through the anterior abdominal wall with the stapled cut end sitting beneath the stoma aperture. The ostomy is matured as a loop stoma. (*Reprinted* with permission, Cleveland Clinic Center for Medical Art & Photography © 2009–2012. All Rights Reserved.)

ileum with a linear stapler; orienting marking sutures are placed, the bowel delivered through the abdominal wall, and the stoma matured in the manner described in the next section for a loop ileostomy.

LOOP ILEOSTOMY

Indications for loop ileostomy are listed in Table 1. The commonest indication for a loop ileostomy is to protect a distal anastomosis. For many years, a loop colostomy was used to protect left-sided anastomoses; however, many data have now emerged to support the superiority of a loop ileostomy in terms of parastomal herniae, appliance leakage, skin problems, and complications at time of ostomy reversal [19–22]. A loop ileostomy is created 12 to 15 cm from the ileocecal valve. When an ileostomy is used to defunction an ileal pouch-anal anastomosis, the ostomy is often more proximal to avoid tension on the pouch-anal anastomosis. Occasionally, it is necessary to divide thin, flimsy adhesions between the terminal ileum, retroperitoneum, and pelvic side-wall to allow a loop of ileum to reach the abdominal wall. Once the appropriate loop of small bowel has been chosen, a Kelly clamp is placed through the mesenteric edge and an umbilical tape passed underneath to encircle the bowel lumen. The proximal and distal limbs of the loop are then marked. We routinely place a 3/0 chromic catgut suture distally and a 3/0 Vicryl suture proximally (brown for the earth [ie, down or distal] and blue for the sky [ie, upward or proximal]). The aperture in the abdominal wall is created as described earlier. A Kelly clamp is then passed through the channel into the abdomen, and the umbilical tape is grasped and gently milked through the abdominal wall by gentle pressure from within the abdomen. We then remove the umbilical tape and place a plastic rod beneath the ostomy through the mesenteric defect created by the umbilical tape. The rod is held in place by 2 small Babcock clamps. Again, it is important to ensure that the ostomy has not twisted and that correct orientation of proximal and distal limbs is confirmed before the abdomen is closed. After closure and covering of the abdominal wound with an appropriate dressing, the ileostomy is opened and matured. Electrocautery is used to open the ileum, at the level of the skin, distally. Approximately 80% of the circumference of the ileum is opened, leaving a bridge of the posterior wall intact between the afferent and efferent limbs. The distal limb of the ostomy, oriented caudally, is secured to the subcuticular portion of the skin with an absorbable suture. Typically, 3 sutures are required on the distal limb. Initially, 3 sutures are also placed on the proximal limb; these full-thickness everting absorbable sutures are passed through the subcuticular portion of the skin, and tagged. The proximal limb of the ostomy is spouted by placing gentle traction on the tagged sutures and everting the serosal surface of the afferent limb. The sutures are then sequentially tied perpendicular to the ostomy (Fig. 3). Two further sutures may be placed between these sutures to complete maturation of the spouted afferent limb of the stoma. A transparent appliance is applied as described earlier, which allows for inspection of the ileostomy in the postoperative period.

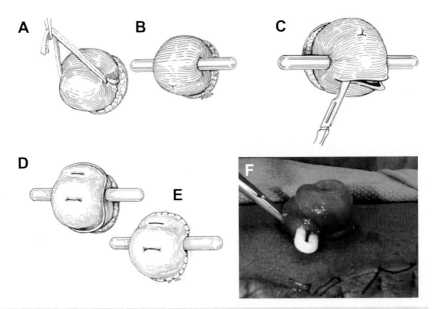

Fig. 3. (A–F) Loop ileostomy. Steps in the creation of an end ileostomy. The ileum is delivered on to the anterior abdominal wall, secured with a glass or plastic rod, opened along the distal limb, and everting sutures are placed. ([A–E] Reprinted with permission, Cleveland Clinic Center for Medical Art & Photography © 2009–2012. All Rights Reserved.)

LAPAROSCOPIC ILEOSTOMY

A minimally invasive approach can be used to construct a defunctioning stoma. Often, the use of laparoscopy is to simply confirm ostomy orientation when essentially creating a trephine ileostomy. Access to the peritoneal cavity is secured using either the Hasson technique or with a Veress needle. After establishment of pneumoperitoneum, the right lower quadrant is addressed. Typically, the distal ileum is sufficiently mobile to allow a segment of small bowel, 12 to 15 cm from the ileocecal valve, to be delivered on to the abdominal wall. If necessary, the ileum is mobilized from the right lower quadrant or lateral pelvic sidewall using sharp scissors dissection. A Babcock grasper is used to identify the segment of small bowel that has been selected for exteriorization. It is crucial to deflate the abdominal cavity before creation of the ileostomy site because the concavity insufflated abdomen may distort the surgeon's perception of the optimal site for ostomy creation. The skin of the abdominal wall is incised, the fascia incised, and the peritoneum exposed as described earlier. The peritoneum is then opened and a Babcock grasper is used to grasp the small bowel and gently deliver it on to the abdominal wall. A rod is then placed beneath the ostomy. Pneumoperitoneum is then reestablished to confirm that the ostomy is correctly oriented. Alternatively, some surgeons orient the afferent and efferent limbs of the small bowel using Vicryl Endoloops (Ethicon

Endo-surgery Inc., Blue Ash, OH, USA); the knot on the Endoloop is secured on the terminal ileal mesentery, and the tail of the sutures are cut long and short to mark the proximal and distal limbs of the ostomy. When using this technique, it remains important to establish pneumoperitoneum and confirm that the ostomy has not twisted. Pneumoperitoneum is then released and the ostomy matured in the usual fashion. Many data support a minimally invasive approach to creation of a defunctioning loop ileostomy [23–25], although it has been suggested that laparoscopic ileostomy may be associated with more frequent complications (obstruction, torsion of the small bowel around the ileostomy) than ileostomies created at time of open surgery [26].

SINGLE-PORT ILEOSTOMY

The advent of single-incision laparoscopic surgery (SILS) has many applications in colorectal surgery. For creation of a loop ileostomy, SILS is a particularly attractive option because it essentially creates the ileostomy at the surgical incision site, hence the term scarless or incisionless surgery. The enterostomal therapist marks the site on the abdominal wall (typically the right lower quadrant) that is most appropriate for siting the ostomy. A disk of skin is excised around the premarked ostomy site. The anterior fascial layer is incised longitudinally, the rectus muscle split, and the peritoneum is exposed. The peritoneum is then incised longitudinally and the SILS port is inserted into the abdominal cavity. CO_2 pneumoperitoneum is then established and the abdominal cavity surveyed. A flexible laparoscope is used because it allows 360° viewing without unnecessary movement of the laparoscope. The additional operating trocars are then used to manipulate the bowel. Typically, we use a 5-mm and a 10-mm trocar. The small bowel is then approached. An ileostomy is best created approximately 15 cm from the ileocecal junction. The orientation of the proximal and distal limbs of the small bowel is then confirmed. As described earlier, the afferent and efferent limbs can be marked by applying Vicryl Endoloops to the mesentery of the bowel and cutting the tail of the sutures long and short to identify afferent and efferent limbs of the small bowel. Alternatively, a Babcock grasper is used to grasp the small bowel and the SILS access device is removed while the Babcock grasper is used to deliver the small bowel on to the anterior abdominal wall. The ileostomy is then matured in the usual fashion.

ILEOSTOMY COMPLICATIONS AND THEIR MANAGEMENT

Many patients suffer a complication related to their ostomy. Frequently, complication rates are underestimated because of the lack of a clear definition as to what constitutes a complication. Complications can be classified as early (perioperative) or late, functional, physiologic, or psychological. Complications related to an ostomy can be minimized by paying careful attention to detail when surgically creating an ostomy. This strategy produces the best outcome for the patient, and a well-functioning ostomy is associated with a superior QoL compared with ileostomates with a poorly functioning stoma. Surgeons often report only structural complications related to the ostomy creation (obstruction, prolapse, retraction, or herniae), whereas most patients with an ostomy have peristomal skin problems at some point in their life with an ostomy. Between 10% and 70% of patients have a complication related to their ostomy [27].

PERISTOMAL SKIN PROBLEMS

Peristomal skin problems are common with a poorly constructed ileostomy. If an ostomy is retracted, the alkaline effluent may not be appropriately pouched and can irritate the surrounding skin. Use of convex appliances and a belt can help to evert or spout a retracting ileostomy. Similarly, suturing the ileal mucosa directly to the skin rather than the subcuticular tissue can lead to mucosal implantation, which can weep (Fig. 4); this can make it difficult to secure the appliance and as a result allow spillage of effluent on to the peristomal skin. Similarly, poorly sited ileostomies, sited in abdominal creases or below the umbilicus in obese patients, are prone to develop skin problems. Obesity is commonly identified as a risk factor for ileostomy complications [28,29] and thus due consideration to preoperative marking must be given in this cohort of patients. It is important that the faceplate is appropriately fitted by an enterostomal therapist. Patient education is also important because an ileostomy needs to be emptied at regular intervals to prevent pooling of small bowel effluent in the base of the pouch, which can irritate the skin. Appropriate input from enterostomal therapy has been implicated in reducing postoperative complications after ileostomy surgery [29]. Older patients may have difficulty with pouching and emptying their ostomy, so family members must also be familiar with ostomy care. Nugent and colleagues [30], in assessing QoL after

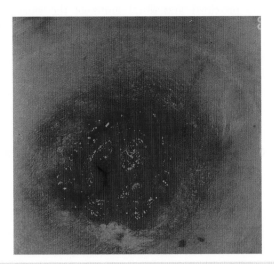

Fig. 4. Mucosal implants surrounding an end ileostomy.

ostomy creation, detail skin problems under or around the ileostomy appliance in 61% of their cohort (n = 141). Of their patients, 57% had difficulty with leakage around the appliance, most of which was caused by failure of the appliance to adhere to the skin. Lefort and colleagues [31] reported peristomal skin problems in 43% of their cohort 1 year after surgery. Law and colleagues [15] in performing a randomized controlled trial comparing defunctioning ileostomy with colostomy after low anterior resection found that only 18.3% of their ileostomy cohort had skin problems 18 months after surgery. Peristomal fungal infections are frequently encountered and appear as peristomal erythema with associated satellite lesions (Figs. 5 and 6). These infections are successfully treated with topical antifungal agents, which are then covered by a sealant, allowed to dry, and the appliance can then be placed. Contact dermatitis typically conforms to the outline of the stoma appliance and is often secondary to an allergic reaction to the constituents of the wafer of the ileostomy device and responds to changing the appliance (Fig. 7). Topical steroids can also be rubbed on the skin but often interfere with appliance adherence. Peristomal ulceration (Figs. 8 and 9) may be seen in association with pyoderma gangrenosum in patients with inflammatory bowel disease. These lesions may be treated with topical, oral, or intralesional steroids depending on the extent of ulceration [32]. The goal of therapy is to keep the ulcerated area dry to allow an appliance to be placed. Application of stoma or antibiotic powder covered by a hydrocolloid usually suffices. Pressure from an ileostomy belt must be avoided. Alternatively, if the ulcer is moist, a foam dressing may be used.

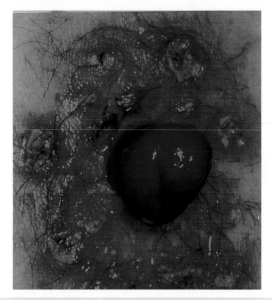

Fig. 5. Peristomal folliculitis.

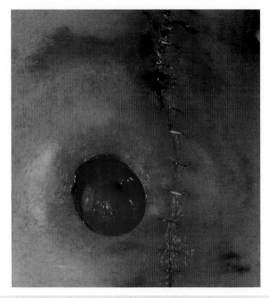

Fig. 6. Peristomal *Candida.*

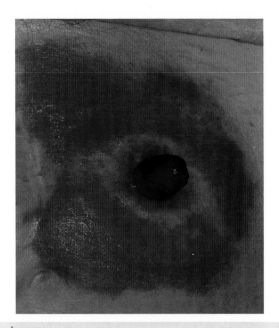

Fig. 7. Contact dermatitis.

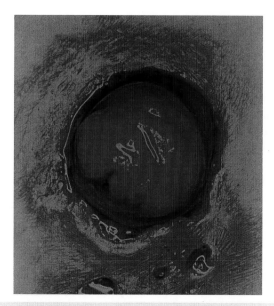

Fig. 8. Peristomal ulceration.

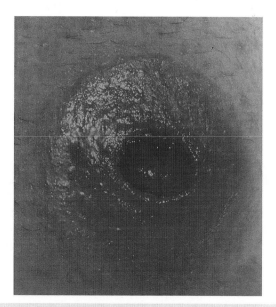

Fig. 9. Skin irritation around a leaking pouch appliance.

More severe disease typically requires further intervention. Data to support immunosuppression with cyclosporine or infliximab are weak [32,33]. Level 1 evidence is lacking, although a prospective randomized controlled trial from the United Kingdom has suggested some benefit from antitumor necrosis factor α therapy to treat pyoderma [34]. These results must be tempered by the small number of patients in the trial (n = 26).

When the pyoderma is severe, surgeons often resite the ostomy, but frequently pyoderma recurs at the new ostomy site. If at all possible, the best management of peristomal pyoderma is to close the ostomy.

ILEOSTOMY ISCHEMIA

Ileostomy ischemia is less common than colostomy ischemia; however, approximately 1% to 5% of patients develop ileostomy ischemia [35]. There are several causes in the development of an ischemic stoma. Classically, the mesentery of the distal ileum is skeletonized for 4 to 5 cm to allow the ileostomy to be delivered through the anterior abdominal wall. In an obese patient, a large abdominal pannus can precipitate ischemia of the ostomy. Similarly, an inadequate opening at the level of the parietal peritoneum or fascia can incarcerate and potentially strangulate the distal ileum. In the early postoperative period, an ischemic stoma warrants further evaluation. A lit, transparent glass rod tube can be inserted into the ileostomy to examine the status of the ileal mucosa. If the mucosa above the fascia is viable, it is appropriate to adopt an expectant approach, paying attention to pouching the ostomy and to patient nutrition. A pediatric gastroscope or ileoscope may also be used to evaluate the ileal mucosa. If there is obvious compromise of blood supply below the level of the fascia, then reintervention to revise the ileostomy is mandatory. In refashioning a stoma in an obese patient, siting the stoma above the umbilicus or performing a loop-end ostomy may be helpful. The stapled distal limb of the ostomy may be secured above the level of the fascia.

HIGH-OUTPUT ILEOSTOMY

Typically, an ileostomy starts to function within 72 hours of surgery [36]. Initial ileostomy output tends to be high, and due care must be paid to ensure that the patient does not become dehydrated, with associated electrolyte imbalance. With resumption of diet, the ileostomy effluent tends to become thicker and lessens in the early postoperative period. Small bowel edema reduces in the first week postoperatively, with a resultant increase in the volume of water absorbed across the small bowel epithelium. Over time, mucosal hypertrophy facilitates small bowel adaptation and this reduces the volume of effluent emitted. If the ostomy output continues to be high in the postoperative period, antidiarrheal agents (described earlier) can be temporarily used. A high-fiber diet can also be beneficial, with low intake of sugar, salt, and fat important in the management of high-output ileostomy. Patients with active Crohn disease or those who have had a small bowel resection may have prolonged problems with high output because of restrictive absorptive capacity. Similarly, if there is a terminal ileal resection, the reflex slowing of gastric emptying and small bowel transit that accompanies absorption of fats and complex carbohydrates is lost. These patients often require prolonged nutritional supplementation with home TPN. Somatostatin has been postulated to be beneficial in patients with high-output secondary to short bowel syndrome; however, these data are historical and no level 1 evidence is available to support its use [37–39].

STOMA RETRACTION

Ileostomy retraction is observed in up to 17% of patients on long-term follow-up [40]. Prevention of this complication is possible at time of ileostomy creation by attention to technical detail. Frequently, retraction occurs in an obese patient undergoing emergency ileostomy creation. Appropriate siting of the stoma, adequate length of ileum delivered through the anterior abdominal wall, absence of tension on the stoma, and an appropriately wide fascial and skin opening at time of ostomy formation are essential. In the obese patient, an end ileostomy is often difficult to create because of a large abdominal pannus. In this setting, we favor a loop-end ileostomy, because it facilitates an adequate length of small bowel delivered on to the anterior abdominal wall without tension on the terminal ileal mesentery. Similarly, it is important to create an appropriately wide fascial opening (2 finger breaths) to deliver the small bowel on to the skin of the abdominal wall. A tight fascial opening can interrupt the blood supply to the ostomy, with necrosis of the tip, which results in sloughing and retraction. In patients with Crohn disease, retraction may signify underlying preileostomy recurrence of disease [41,42]. Local revision of a retracted ileostomy is usually feasible. Access to the peritoneal cavity is generally required to deliver additional length of small bowel through the stoma aperture to facilitate adequate length of ileum for eversion. Sutures may be placed between the cut edge of the small bowel mesentery and the peritoneum to fix the ileum in place. Similarly, the Constantino suture placed between the serosa of the ileum and fascia of Scarpa may fix the stoma above the fascia, allowing normal fibrosis to occur during the postoperative period, preventing retraction. Occasionally, it may not be possible to perform a local revision (dense intra-abdominal adhesions, Crohn recurrence in the preileostomy small bowel) and a minilaparotomy may be necessary.

STOMA PROLAPSE/HERNIAE

Stoma prolapse occurs in 1% to 3% of ileostomies [43–45]. Some surgeons advocate suturing the cut edge of the terminal ileal mesentery to the peritoneum to prevent small bowel prolapsing through the stoma aperture; however, this is not always successful. Typically, prolapse occurs more frequently in obese patients, in those with parastomal herniae, and at previously used ostomy sites. Patients present with concerns regarding the appearance of the ostomy, and repair is often performed for cosmetic purposes. However, repair is generally mandated to prevent an obstruction of the prolapsed/herniated small bowel at the level of the stoma aperture. In addressing stoma prolapse, it is essential to attend to the associated parastomal hernia that is inevitably present. Local repair with reduction of the hernia and closure of the fascial defect with simple sutures are associated with a high recurrence rate of up to 60% [46,47]. Laterally, mesh repair is in vogue for management of parastomal prolapse and herniation. This procedure can be performed locally with the placement of an onlay mesh (anterior to the fascia) or preperitoneal, sublay mesh to strengthen the anterior abdominal wall musculature.

The laparoscopic approach can also be used with a variety of meshes (dual mesh composed of polytetrafluoroethylene, which has an antiadhesive layer on the visceral side, is the commonest used mesh) are used to prevent recurrent parastomal herniation. These meshes have a central keyhole with a slit to encircle the ostomy as it exits the abdominal cavity and can be fixed in place with absorbable sutures or tacking staples. Alternatively, a modified Sugar-baker technique can be used. by which the mesh is placed against the medial aspect of the hernial defect (without encircling the small bowel) and secured in place. A paucity of data exists on the benefits of laparoscopic versus open surgery for parastomal hernia. The use of prophylactic mesh placement at time of index stoma formation is gaining popularity, with several groups showing a reduction in parastomal herniae [48]. Stenosis, fistula formation, and mesh infection remain a concern and no level 1 evidence is available to support their use. Frequently, relocation of the stoma is required; this brings additional risk of parastomal hernia development at the site of the new ostomy.

SMALL BOWEL OBSTRUCTION
Bowel obstruction after ileostomy creation is relatively common, affecting up to 25% of ileostomates during their lifetime [49,50]. Frequently, these episodes correspond to a food bolus obstruction proximal to the terminal portion of the small bowel. Most respond to nonoperative management with intravenous fluid resuscitation, nasogastric decompression, and adopting an expectant policy. Double-contrast computed tomography (CT) is the diagnostic modality of choice and can be useful in predicting the need for surgical intervention [51–53]. Alternatively, a water-soluble contrast study can be used, because it has the dual capacity to be both diagnostic and therapeutic [54–56]. In the early postoperative period, the finding of small bowel obstruction should raise the suspicion of a twist in the ileostomy at creation or volvulus around the ileos-tomy [26]. Volvulus around an ileostomy has been implicated in laparoscopic ileostomy creation; this problem can be circumvented during open surgery by plicating the cut edge of the ileal mesentery to the peritoneum, closing the lateral space. Both of these problems require immediate surgical exploration. Later obstruction in patients with an ileostomy may occur at the fascial level or within the abdominal cavity. Intra-abdominal obstruction is most likely to occur secondary to an adhesive band, prestomal Crohn disease, or food bolus obstruction. Radiologic investigation is as described. If the patient seems hemo-dynamically compromised, with signs of sepsis or peritonitis, laparotomy is mandatory to release a band obstruction and maintain blood supply to the

small intestine. Some surgeons advocate a minimally invasive approach to small bowel obstruction [57,58]. In the era of widespread use of laparoscopic surgery, access to the peritoneal cavity by laparoscopy may be possible. However, these patients have often had multiple complex abdominal operations, and no randomized controlled trials exist to support the laparoscopic approach to small bowel obstruction. If a bolus obstruction is suspected, a contrast study through the ileostomy may dislodge the food bolus and relieve the obstruction. Ileostomy injection or CT enterography may be beneficial in uncovering recurrent ileal Crohn disease as the cause of an obstructed small bowel in patients with a preexisting diagnosis of Crohn disease. Generally, medical therapy and endoscopic intervention in this subset of patients fail; after carefully correcting nutritional and hematologic abnormalities, surgery is undertaken.

LOOP JEJUNOSTOMY

Loop jejunostomy is rarely indicated but is a vital part of the colorectal surgeon's armamentarium. When dealing with the abdominal catastrophe in a patient with severe intra-abdominal sepsis secondary to anastomotic leak, inadvertent small bowel injury, enterocutaneous fistula (ECF), or severe small bowel inflammation (Crohn disease or radiation injury) a proximal diverting jejunostomy may be created in the left upper quadrant to divert the enteric contents away from the area of injury. This procedure is typically performed in the emergency setting, in a patient who has undergone recent surgery and suffered a dramatic complication, classically an anastomotic leak. Proximal diversion should be accompanied, when possible, with drainage of downstream sepsis. Access to the abdominal cavity may be difficult via a previous midline incision so we occasionally use a left upper quadrant subcostal incision. This strategy allows identification of the ligament of Treitz and permits the surgeon to select as distal a portion of jejunum as is technically possible for creation of the stoma. The stoma is created in the usual manner. We routinely wait a minimum of 6 months before closing these ostomies because patients are generally very ill with significant intra-abdominal sepsis when a jejunostomy is necessary. In the elective setting, we use a loop jejunostomy to defunctionalize a small bowel anastomosis in a patient at high risk of leak (eg, Crohn disease with short bowel syndrome and poor nutrition or a patient having an extensive surgery to take down an ECF). Postoperatively, these patients typically have a high-output stoma, and care must be taken to monitor electrolytes and renal function. Supplementation with TPN is mandatory, and the intestinal rehabilitation team play a crucial role in managing these patients.

QoL AFTER ILEOSTOMY SURGERY

Most patients have a good QoL with an ileostomy. Often, the expression of dissatisfaction with QoL in patients with an ileostomy reflects frustration at the activity of the underlying disease process. In those patients who express concerns regarding suboptimal QoL, social restrictions, psychosexual issues, and fear of the ostomy appliance leaking seem to be the major limiting factors [59–61]. Up to half of all patients with an ileostomy report mild to moderate restrictions, with 10% reporting major restrictions [62,63]. However, a well-constructed ileostomy provides a superior QoL compared with a poorly functioning ileal pouch or low rectal anastomosis, with their attendant incontinence, pruritus, and odor [64,65]. The predominant social issue in patients with an ileostomy is sexual relationships, and is more frequently observed in women and those with preexisting low self-esteem [66,67]. However, it seems that QoL improves over time as patients become accustomed to life with an ostomy [68]. Critical to this acceptance seems to be the attention of ostomy care nurses in the initial postoperative care period, facilitating patient education and direction [62].

COLOSTOMY: INDICATIONS, CONSTRUCTION, AND MANAGEMENT

Indications for colostomy are listed in Table 2. Like an ileostomy, a colostomy may be constructed as an end, loop, or loop-end loop stoma. An end colostomy is typically constructed in patients in whom a restorative procedure is not possible, for example a very low rectal cancer necessitating an abdominoperineal resection of the rectum. Frequently, an end colostomy is necessary in older, infirm patients who would not tolerate a coloanal anastomosis or the impact of potential anastomotic complications. Occasionally, multiparous elderly women are unable to have a coloanal anastomosis after low anterior resection because of poor sphincter function, and a colostomy is preferred in this scenario. In the emergent situation, an end colostomy may be used. Hinchey 4 diverticulitis (fecal peritonitis) necessitates a Hartmann procedure, which involves resection of the diseased segment of sigmoid colon with a left lower quadrant left colonic end colostomy. In this scenario, it is thought unsafe to undertake a primary colorectal anastomosis in the presence of fecal contamination of the abdominal cavity, although some investigators advocate a colorectal anastomosis with proximal diverting loop ileostomy [69–71]. Data from a prospective European multicenter, international randomized controlled trial are eagerly awaited to help clarify this area of controversy [72]. An end colostomy is also used in patients with fecal incontinence after failed sphincter

Table 2	
Indications for colostomy	
Defunctioning loop colostomy	End or loop-end colostomy
Low rectal/coloanal anastomosis	Abdominoperineal resection
Relief of distal obstruction	Low anterior resection in patient not suitable
Rectal trauma/sphincter injury	for coloanal anastomosis
Fecal incontinence	Hartmann's procedure
Turnbull blowhole colostomy	Fecal incontinence
Complex rectovaginal, rectourethral fistula	Radiation proctitis
Necrotizing fasciitis of perineum	
Fournier gangrene	

reconstruction or neosphincter/sacral nerve stimulation surgery. Similarly, an end stoma is used for patients with severe radiation proctitis who have failed nonoperative management; however, this is rarely necessary. A loop colostomy is used to defunction a low rectal anastomosis or to divert the fecal stream from a distal obstruction, pelvic sepsis, or rectal/sphincter injury. Most surgeons prefer to defunction a low rectal anastomosis with a loop ileostomy rather than a loop colostomy because many data exist to suggest that stoma-related complications and incisional herniae are more frequent after construction of a loop colostomy [20,21,73]. Also, there is a risk of injury to the marginal artery when constructing a loop colostomy, which may interfere with the blood supply to the colonic conduit used for colorectal anastomosis. A loop colostomy may be necessary to defunction a distal obstructing tumor in patients with a competent ileocecal valve when a staged resection is preferable. Occasionally, when operating on a patient with fecal peritonitis who is hemodynamically unstable (on significant vasopressor support), an expedited operation with drainage of the peritoneal cavity and a proximal diverting transverse loop colostomy without resection of the diseased colon are necessary. Although uncommon, it is an approach that may benefit a critically ill, unstable patient, and the surgeon must be aware of this option. A loop colostomy is also of value to divert the fecal stream from pelvic or perineal sepsis encountered with Fournier gangrene or necrotizing fasciitis of the perineum. Complex rectal fistulae, involving the vagina or urethra in patients with a previous history of pelvic irradiation or previous surgery, may require intricate surgical repair that benefits from fecal diversion to allow optimal chance of healing. In patients with rectovaginal fistulae secondary to Crohn disease, we prefer to use a defunctioning loop ileostomy.

COLOSTOMY PHYSIOLOGY

Typically, the contents of a left-sided colostomy are semisolid, and the patient empties the colostomy bag once a day. The colon functions to absorb a significant proportion of water that crosses the ileocecal valve, such that the contents of the left colon are relatively solid. Transverse loop colostomies may emit contents that are slightly more liquid but generally are relatively well formed and require emptying only once daily. The more proximal the colostomy, the less the surface area of colon in circuit to absorb water and the more liquid the contents are. Right-sided colostomies are uncommon. The main problem experienced by patients with a right-sided colostomy is that the contents are malodourous, because of the effects of colonic bacteria. This situation can be particularly bothersome if the patient has Crohn disease of the small bowel and right colon.

CREATION OF AN END COLOSTOMY

An end colostomy is generally created in the left lower quadrant. The patient should be seen preoperatively by the enterostomal therapist to mark the appropriate site on the abdominal wall that suits the individual patient. Once the decision is taken to make an end colostomy, it is necessary to ensure that an adequate length of left colon has been mobilized to allow the cut end of the colon to be delivered through the abdominal wall in a tension-free fashion. It is crucial that the blood supply to the left colon is good to ensure vascularity of the distalmost portion of the colon, which is delivered through the skin aperture. Occasionally, it is necessary to mobilize the splenic flexure to allow for adequate length and mobility to deliver the colon on to the skin surface. The stoma site is then prepared. First, the surgeon grasps the anterior fascial layer with a Kocher clamp and places a second clamp on the subcutaneous portion of the skin, retracting both clamps toward the midline. A dry, folded sponge is then placed in the abdominal cavity against the abdominal wall where the colostomy is sited. A disk of skin is then excised in the left lower quadrant at the preordained ostomy site. Two small right-angle retractors are held by the first assistant and used to provide retraction. The anterior fascial layer is divided longitudinally with the electrocautery. The rectus muscles are split with Mayo scissors or a Kelly clamp, taking care to avoid the inferior epigastric vessels. The right-angle retractors are then used to retract the muscle, allowing access to the parietal peritoneum. The operating surgeon then places upward tension on the sponge held in the left hand while incising the peritoneum longitudinally with the electrocautery. The sponge becomes visible on entering the abdominal cavity and prevents injury to underlying bowel. The stoma aperture should be sufficient to permit 2 fingers, but occasionally in an obese patient or when large bowel obstruction is encountered a larger aperture may be needed. A Babcock clamp is then passed through the aperture from outside, and the cut end of the colon is grasped. Gentle pressure from within the abdominal cavity is necessary to deliver the colon through the abdominal wall. It is important that excess force is not used during this step, because it can tear the bowel wall or injure its blood supply. Care must be taken to ensure correct orientation of the colon before delivery through the anterior abdominal wall. Once delivered on to the surface of the skin, the bowel is held in place with a small Kocher clamp. We like to deliver 2 to 3 cm of well-vascularized colon on to the skin surface to allow excision of the staple line that has been manipulated during delivery of the colon and to permit construction of a spout on the colostomy, if desired. In obese patients, it may be difficult to deliver the colon through a large abdominal pannus. This situation may be circumvented by inserting an Alexis wound protector, lubricated in sterile water, through the stoma aperture into the abdomen and delivering the colon through the wound protector. The Alexis wound protector device is then divided in the abdominal cavity with heavy scissors and the 2 ends removed. Some surgeons overcome the problem of a large abdominal pannus by dissecting the anterior fascial layer from the overlying fat and delivering the colostomy to fascial level as a first step. The opening in the abdominal wall fat is then fashioned and can be as large as necessary to facilitate delivery of the colon on to the skin surface. In extreme obesity, it is often necessary to construct a loop-end colostomy. We do not routinely close the lateral mesenteric defect. After the midline abdominal wound has been closed, we secure the colostomy with a 3/0 absorbable suture. Although most colostomies are flush with the skin, some investigators advocate leaving a 1-cm to 2-cm spout on the colostomy because it facilitates easy placement of the colostomy appliance; in some patients, weight gain that ensues with recovery from illness may result in colostomy retraction.

CREATION OF A LOOP COLOSTOMY

A loop colostomy is generally fashioned in the left lower quadrant (sigmoid loop colostomy) or in the upper quadrant of the abdominal cavity (transverse loop colostomy). A loop colostomy can be created at open surgery or using a minimally invasive technique. Occasionally, a trephine loop colostomy can be constructed in a thin patient. When performing a trephine loop colostomy in the left lower quadrant, a disk of skin is excised from the anterior abdominal wall at the preferred stoma site. Access to the peritoneal cavity is as described earlier. In a thin patient, it may not be necessary to mobilize the sigmoid colon, and it may be easy to deliver the colon through the stoma aperture. A rod may be placed beneath the mobile colon on the anterior abdominal wall, and the colostomy is created by making a transverse incision with electrocautery along the colon just cephalad to the point at which the colon meets the skin at the inferior aspect of the skin aperture. The distal end is sutured with a 3/0 absorbable suture and the proximal portion is matured with slight eversion (Figs. 10–13). The rod is removed by the enterostomal therapist 4 to 5 days after surgery. When creating a trephine transverse loop colostomy, it is often useful to identify the position of the transverse colon preoperatively. This position can be

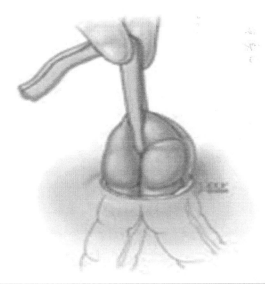

Fig. 10. Delivery of loop colostomy through the anterior abdominal wall. (*Reprinted* with permission, Cleveland Clinic Center for Medical Art & Photography © 2009–2012. All Rights Reserved.)

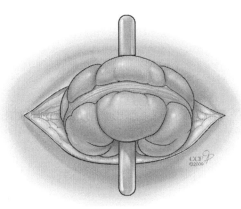

Fig. 11. Loop colostomy. A glass rod placed through the colon mesentery. (*Reprinted* with permission, Cleveland Clinic Center for Medical Art & Photography © 2009–2012. All Rights Reserved.)

identified by taping a coin to the patient's anterior abdominal wall in the upper quadrant of the abdomen and obtaining a plain abdominal radiograph with the patient in the supine position. This strategy allows the surgeon to visualize the transverse colon relative to the marker on the abdominal wall and plan the appropriate incision site. At surgery, the coin is removed, but its position should be marked with an atraumatic needle or indelible ink marker. In the thin patient, it is easy to deliver the transverse colon on to the anterior abdominal wall. The omentum is carefully dissected off the colon and returned to the abdominal

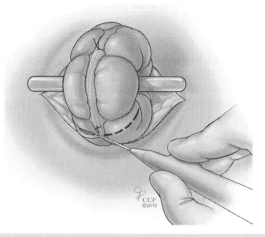

Fig. 12. Incising the distal portion of the loop colostomy with electrocautery. (*Reprinted* with permission, Cleveland Clinic Center for Medical Art & Photography © 2009–2012. All Rights Reserved.)

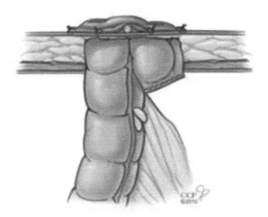

Fig. 13. The loop-end colostomy with the stapled distal end of colon within the abdomen. (*Reprinted* with permission, Cleveland Clinic Center for Medical Art & Photography © 2009–2012. All Rights Reserved.)

cavity before creating the stoma. At open surgery, it is important to pay attention to stoma orientation and ensure that the stoma can be delivered on to the anterior abdominal wall in a tension-free manner. The proximal and distal limbs of the stoma are marked with a blue (Vicryl) and a brown (chromic) suture to ensure correct orientation. Typically, it is necessary to mobilize the colon to allow sufficient length for a tension-free stoma. The white line of Toldt is divided and the colonic mesentery is dissected off the retroperitoneum. Appropriate care must be taken to identify and preserve the left ureter and gonadal vessels. It is usually not necessary to mobilize the splenic flexure when creating a sigmoid loop colostomy, but if necessary the lateral attachments of the splenic flexure may be divided, with liberation of the colon from the left upper quadrant. If this strategy does not provide sufficient length, it may be necessary to divide the inferior mesenteric artery and vein to allow sufficient mobility for ostomy creation. If this strategy fails, liberating the peritoneal attachments at the base of the colonic mesentery provides extra length to allow the ostomy to reach. The opening in the anterior abdominal wall was described earlier, and the opening should permit 2 fingers. Once the colon is delivered to the anterior abdominal wall, the abdomen is lavaged with sterile saline and the abdominal wall closed in the usual fashion. Before opening the colon, we cover the stapled incision with a sterile blue towel. The bowel is then opened as described and the colon secured to the subcutaneous tissues with a 3/0 absorbable suture. In the postoperative period, it is important to remove the ostomy appliance and directly visualize the ostomy to ensure viability, fixation, and that the stoma has not retracted. As the colostomy begins to work, diet is advanced as appropriate.

A loop-end colostomy is made using the same steps as were described for a loop-end ileostomy (see Fig. 13).

LAPAROSCOPIC LOOP COLOSTOMY

Laparoscopy has allowed us to access the peritoneal cavity to facilitate ostomy creation. However, often these patients have had multiple, complex abdominal surgeries, and caution must be exercised when opting for a minimally invasive approach. Access to the peritoneal cavity is by the Hasson technique or with a Veress needle, allowing the establishment of pneumoperitoneum. We generally use 2 5-mm operating trocars to mobilize the bowel. If a transverse loop colostomy is being created, we dissect the omentum from the transverse colon and create a stoma along the proximal transverse colon. We find that minimal mobilization is necessary for these stomas. An electrothermal coagulation device may be used to dissect the omentum from the transverse colon and to mobilize the colon, if necessary. Before excising a disk of skin from the anterior abdominal wall to create the stoma aperture, we release the gas from the abdominal cavity, such that the positioning of the stoma is appropriate. Also, release of pneumoperitoneum allows us to gauge more accurately if the stoma can reach the anterior abdominal wall in a tension-free manner. When approaching the left colon to create a sigmoid loop colostomy, we incise the white line of Toldt with the electrocautery or with an electrothermal coagulation device such as a LigaSure (Covidien Inc, Mansfield, MA, USA) or harmonic scalpel (Ethicon Endo-surgery Inc., Blue Ash, OH, USA). The colon is then liberated from its retroperitoneal attachments in the same manner as at open surgery to allow it to reach the proposed stoma site without tension. Once the surgeon is satisfied that the bowel will reach the abdominal wall without tension, the desired segment of colon is held with an atraumatic grasper. Pneumoperitoneum is released and the stoma aperture created. The laparoscopic grasping device holding the colon is then gently manipulated to allow identification of the colon through the stoma aperture. Then a Babcock grasper is used to grasp the colon, the laparoscopic grasping instrument is released, and the stoma delivered through the opening with gentle manipulation, rocking the colon backward and forward with the Babcock until it is delivered on to the skin. Once the stoma has been matured, pneumoperitoneum is reestablished to ensure correct orientation. A sigmoid end colostomy can also be created laparoscopically; this is done in the same manner with intracorporeal division of the colon using an Endo GIA stapling device, or the colon may be divided on the anterior abdominal wall. The distal segment of colon is then returned to the abdominal cavity or may be implanted subcutaneously, with the proximal end opened and secured to the abdominal wall as an end colostomy.

TURNBULL BLOWHOLE COLOSTOMY

The Turnbull blowhole colostomy technique was first described by Dr Rupert Turnbull at the Cleveland Clinic in 1953 for the management of patients with toxic colitis. This technique was devised to manage patients with toxic colitis in whom a resection was believed to be contraindicated because of the risk of injury to a paper-thin colon with a high risk of peritoneal contamination and subsequent mortality. The abdominal cavity is entered through a lower midline incision and the distal ileum is identified for a loop ileostomy. The proximal and distal limbs are appropriately marked, as described. A stoma aperture is created in the right lower quadrant and the ileum delivered on to the anterior abdominal wall. The midline incision is then closed and the loop ileostomy created. An incision is then made in the left upper quadrant over the grossly distended transverse colon. Care must be taken to minimally handle the grossly inflamed colon. After the fascia has been opened and the colon identified, the serosal surface of the colon is circumferentially sutured to the fascia with interrupted absorbable sutures. This strategy isolates the colon above the fascia and the colon is incised longitudinally. With great care, the colon is secured to the skin with full-thickness absorbable sutures. This technique, albeit rarely necessary, may be of value in a very sick patient unlikely to tolerate a resection (Figs. 14–17) [74]. It has previously been successfully reported for the management of severe toxic colitis in pregnancy, with successful delivery of the fetus at term and interval ileal pouch-anal construction for the 2 mothers involved [75].

COMPLICATIONS OF COLOSTOMY

After creation of a colostomy, complications can be classified as early, late, or related to closure/reversal of the stoma. Early complications include colostomy ischemia, retraction, ileus, wound sepsis, and skin irritation. In the longer-term, most complications of a colostomy are related to stoma prolapse or parastomal herniation. These problems when encountered are difficult to manage, and

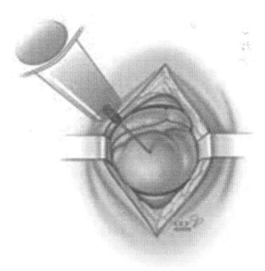

Fig. 14. The Turnbull blowhole colostomy. The distended transverse colon is delivered into the wound and decompressed with a trephine needle. (*Reprinted* with permission, Cleveland Clinic Center for Medical Art & Photography © 2009–2012. All Rights Reserved.)

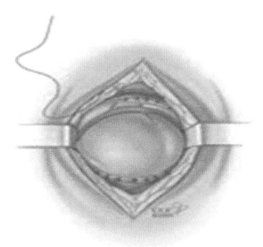

Fig. 15. The Turnbull blowhole colostomy. The serosal surface of the transverse colon is sutured to the anterior abdominal wall fascia. (*Reprinted* with permission, Cleveland Clinic Center for Medical Art & Photography © 2009–2012. All Rights Reserved.)

often patients have multiple procedures to address the issue. Multiple randomized controlled trials have reported that loop colostomy is associated with a higher incidence of parastomal hernia than loop ileostomy [19–21]. The surgical management of parastomal herniae is subject to much debate. Local sutured repair of the abdominal wall defect is rarely successful and is associated

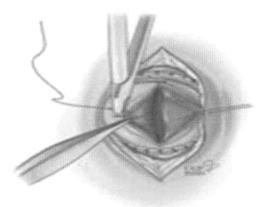

Fig. 16. The Turnbull blowhole colostomy. The colon is opened longitudinally and the cut edges sutured to the skin. (*Reprinted* with permission, Cleveland Clinic Center for Medical Art & Photography © 2009–2012. All Rights Reserved.)

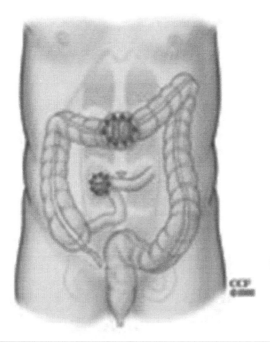

Fig. 17. The completed Turnbull blowhole colostomy with diverting loop ileostomy. *(Reprinted with permission, Cleveland Clinic Center for Medical Art & Photography © 2009–2012. All Rights Reserved.)*

with a high recurrence rate approaching 50% [76]. Multiple investigators have described the technique of mesh repair of paracolostomy herniae and report a recurrence rate of 15% [47,77,78]; however, the study numbers are small, with poor longevity at follow-up. These procedures can be performed as an open repair or laparoscopically with synthetic or biologic mesh. Many observers have advocated using prophylactic mesh placement at the time of colostomy construction to prevent herniation [48,79,80]. However, there is no level 1 evidence to support routine use of prophylactic mesh at the time of index surgery. Frequently, these patients require stoma relocation, and it is critical to take care in creating an appropriately sized fascial and skin opening at the time of index surgery to prevent this complication.

SUMMARY

The ability to appropriately construct and care for an ostomy is crucial to good colorectal surgical practice. Enterostomal therapy is critical to the successful management of ostomies and their complications. Although associated with morbidity, a well-constructed ostomy can provide our patients with a good, durable QoL.

References

[1] Cataldo PA. Intestinal stomas: 200 years of digging. Dis Colon Rectum 1999;42(2): 137–42.
[2] McGarity WC. The evolution of continence following total colectomy. Am Surg 1992; 58(1):1–16.
[3] Brooke BN. The management of an ileostomy, including its complications. Lancet 1952;2(6725):102–4.
[4] Kramer P, Kearney MM, Ingelfinger FJ. The effect of specific foods and water loading on the ileal excreta of ileostomized human subjects. Gastroenterology 1962;42:535–46.
[5] Brooke BN. Ileostomy chemistry. Dis Colon Rectum 1958;1(1):3–14.
[6] Ladas SD, Isaacs PE, Murphy GM, et al. Fasting and postprandial ileal function in adapted ileostomates and normal subjects. Gut 1986;27(8):906–12.
[7] Kennedy HJ, Al-Dujaili EA, Edwards CR, et al. Water and electrolyte balance in subjects with a permanent ileostomy. Gut 1983;24(8):702–5.
[8] Thomson TJ, Runcie J, Khan A. The effect of diet on ileostomy function. Gut 1970;11(6): 482–5.
[9] Burch J. Nutrition for people with stomas. 2: an overview of dietary advice. Nurs Times 2008;104(49):26–7.
[10] DuPont AW, Sellin JH. Ileostomy diarrhea. Curr Treat Options Gastroenterol 2006;9(1): 39–48.
[11] Newton CR. Effect of codeine phosphate, Lomotil, and Isogel on iileostomy function. Gut 1978;19(5):377–83.
[12] Duerksen DR, Fallows G, Bernstein CN. Vitamin B_{12} malabsorption in patients with limited ileal resection. Nutrition 2006;22(11–12):1210–3.
[13] Ishii G, Nakajima K, Tanaka N, et al. Clinical evaluation of urolithiasis in Crohn's disease. Int J Urol 2009;16(5):477–80.
[14] Evan AP, Lingeman JE, Worcester EM, et al. Renal histopathology and crystal deposits in patients with small bowel resection and calcium oxalate stone disease. Kidney Int 2010;78(3):310–7.
[15] Arumugam PJ, Bevan L, Macdonald L, et al. A prospective audit of stomas–analysis of risk factors and complications and their management. Colorectal Dis 2003;5(1):49–52.
[16] Gulbiniene J, Markelis R, Tamelis A, et al. Tinkamai parinktos stomos vietos bei jos prieziuros reiksme pacientu gyvenimo kokybei [The impact of preoperative stoma siting and stoma care education on patient's quality of life]. Medicina (Kaunas) 2004;40(11):1045–53 [in Lithuanian].
[17] Millan M, Tegido M, Biondo S, et al. Preoperative stoma siting and education by stoma-therapists of colorectal cancer patients: a descriptive study in twelve Spanish colorectal surgical units. Colorectal Dis 2010;12(7 Online):e88–92.
[18] Unti JA, Abcarian H, Pearl RK, et al. Rodless end-loop stomas. Seven-year experience. Dis Colon Rectum 1991;34(11):999–1004.
[19] Gooszen AW, Geelkerken RH, Hermans J, et al. Temporary decompression after colorectal surgery: randomized comparison of loop ileostomy and loop colostomy. Br J Surg 1998;85(1):76–9.
[20] Edwards DP, Leppington-Clarke A, Sexton R, et al. Stoma-related complications are more frequent after transverse colostomy than loop ileostomy: a prospective randomized clinical trial. Br J Surg 2001;88(3):360–3.
[21] Tilney HS, Sains PS, Lovegrove RE, et al. Comparison of outcomes following ileostomy versus colostomy for defunctioning colorectal anastomoses. World J Surg 2007;31(5): 1142–51.
[22] Klink CD, Lioupis K, Binnebosel M, et al. Diversion stoma after colorectal surgery: loop colostomy or ileostomy? Int J Colorectal Dis 2011;26(4):431–6.
[23] Swain BT, Ellis CN Jr. Laparoscopy-assisted loop ileostomy: an acceptable option for temporary fecal diversion after anorectal surgery. Dis Colon Rectum 2002;45(5):705–7.

[24] Young CJ, Eyers AA, Solomon MJ. Defunctioning of the anorectum: historical controlled study of laparoscopic vs. open procedures. Dis Colon Rectum 1998;41(2):190–4.

[25] Hollyoak MA, Lumley J, Stitz RW. Laparoscopic stoma formation for faecal diversion. Br J Surg 1998;85(2):226–8.

[26] Ng KH, Ng DC, Cheung HY, et al. Obstructive complications of laparoscopically created defunctioning ileostomy. Dis Colon Rectum 2008;51(11):1664–8.

[27] Colwell JC, Goldberg M, Carmel J. The state of the standard diversion. J Wound Ostomy Continence Nurs 2001;28(1):6–17.

[28] Nybaek H, Bang Knudsen D, Norgaard Laursen T, et al. Skin problems in ostomy patients: a case-control study of risk factors. Acta Derm Venereol 2009;89(1):64–7.

[29] Duchesne JC, Wang YZ, Weintraub SL, et al. Stoma complications: a multivariate analysis. Am Surg 2002;68(11):961–6 [discussion: 6].

[30] Nugent KP, Daniels P, Stewart B, et al. Quality of life in stoma patients. Dis Colon Rectum 1999;42(12):1569–74.

[31] Lefort MM, Closset J, Sperduto N, et al. The definitive stoma: complications and treatment in 50 patients. Acta Chir Belg 1995;95(1):63–6.

[32] Kiran RP, O'Brien-Ermlich B, Achkar JP, et al. Management of peristomal pyoderma gangrenosum. Dis Colon Rectum 2005;48(7):1397–403.

[33] Poritz LS, Lebo MA, Bobb AD, et al. Management of peristomal pyoderma gangrenosum. J Am Coll Surg 2008;206(2):311–5.

[34] Brooklyn TN, Dunnill MG, Shetty A, et al. Infliximab for the treatment of pyoderma gangrenosum: a randomised, double blind, placebo controlled trial. Gut 2006;55(4): 505–9.

[35] Shellito PC. Complications of abdominal stoma surgery. Dis Colon Rectum 1998;41(12): 1562–72.

[36] Tang CL, Yunos A, Leong AP, et al. Ileostomy output in the early postoperative period. Br J Surg 1995;82(5):607.

[37] Spiliotis J, Tambasis E, Christopoulou A, et al. Sandostatin as a "hormonal" temporary protective ileostomy in patients with total or subtotal colectomy. Hepatogastroenterology 2003;50(53):1367–9.

[38] Mulvihill SJ. Perioperative use of octreotide in gastrointestinal surgery. Digestion 1993;54(Suppl 1):33–7.

[39] Kusuhara K, Kusunoki M, Okamoto T, et al. Reduction of the effluent volume in high-output ileostomy patients by a somatostatin analogue, SMS 201-995. Int J Colorectal Dis 1992;7(4):202–5.

[40] Leong AP, Londono-Schimmer EE, Phillips RK. Life-table analysis of stomal complications following ileostomy. Br J Surg 1994;81(5):727–9.

[41] Ecker KW, Gierend M, Kreissler-Haag D, et al. Reoperations at the ileostomy in Crohn's disease reflect inflammatory activity rather than surgical stoma complications alone. Int J Colorectal Dis 2001;16(2):76–80.

[42] Scaglia M, Delaini GG, Hulten L. Le complicanze a lungo termine dell'ileostomia in pazienti affetti da morbo di Crohn e colite ulcerativa [The long-term complications from ileostomy in patients with Crohn's disease and ulcerative colitis]. Chir Ital 1992;44(5–6):211–22 [in Italian].

[43] Park JJ, Del Pino A, Orsay CP, et al. Stoma complications: the Cook County Hospital experience. Dis Colon Rectum 1999;42(12):1575–80.

[44] Robertson I, Leung E, Hughes D, et al. Prospective analysis of stoma-related complications. Colorectal Dis 2005;7(3):279–85.

[45] Garcia-Botello SA, Garcia-Armengol J, Garcia-Granero E, et al. A prospective audit of the complications of loop ileostomy construction and takedown. Dig Surg 2004;21(5–6): 440–6.

[46] Rubin MS, Schoetz DJ Jr, Matthews JB. Parastomal hernia. Is stoma relocation superior to fascial repair? Arch Surg 1994;129(4):413–8 [discussion: 418–9].

[47] Rieger N, Moore J, Hewett P, et al. Parastomal hernia repair. Colorectal Dis 2004;6(3): 203–5.

[48] Janes A, Cengiz Y, Israelsson LA. Preventing parastomal hernia with a prosthetic mesh: a 5-year follow-up of a randomized study. World J Surg 2009;33(1):118–21 [discussion: 122–3].

[49] Marcello PW, Roberts PL, Schoetz DJ Jr, et al. Obstruction after ileal pouch-anal anastomosis: a preventable complication? Dis Colon Rectum 1993;36(12):1105–11.

[50] Francois Y, Dozois RR, Kelly KA, et al. Small intestinal obstruction complicating ileal pouch-anal anastomosis. Ann Surg 1989;209(1):46–50.

[51] Schwenter F, Poletti PA, Platon A, et al. Clinicoradiological score for predicting the risk of strangulated small bowel obstruction. Br J Surg 2010;97(7):1119–25.

[52] Hwang JY, Lee JK, Lee JE, et al. Value of multidetector CT in decision making regarding surgery in patients with small-bowel obstruction due to adhesion. Eur Radiol 2009;19(10): 2425–31.

[53] Qalbani A, Paushter D, Dachman AH. Multidetector row CT of small bowel obstruction. Radiol Clin North Am 2007;45(3):499–512, viii.

[54] Branco BC, Barmparas G, Schnuriger B, et al. Systematic review and meta-analysis of the diagnostic and therapeutic role of water-soluble contrast agent in adhesive small bowel obstruction. Br J Surg 2010;97(4):470–8.

[55] Tresallet C, Lebreton N, Royer B, et al. Improving the management of acute adhesive small bowel obstruction with CT-scan and water-soluble contrast medium: a prospective study. Dis Colon Rectum 2009;52(11):1869–76.

[56] Abbas S, Bissett IP, Parry BR. Oral water soluble contrast for the management of adhesive small bowel obstruction. Cochrane Database Syst Rev 2007;3:CD004651.

[57] O'Connor DB, Winter DC. The role of laparoscopy in the management of acute small-bowel obstruction: a review of over 2,000 cases. Surg Endosc 2012;26(1):12–7.

[58] Cirocchi R, Abraha I, Farinella E, et al. Laparoscopic versus open surgery in small bowel obstruction. Cochrane Database Syst Rev 2010;2:CD007511.

[59] Sprangers MA, Taal BG, Aaronson NK, et al. Quality of life in colorectal cancer. Stoma vs. nonstoma patients. Dis Colon Rectum 1995;38(4):361–9.

[60] Charua-Guindic L, Benavides-Leon CJ, Villanueva-Herrero JA, et al. Quality of life in ostomized patients. Cir Cir 2011;79(2):149–55.

[61] Camilleri-Brennan J, Steele RJ. Objective assessment of quality of life following panproctocolectomy and ileostomy for ulcerative colitis. Ann R Coll Surg Engl 2001;83(5):321–4.

[62] Karadag A, Mentes BB, Uner A, et al. Impact of stomatherapy on quality of life in patients with permanent colostomies or ileostomies. Int J Colorectal Dis 2003;18(3):234–8.

[63] McLeod RS, Lavery IC, Leatherman JR, et al. Patient evaluation of the conventional ileostomy. Dis Colon Rectum 1985;28(3):152–4.

[64] Das P, Smith JJ, Tekkis PP, et al. Quality of life after indefinite diversion/pouch excision in ileal pouch failure patients. Colorectal Dis 2007;9(8):718–24.

[65] Tan HT, Morton D, Connolly AB, et al. Quality of life after pouch excision. Br J Surg 1998;85(2):249–51.

[66] Kilic E, Taycan O, Belli AK, et al. Kalici ostomi ameliyatinin beden algisi, benlik saygisi, es uyumu ve cinsel islevler uzerine etkisi [The effect of permanent ostomy on body image, self-esteem, marital adjustment, and sexual functioning]. Turk Psikiyatri Derg 2007;18(4): 302–10 [in Turkish].

[67] Turns D. Psychosocial issues: pelvic exenterative surgery. J Surg Oncol 2001;76(3): 224–36.

[68] Marquis P, Marrel A, Jambon B. Quality of life in patients with stomas: the Montreux Study. Ostomy Wound Manage 2003;49(2):48–55.

[69] Zingg U, Pasternak I, Dietrich M, et al. Primary anastomosis vs Hartmann's procedure in patients undergoing emergency left colectomy for perforated diverticulitis. Colorectal Dis 2010;12(1):54–60.

[70] Salem L, Flum DR. Primary anastomosis or Hartmann's procedure for patients with diverticular peritonitis? A systematic review. Dis Colon Rectum 2004 Nov;47(11):1953–64.

[71] Constantinides VA, Heriot A, Remzi F, et al. Operative strategies for diverticular peritonitis: a decision analysis between primary resection and anastomosis versus Hartmann's procedures. Ann Surg 2007;245(1):94–103.

[72] Swank HA, Vermeulen J, Lange JF, et al, Dutch Diverticular Disease (3D) Collaborative Study Group. The ladies trial: laparoscopic peritoneal lavage or resection for purulent peritonitis and Hartmann's procedure or resection with primary anastomosis for purulent or faecal peritonitis in perforated diverticulitis (NTR2037). BMC Surg 2010;10:29.

[73] Rondelli F, Reboldi P, Rulli A, et al. Loop ileostomy versus loop colostomy for fecal diversion after colorectal or coloanal anastomosis: a meta-analysis. Int J Colorectal Dis 2009;24(5): 479–88.

[74] Remzi FH, Oncel M, Hull TL, et al. Current indications for blow-hole colostomy: ileostomy procedure. A single center experience. Int J Colorectal Dis 2003;18(4):361–4.

[75] Ooi BS, Remzi FH, Fazio VW. Turnbull-Blowhole colostomy for toxic ulcerative colitis in pregnancy: report of two cases. Dis Colon Rectum 2003;46(1):111–5.

[76] Cheung MT, Chia NH, Chiu WY. Surgical treatment of parastomal hernia complicating sigmoid colostomies. Dis Colon Rectum 2001;44(2):266–70.

[77] Slater NJ, Hansson BM, Buyne OR, et al. Repair of parastomal hernias with biologic grafts: a systematic review. J Gastrointest Surg 2011;15(7):1252–8.

[78] Stelzner S, Hellmich G, Ludwig K. Repair of paracolostomy hernias with a prosthetic mesh in the intraperitoneal onlay position: modified Sugarbaker technique. Dis Colon Rectum 2004;47(2):185–91.

[79] Vijayasekar C, Marimuthu K, Jadhav V, et al. Parastomal hernia: is prevention better than cure? Use of preperitoneal polypropylene mesh at the time of stoma formation. Tech Coloproctol 2008;12(4):309–13.

[80] Helgstrand F, Gögenur I, Rosenberg J. Prevention of parastomal hernia by the placement of a mesh at the primary operation. Hernia 2008;12(6):577–82.

Zero Surgical Site Infections
Is It Possible?

C. Daniel Smith, MD

Department of Surgery, Mayo Clinic in Florida, 4500 San Pablo Road, Jacksonville, FL 32224, USA

Keywords
• Surgery • Surgical infection • Quality improvement • Outcomes
• Surgical complications • Complications

Key Points
• Surgical site infection (SSI) accounts for a significant number of postoperative complications with associated cost.
• Actions centered around process improvement and standardizing patient care promises to significantly reduce SSI.
• An SSI bundle was developed and implemented resulting in a significant reduction in SSIs.
• Strong executive leadership, communication and transparency, multidisciplinary involvement, and eliminating competing incentives are keys to successful implementation of an SSI bundle.

BACKGROUND

Surgical site infections (SSIs) present a significant burden to US health care. It is estimated that there are approximately 300,000 SSIs per year in the United States. This number accounts for 17% of all health care acquired infections (HAIs) and is second only to urinary tract infections as a cause for HAIs in US hospitals [1]. SSIs accounts for 3% of hospital mortalities, and patients with an SSI are at a 2 to 11 times higher risk of death when compared with those without an SSI [2]. Looking at this differently, 75% of deaths among patients with SSIs are directly attributable to the SSIs. Additionally, patients with SSIs may experience significant long-term disabilities.

As already stated, this represents a significant burden to the overall health care system. For example, those who suffer from SSIs will experience an additional 7- to 10-day hospital length of stay when compared with those without SSIs. It is estimated that this results in an incremental cost of care between $3200 and $9000 per SSI. In the overall health care system, this represents up to an $8

E-mail address: smith.c.daniel@mayo.edu

0065-3411/12/$ – see front matter
doi:10.1016/j.yasu.2012.04.006

billion to $10 billion annual incremental health care expenditure [3]. This esti-
mate is probably conservative because these calculations are based on inpatient
costs at the time of the index operation and often do not account for the
additional cost of readmission, postdischarge outpatient care, and long-term
disabilities.

When considering SSI prevention, it is important to define what constitutes
an SSI, understand the classification systems and reporting structure around
SSIs, and then assess interventions that have been proven to decrease the
SSIs, including current recommendations from national health organizations.

SSI DEFINED
By definition, an SSI is an infection that develops within 30 days after an operation or within 1 year if an implant was placed and the infection seems to be
related to the surgery [4].

SSI CLASSIFICATION
Prevention strategies
When considering prevention strategies, one can break them into core and
supplemental prevention strategies (Table 1). Core strategies are defined as those
that have high levels of scientific evidence of effectiveness and have demonstrated feasibility of implementation. Supplemental strategies have some evidence
that support their impact on SSI prevention and have variable levels of feasibility
with regard to implementation (Tables 2 and 3).

One of the most challenging aspects of quality improvement is the identification of best practices. Multiple agencies, including the US Department of Health
and Human Services (HHS), Hospital Infection Control Practices Advisory
Committee, Institute for Healthcare Improvement, Infectious Disease Society
of America, and the Surgical Care Improvement Project (SCIP), have published

Table 1
Classification of operative wounds

Classification	Criteria
Clean	Elective, not emergency, nontraumatic, primarily closed; no acute inflammation; no break in technique; respiratory, gastrointestinal, biliary, and genitourinary tracts not entered
Clean-contaminated	Urgent or emergency case that is otherwise clean; elective opening of respiratory, gastrointestinal, biliary, or genitourinary tract with minimal spillage (eg, appendectomy) not encountering infected urine or bile; minor technique break
Contaminated	Nonpurulent inflammation; gross spillage from gastrointestinal tract; entry into biliary or genitourinary tract in the presence of infected bile or urine; major break in technique; penetrating trauma <4 h old; chronic open wounds to be grafted or covered
Dirty	Purulent inflammation (eg, abscess); preoperative perforation of respiratory, gastrointestinal, biliary, or genitourinary tract; penetrating trauma >4 h old

Table 2
Core strategies

Preoperative	
Antimicrobial administration	Procedure-specific antibiotic administered 1 h before incision
Remote infections	Identify and, when possible, postpone operation or treat infection
Operative site preparation	Leave hair at operative site or clip rather than shave if hair removal necessary
Skin preparation	Use antiseptic agent and technique
Bowel preparation	In colorectal cases, use mechanical bowel prep and nonabsorbable intraluminal antimicrobial
Intraoperative	
Operating room traffic	Limit traffic through operating room to only essential traffic
Patient temperature	Maintain normothermia throughout operation
Postoperative	
Temperature	Maintain normothermia in immediate postoperative period
Wound care	Maintain sterile wound coverage for 24–48 h
Blood glucose	Maintain blood glucose level <200 mg/dL (test at 6:00 AM each day)
Antimicrobial administration	Discontinue after 24 h (48 h for cardiac surgery)

guidelines and recommendations for the prevention of SSIs. Literature demonstrating direct cause-and-effect relationships for a specific intervention is scarce, and there are few category IA recommendations. However, there is evidence that the implementation of bundles of elements can reduce the number of SSIs [5–7].

SURGICAL CARE IMPROVEMENT PROJECT

In 2006, the SCIP was implemented with the goal of reducing surgical complications [5]. A significant component of this nationwide quality-improvement initiative focused on reducing postoperative SSIs. The project was based on

Table 3
Supplemental strategies

Preoperative	
Nasal colonization screening	Screen for and decolonize *Staph aureus* carriers selectively (cardiac, orthopedic, neurosurgery, implant cases) with mupirocin therapy
Blood glucose	Maintain tight glucose control on postoperative day 1 and 2 for select procedures (eg, arthroplasties, spinal fusions)
Intraoperative	
Antimicrobial administration	Redose antimicrobial at 3-h intervals
Antimicrobial administration	Adjust dose of antimicrobials if patients' BMI >30
Oxygen administration	Use FIO_2 of at least 50% intraoperatively and immediately postoperatively
Postoperative	
SSI Rates	Provide surgeon-specific feedback on SSI rates to surgeons

Abbreviations: BMI, body mass index; FIO_2, fraction of inspired oxygen.

the concept that compliance with a bundle of interventions would reduce SSIs, and much of the bundle was drawn from the previously mentioned core and supplemental strategies (Table 4).

The SCIP has been implemented by the Centers for Medicare and Medicaid Services and endorsed by numerous stakeholders as a valid measure of surgical quality. Hospital adherence to SCIP measures is publically reported with the intent to guide patients and payers to the best hospitals for their surgical care. Numerous studies have demonstrated that adherence to the SCIP measures has improved over the implementation period but only a few assessed whether adherence has resulted in improved surgical outcomes. Although these studies demonstrate that SCIP implementation has achieved substantial improvements in adherence, there is minimal evidence to support that SCIP adherence improves surgical outcomes at the patient or hospital level. The current literature is limited by the lack of patient-level data for both adherence and outcomes as well as a valid measure for SSI outcome.

Several recent studies have called into question the effectiveness of the adherence to SCIP measures at actually decreasing or preventing SSIs [8–11]. A recent study by Hawn and colleagues [8] performed across 112 Veterans Affairs hospitals and involving a total of 60,853 operations found that the implementation of the SCIP infection-prevention measures did not yield measurable improvement in SSIs at the patient or hospital level or an improvement in adjusted SSI rates over the implementation period. The investigators concluded that "although the processes measured are best practices and should continue, they might be too simplistic or blunt to discriminate hospital quality." Indeed others have reported similar findings and concerns. Although adherence to SCIP measures assures that processes are followed that intuitively make sense with regard to process improvement and hospital-wide coordination of processes, as a true SSI reduction strategy, SCIP has thus far failed to demonstrate a causal relationship to SSI reduction.

AN SSI REDUCTION PROCESS AND BUNDLE
The author's group hypothesized that the development of an organized structure to facilitate rapid development and diffusion of multiple infection-prevention strategies

Table 4
SCIP measures

Measure	Details
SCIP-inf 1	Prophylactic antibiotic received within 1 h before surgical incision
SCIP-inf 2	Prophylactic antibiotic selection for surgical patients
SCIP-inf 3	Prophylactic antibiotics discontinued within 24 h after surgery end time
SCIP-inf 4	Cardiac surgery patients with controlled 6:00 AM postoperative blood glucose
SCIP-inf 6	Surgery patients with appropriate hair removal
SCIP-inf 9	Urinary catheter removed on postoperative day 1 or postoperative day 2 with day of surgery being day zero
SCIP-inf 10	Surgery patients with perioperative temperature management

simultaneously would result in lower rates of SSIs [12]. To this end, a multidisciplinary team was formed to develop interval SSI reduction targets and the framework to identify gaps, improve performance, measure compliance, and assess the impact of the interventions. To affect this, a partnership between surgical leadership, hospital administration, quality management services, and infection control was created resulting in the creation of an SSI reduction steering committee that reported directly to the chief executive officer. The SSI reduction steering committee met weekly to set priorities, allocate resources, and review progress.

From an extensive review of the medical literature and published guidelines, a list of modifiable risk factors was generated and reviewed for strength of evidence and feasibility: an SSI bundle (Table 5). A gap analysis was completed

Table 5
SSI bundle

Preoperative
  Identify and treat all infections remote to the surgical site before an elective operation
  Encourage smoking cessation within 30 d before the procedure
  Avoid immunosuppressive medications in the perioperative period if possible
  Perform preoperative antiseptic skin cleansing
  Mechanical preparation of the colon for colorectal surgery patients
  Administer nonabsorbable oral antimicrobial agents on the day before the operation
  Screen and decolonize *Staphylococcus aureus* carriers undergoing elective procedures
Holding
  Only remove hair that will interfere with the operation
  Remove hair immediately before the operation with clippers (SCIP 6)
Intraoperative
  Select the appropriate antibiotic based on the surgical procedure (SCIP 2)
  Increase dosing of prophylactic antimicrobial agent for patients who are morbidly obese.
  Administer prophylactic antimicrobial agents IV on time (SCIP 1)
  Use an appropriate antiseptic agent for skin preparation
  Maintain therapeutic levels of the prophylactic antimicrobial agent throughout the operation
  Use at least a 50% fraction of inspired oxygen for select procedures
  Keep operating room doors closed during surgery
  Maintain perioperative normothermia (SCIP 9)
  Adhere to standard principles of operating room asepsis
  Optimize ventilation, environmental cleaning, and sterilization of surgical equipment
  Minimize flash sterilization
Postoperative
  Adequately control serum blood glucose levels in patients with diabetes (SCIP 4)
  Protect primary-closure incisions with a sterile dressing for 24–48 h postoperatively
  Discontinue the prophylactic antimicrobial agent within 24 h of surgery (SCIP 3)
Surgeon technique
  Use appropriate antiseptic agent to perform preoperative surgical scrub for surgical team members
  Handle tissue carefully and eradicate dead space
  Minimize operative time as much as possible
Transparency
  Feedback surgeon-specific infection rates

Abbreviation: IV, intravenously.

to identify and prioritize opportunities for practice improvement. Results from the gap analysis were used to develop specific targets for improvement. Each target was assigned a multidisciplinary workgroup lead by a performance-improvement (PI) coach and tasked with identifying and testing potential solutions. Care was taken to ensure that the workgroup represented all members of the health care team who performed in or would be impacted by the practice improvement they were charged to develop. For example, the hand-hygiene workgroup was comprised of outpatient, holding, and postoperative care unit nurses; an anesthesiologist; and a surgeon.

Over the past 2 years, this SSI bundle was set in place. Over this same time period, there was a reduction in the total number of infections and the rate of SSIs (Figs. 1 and 2; Table 6).

A cost analysis based on cost estimates as outlined by Scott [3] reveals a cost savings of $668,352 to $1,634,944 over this period.

This experience is not powerful enough to conclude that the specific interventions that were targeted lead directly to SSI reduction; however, there is a clear trend downward that occurred contemporaneously with this work. There are currently few studies that directly link a specific intervention to SSI reduction; however, several suggest that bundled interventions may lead to improvements. Although the individual interventions may not directly impact the rate of infection, the ability to demonstrate adherence to multiple strategies to mitigate risk may. In a recent study, the aggregated measure of SCIP adherence was associated with decreases in postoperative infection rates [7].

SSI REDUCTION LESSONS

The methodology selected for this improvement project focused on the identification of best practices, gap analysis, and targeted interventions to close those

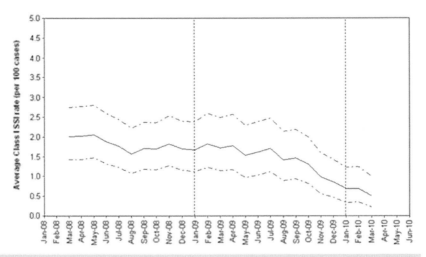

Fig. 1. Class I surgical site infection rates (January 2008 to June 2010, rolling 12-month average).

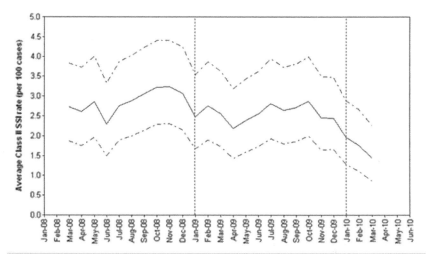

Fig. 2. Class 2 surgical site infection rates (January 2008 to June 2010, rolling 12-month average).

gaps (Box 1). Although it sounds simple, the size of the organization and the number of interventions identified resulted in a massive PI effort. Historically, process improvement was the purview of a small group of experts working in isolation. One of the key features of this successful implementation was the alliance formed between the data collection and reporting groups (infection control, quality management services), the PI and content experts (infectious disease, surgical quality committee), and the frontline health care providers. The strategies for improvement were developed with the content experts, gap analysis and data extraction originated from the quality-improvement experts, and opportunities were identified and assigned to frontline groups.

Table 6
SSI reduction

	2008	2009	2010	2008–2010 change (%)
Number of infections				
Class I	47	49	8	—
Class II	43	60	18	—
Total	90	109	26	—
Number of cases				
Class I	2634	3143	1573	—
Class II	1526	2353	1253	—
Overall	4160	5496	2826	—
Class I SSI rate	1.78	1.56	0.51	(71)
Class II SSI rate	2.82	2.55	1.44	(49)
Overall SSI rate	2.16	1.98	0.92	(57)

Box 1: Keys to success

- Methodology embedded in organization's existing quality and safety structure
- Executive-leadership driven
- Leverage information technology (electronic medical record)
- Communication and transparency
- Multidisciplinary team–based development and deployment
- No competing or conflicting individual financial incentives

Those groups, coached by PI experts, then developed strategies to align the author's practice with the recommendations and sent them back to the surgical quality committee for endorsement and then disseminated the solutions to the rest of the practice. The SSI reduction steering committee was available to assist with the allocation of resources if needed for implementation and dissemination. It was this continuous-flow loop that allowed the simultaneous practice changes demonstrated in this project. This volume of interventions would take years to deploy if developed in isolation and implemented in sequence.

Strong executive leadership and support was key to the successful rapid practice improvements required in this project. The clear message that HAIs are preventable and the challenge to get to zero as quickly as possible provided the foundation for the project and facilitated alignment of the practice in working toward that clearly stated goal. The ongoing engagement of leadership throughout served to emphasize its importance and keep the momentum moving forward. Frontline workers were engaged and empowered to address a specific issue directly impacting their daily activities. Because they identified barriers, performed the rapid tests of change, and identified solutions together, they were able to be champions and experts in the rapid dissemination phase of each intervention. This success created buy-in and ownership, which was crucial to the integration of the improvements into daily practice. It was to the advantage of the author's group to be operating in a fully integrated practice focused on the needs of the patients and free of any potential conflicting financial incentives tied to provider productivity. This project aligned with the group's embedded organizational culture allowing for rapid buy-in at all levels.

Another key strategy was to leverage the electronic medical record wherever possible to make it easy to perform a task correctly but difficult to make an error. This approach was used in multiple areas but is most visible to the clinician in the SCIP metrics. Order sets were designed to match SCIP 2 recommendations for appropriate antibiotic use and eliminated all other options. An alert was created for SCIP 3 that notifies a provider when they are about to continue an antibiotic past the recommended perioperative timeframe and forces documentation of the justification for doing so. These 2 interventions have dramatically improved the compliance with the guidelines and enabled the clinician to provide the documentation required to avoid a publically reported defect.

Transparency was another key feature of this project. The author's group was challenged to make this effort as transparent as possible to patients, visitors, and staff members. Scorecards were developed that displayed monthly audits of specific performance metrics and the overall infection rates by service and by month. These scorecards were posted in the surgical hallways, patient-care areas, and in the boardroom. Surgeon-specific rates were calculated annually, and members of the steering committee met regularly with surgical groups to share knowledge and identify barriers and opportunities.

The challenges that were faced that are not likely unique to this institution included the presence of learners, an evolving electronic medical record, and the difficulty identifying clear ownership for particular interventions. Many of the identified improvements require residents or fellows in the process. The institution has tried to integrate them into workgroups, but the constant turnover of learners represents an ongoing opportunity for which a reliable solution has not been developed. As this project progressed, the electronic medical record underwent multiple upgrades and system changes. It was challenging to continuously assess the impact of each upgrade to the processes that were already in place as well as those that were in development. Several interventions were targeted toward risk mitigation in the preoperative phase of care. Initially, it was difficult identifying which interventions belonged to the surgeon and which would be better performed by the medical specialists providing clearance for surgery. The development of the preoperative evaluation clinic allowed the team to centralize these activities and improve compliance by limiting the number of providers engaged in the process.

References

[1] Klevens RM, Edwards JR, Richards CL Jr, et al. Estimating health care-associated infections and deaths in U.S. hospitals, 2002. Public Health Rep 2007;122(2):160–6.

[2] Kirkland KB, Briggs JP, Trivette SL, et al. The impact of surgical-site infections in the 1990s: attributable mortality, excess length of hospitalization, and extra costs. Infect Control Hosp Epidemiol 1999;20(11):725–30.

[3] Scott RD. The direct medical costs of healthcare-associated infections in U.S. hospitals and the benefits of prevention April 1, 2010. Available at: http://www.cdc.gov/ncidod/dhqp/pdf/Scott_CostPaper.pdf. Accessed July 1, 2010.

[4] Mangram AJ, Horan TC, Pearson ML, et al. Guideline for prevention of surgical site infection, 1999. Centers for Disease Control and Prevention (CDC) Hospital Infection Control Practices Advisory Committee. Am J Infect Control 1999;27(2):97–132 [quiz: 133–4; discussion: 96].

[5] Bratzler DW, Hunt DR. The surgical infection prevention and surgical care improvement projects: national initiatives to improve outcomes for patients having surgery. Clin Infect Dis 2006;43(3):322–30.

[6] Dellinger EP, Hausmann SM, Bratzler DW, et al. Hospitals collaborate to decrease surgical site infections. Am J Surg 2005;190(1):9–15.

[7] Stulberg JJ, Delaney CP, Neuhauser DV, et al. Adherence to surgical care improvement project measures and the association with postoperative infections. JAMA 2010;303(24):2479–85.

[8] Hawn MT, Vick CC, Richman J, et al. Surgical site infection prevention: time to move beyond the surgical care improvement program. Ann Surg 2011;254(3):494–9 [discussion: 499–501].

[9] Edmiston CE, Spencer M, Lewis BD, et al. Reducing the risk of surgical site infections: did we really think SCIP was going to lead us to the promised land? Surg Infect 2011;12(3): 169–77.

[10] Dixon E, Cheadle WG, Khadaroo RG, et al. Preventing postoperative surgical site infection. J Am Coll Surg 2011;212(3):418–20.

[11] Anthony T, Murray BW, Sum-Ping JT, et al. Evaluating an evidence-based bundle for preventing surgical site infection: a randomized trial. Arch Surg 2011;146(3):263–9.

[12] Thompson KM, Oldenburg WA, Deschamps C, et al. Chasing zero: the drive to eliminate surgical site infections. Ann Surg 2011;254(3):430–6 [discussion: 436–7].

Does Simulation Training Improve Outcomes in Laparoscopic Procedures?

Benjamin Zendejas, MD, MSc, Roberto Hernandez-Irizarry, BS, David R. Farley, MD*

Department of Surgery, College of Medicine, Mayo Clinic, 200 First Street, Southwest, Rochester, MN 55905, USA

Keywords
• Simulation • Laparoscopy • Education • Outcomes

Key Points
• Clear evidence supports that the training of surgeons with technology-enhanced simulation improves outcomes in laparoscopic procedures. However, most of this evidence comes from studies that compare simulation with a no-intervention or control group.
• Evidence suggests that the effectiveness of technology-enhanced simulation rests upon the strength of the instructional design features embedded in the educational intervention, and not on the type of simulator used (ie, high versus low fidelity).
• Studies that actively compare simulation modalities head to head are needed to help us understand when, how, to whom, and in what intervals is simulation most effective.

Yes, simulation does improve outcomes in laparoscopic procedures. The authors are biased surgeons and researchers with affection for simulation, but the emerging data speak for themselves. Repetition is the mother of learning, and it should be intuitive to say that simulation works, so does practicing operative techniques on animals and operating on cadavers. Operating on human patients under the tutelage of master surgeons is the ultimate learning experience, but the road to mastery in surgery is long, and simulation must take its place with lectures, cadaver dissection, and live surgery as facilitators on this journey. In this brief review, the authors discuss the most recent and relevant data on simulation-based curricula measured against patient outcomes and operating room (OR) performance; there is a heavy slant toward the performance of minimally invasive surgery.

*Corresponding author. E-mail address: farley.david@mayo.edu

0065-3411/12/$ – see front matter
doi:10.1016/j.yasu.2012.03.004

Since the early days of the laparoscopic revolution, several challenges between surgeons and laparoscopy became evident: altered tactile feedback, a different set of instruments, the fulcrum effect, increased distance from the surgical field, and differences in depth perception secondary to viewing a 2-dimensional screen. Such challenges became clinically relevant when an increase in the incidence of bile duct injuries in the setting of laparoscopic cholecystectomy was immediately evident in the early 1990s [1], mostly because of the quick and unstructured adoption of laparoscopy at weekend courses without formal training.

As time progressed and the challenges of the laparoscopic view toward operative procedures evolved and matured, it became evident that a unique set of advanced skills was required to embark on laparoscopic surgery. But for surgical educators, the training of surgeons in laparoscopy posed additional challenges. The increased public awareness of patient safety [2], the ethical dilemma of practicing on patients, increased costs from delays in OR time from teaching learners [3], and different intraoperative teaching dynamics (ie, the lack of direct instrument control from the supervising surgeon when the surgical trainee performs a laparoscopic procedure) have led surgeons and educators to seek a safer, cheaper, and more structured environment for repeated practice toward proficiency. Animal and cadaver models have been used for centuries for the training of surgical techniques, including laparoscopic surgery. Within this rational context, however, animal protection groups, country regulations, health concerns, costs, and specialized upkeep requirements became obstacles that, coupled with the technologic boom of the start of the twenty-first century, led the way for the emergence of technology-enhanced simulation. Technology-enhanced simulation has been defined as an educational tool or device with which the learner physically interacts to mimic an aspect of clinical care for the purpose of teaching or assessment [4]. Because of the characteristics of laparoscopic surgery, technology-enhanced simulation quickly became a great fit for the training of laparoscopic surgery *outside* of the clinical environment.

Intuitively, one would expect a benefit from such an educational intervention teaching basic skills in this new laparoscopic world when compared with a control group receiving no active intervention. It seems that only after several hundred no-intervention comparison studies, we now have strong evidence to support the effectiveness of simulation for the training of health professionals [4] and now surgeons [5].

Learning or skill acquisition can be measured at different levels. Evidence and logic supports the notion that repeated practice on a simulator leads to improvement of performance on the same simulator over time [4]; this outcome has been shown repeatedly. But the ultimate goal of surgical simulation training is the transfer of skills learned in the simulation environment to the clinical setting and ultimately with improvements in objective criteria in clinical outcomes. Studies that seek to evaluate the transfer of such skills are often termed transferability studies [6]. The transfer of learning has frequently been measured on a different simulator, usually a more realistic one, such as an animal model [7]. However, in an effort to address the often-touted question of whether simulation training leads to improved outcomes in laparoscopic procedures, this review focuses only on studies that have taken skill assessment after laparoscopic simulation training to the next level: the OR and eventually patient outcomes.

APPRAISAL OF EVIDENCE

This review is based on a recent appraisal of the literature on technology-enhanced simulation for the training of health professionals. A detailed description of the methods and search strategy has been described previously [4]. Briefly, the authors systematically searched the databases of MEDLINE, EMBASE, CINAHL, ERIC, PsychINFO, and Scopus as well as key journals and previous review bibliographies through May 2011. For the purpose of this review, the authors focused on studies that evaluated the role of simulation for the training of health professionals (at any stage in training) in laparoscopic surgery and assessed outcomes in the clinical setting. Studies were categorized according to their comparison arm as no intervention, other instructional modality, or simulation. According to Kirkpatrick's [8] classification, study outcomes were classified as either behaviors with patients (time and process measures) or effects on patients. Outcomes are presented as standardized mean differences (Hedges' g effect size) and determinations of significance that emphasize Cohen's classifications of effect size: less than 0.2 = negligible; 0.2 to 0.49 = small; 0.5 to 0.8 = moderate; greater than 0.8 = large, with positive numbers favoring the intervention [9].

EVIDENCE OF TRANSFERABILITY

From a pool of 10,903 articles screened, the authors identified 967 comparative studies of simulation-based training. From these, only 17 studies (1.8%) compared simulation for the training of laparoscopic surgery and evaluated outcomes in the clinical setting (Table 1). Fifteen studies had a no-intervention comparison and 2 compared simulation against another simulation modality. No study compared simulation with another method of instruction (ie, lecture, video, e-media) for the purpose of laparoscopic surgery training [10]. All but one study [11] demonstrated evidence to support the transferability of laparoscopic skills learned in a simulated environment to the OR.

Simulation versus no intervention

The first study to demonstrate the transfer of laparoscopic skills acquired in the simulated setting to the OR was published in 2000 by Scott and colleagues [12] from the University of Texas Southwestern Medical Center (UTSW). They randomized 27 junior level general surgery residents to either practice 5 laparoscopic tasks on a video-trainer type simulator for 30 minutes for 10 consecutive days or to a control group who were not simulation trained. Operative performance was assessed with a global rating scale in the OR during a laparoscopic cholecystectomy at baseline and at 1 month after training. Study results showed that residents who had undergone simulation training were judged to be superior by the blinded supervising surgeons when compared with their control counterparts as demonstrated by greater performance ratings.

Table 1
Characteristics and outcomes of transferability studies

Citation	Intervention	Simulator	Comparison	Trainee level	N	Specialty	Task/procedure assessed	Outcome, effect size[a]
SIM vs No-Intervention Comparisons								
Zendejas B et al [5], 2011	Training to mastery of cognitive and surgical skills with feedback	Commercial video trainer	NI	PGY 1–5	50	General surgery	Lap TEP inguinal hernia repair	Process, 1; Time, 1.1; Patient effects, 1.1
Yang B et al [24], 2010	Skills training for 10 repetitions per d for 5 d	Homemade video trainer	NI	MD	5	Urology	Retroperitoneal lap dismembered pyeloplasty	Time, 5.6
Sroka G et al [15], 2010	Proficiency-based FLS training	Commercial video trainer	NI	PGY 1–3	19	General surgery	Lap cholecystectomy	Process, 2.3
Calatayud D et al [16], 2010	Warm-up vs no warm-up	VR LapSIM	NI	PG	10	General surgery	Lap cholecystectomy	Process, 0.56
Mohan, PVR & Chaudhry [19], 2009	2 skills practice sessions, 3 mo apart	Commercial video trainer	NI	PG	24	General surgery	Lap cholecystectomy	Process, 1.7
Larsen CR et al [22], 2009	Practice on 2 tasks and 1 procedure until mastery	LapSIM	NI	PGY 1–2	24	OB&GYN	Lap salpingectomy	Process, 1.7; Time, 1.7
Hogle NJ et al [11], 2009	Train to level 3 on simulator	VR LapSIM	NI	PGY 1	12	General surgery	Lap cholecystectomy	Process, 0.2
Van Sickle KR et al [23], 2008	Train to mastery with feedback	MIST-VR and homemade video trainer	NI	PGY 3,5,6	22	General surgery	Lap intracorporeal knot during Nissen fundoplication	Process, 1; Time, 1.2
Cosman PH et al [18], 2007	Train to mastery of cut and clip task	LapSim	NI	PG	10	General surgery	Lap cholecystectomy clip application	Process, 1.5; Time, 1.3

Study	Intervention	Simulator		PGY	N & Specialty	Procedure	Outcome
Banks EH et al [21], 2007	1-h lecture then 2-h of practice on pigs feet, knot board, and 2 laparoscopy simulators	Commercial video trainer	NI	PGY 1	20 OB&GYN	Lap tubal ligation	Process, 1.5
Ahlberg G et al [17], 2007	6 tasks at 3 levels of difficulty; supervised practice, human + VR feedback after each task; repeat until mastery: 1-h training blocks	LapSim	NI	PGY 1–2	13 General surgery	Lap cholecystectomy	Process, 1.3; Time, 1.2
Grantcharov TP et al [20], 2004	10 repetitions of 6 tasks	MIST-VR	NI	PG	16 General surgery	Lap cholecystectomy dissection of GB from fossa	Process, 1.8; Time, 1.3
Seymour NE et al [14], 2002	1 task manipulate and diathermy, repeat until mastery; 1-h sessions	MIST-VR	NI	PGY 1–4	16 General surgery	Lap cholecystectomy dissection of GB from fossa	Process, 1.6; Time, 0.3
Hamilton EC et al [13], 2001	Video and 10 × 30-min supervised sessions: 5 with interactive CD-ROM and 5 on simulator	Homemade video trainer	NI	PGY 3–4	21 General surgery	Lap TEP inguinal hernia repair	Process, 0.5
Scott DJ et al [12], 2000	30 min × 10 sessions on box trainer; no supervision or feedback; could select any of 5 tasks	Video trainer	NI	PGY 2–3	27 General surgery	Lap cholecystectomy	Process, 1.1

(continued on next page)

Table 1
(continued)

Citation	Intervention	Simulator	Comparison	Trainee level	N	Specialty	Task/procedure assessed	Outcome, effect size[a]
SIM vs SIM Comparisons								
Gauger PG et al [25], 2010	Training with proficiency targets	LapSim	No proficiency targets	PGY 1	14	General surgery	Lap cholecystectomy	Process, 0.7
Hamilton EC et al [27], 2002	10 × 30-min sessions on MIST-VR vs video trainer	MIST-VR	Video trainer	PGY 1–2	50	General surgery	Lap cholecystectomy	Process, 1.5

Abbreviations: FLS, Fundamentals of Laparoscopic Skills program; GB, gallbladder; Lap, laparoscopic; MD, practicing physician/surgeon; NI, no-intervention comparison group (pretest, posttest single group, or a control group); OB&GYN, obstetrics and gynecology; PG, resident, postgraduate without year specified; PGY, resident, postgraduate year level 1 through 5 (when specified); TEP, totally extraperitoneal; VR, virtual reality.

[a]Outcomes were classified as either behaviors with patients (time and process measures, such as performance or errors) or effects on patients. Outcomes are presented as standardized mean differences (Hedges g effect size) and determinations of significance emphasize Cohen's effect size classifications: <0.2 = negligible; 0.2–0.49 = small; 0.5–0.8 = moderate, >0.8 = large, with positive numbers favoring the intervention.

Subsequently, the same group from UTSW with a similar study design replicated their previous findings for totally extraperitoneal (TEP) inguinal hernia repairs [13]. Again, with greater global ratings of performance, general surgery residents who practiced on a video-trainer–type simulator were judged by blinded faculty to be superior to their control counterparts during an actual TEP repair.

Later, Seymour and colleagues [14] were the first to demonstrate a positive transfer to the OR from virtual reality (VR) training in laparoscopic cholecystectomy. A notable difference in this learning effort was its proficiency-based training regimen that required residents to train until they met certain training benchmarks, regardless of the time needed, as opposed to the previously used fixed-time regimens. Sixteen general surgery residents from postgraduate years 1 through 4 were randomized to a VR training group or a control group. The training group practiced until proficiency on the manipulate and diathermy task of the Minimally Invasive Surgical Trainer - Virtual Reality (MIST-VR [Mentice, Gothenburg, Sweden]) simulator, and then all of the participants' performance was assessed in the OR during the gallbladder dissection phase of a laparoscopic cholecystectomy. The assessment of operative performance was also novel in nature. With blinded video review, a sophisticated error-scoring matrix counted the number of predefined errors of dissection on a minute-by-minute basis. Results convincingly demonstrated up to 5 times fewer errors and 29% faster operative times during the gallbladder dissection phase of a laparoscopic cholecystectomy for residents trained under simulation conditions when compared with those who were not.

Additional studies evaluated the effects of simulation-based training for laparoscopic cholecystectomy [15–20] as well as other operations, such as tubal ligation [21], salpingectomy [22], intracorporeal knot tying during a Nissen fundoplication [23], and even a retroperitoneal dismembered pyeloplasty [24]. All of these studies demonstrated in one way or another improvement in performance and a decrease in operative time and intraoperative errors after laparoscopic simulation-based training.

In contradistinction, a series of experiments reported by Hogle and colleagues [11] failed to find any significant transfer effect from simulation training of laparoscopic surgery. Twelve interns were randomized to either receive training on the LapSim (Surgical Science, Gothenburg, Sweden) VR simulator for a specified time period or to no training. Trainees were required to reach level 3 in 7 tasks that included camera navigation, instrument navigation, coordination, lifting, grasping, cutting, and clip applying. Unblinded expert surgeons evaluated each trainee's laparoscopic skills through global rating scales, and the results showed no statistical difference between the 2 groups. They postulated that small sample sizes, nonchallenging training regimens, or ineffective assessment methods could have been implicated.

Most studies evaluated the effects of simulation training on naïve (usually junior level) surgery trainees. However, one study by Van Sickle and colleagues [23] evaluated laparoscopic suturing in 22 senior surgical residents and one study by Yang and colleagues [24] evaluated surgeons in practice. Using a plastic clay model, the latter group provided intensive training to 5 laparoscopic surgeons on uteropelvic anastomoses. Results showed that the mean operative time decreased, with an increase in self-confidence. Additionally, several other studies have shown that regardless of the type of the simulator used (either a video trainer [5,13,15,19,21,24] or a VR-type simulator [14,16,17,20,22,25]), an objective measurable transfer to the OR can be achieved, suggesting that the curricular design may be more important than the type of simulator used.

Most studies have evaluated the effect of asynchronous training in the simulation center and assessment in the OR. Nonetheless, Calatayud and colleagues [16] evaluated the benefits of a 15-minute VR preoperative warm-up immediately before a laparoscopic cholecystectomy in 8 general surgery residents. With a randomized crossover design (ie, each surgeon served as their own control), these investigators showed a 9-point difference in improvement in median global ratings of performance (scale 7–35) when warm-up was present.

To the authors' knowledge, their group was the first to report objective improvements in clinically relevant patient outcomes after simulation-based training of laparoscopic inguinal hernia repairs [5,26]. In brief, the authors developed a curriculum rooted in mastery learning theory [5] for the training of the laparoscopic TEP inguinal hernia repair. Similar to proficiency-based training, mastery learning is a variant of competency-based education in which learners train repeatedly until they have demonstrated mastery of essential knowledge and skills rather than following a training regimen of a fixed duration of time. What sets mastery learning apart from proficiency-based training is the coupling of endpoints in both knowledge-based and skills-based training and the level at which the bar is set, which is typically higher, because mastery training endpoints are set to expert levels of performance. Hence, the authors' curriculum contained components of both cognitive and skills training. After a baseline assessment of OR skills, general surgery residents at all levels of training were randomized to a simulation-based training or to a nonintervention control group. Participants in the simulation arm trained until they met the mastery training endpoints, which included passing an online multiple-choice test of knowledge and being able to perform a technically correct simulated TEP repair on a video-trainer–type simulator under the expert-defined benchmark time without errors. Training sessions were 1 hour or 10 simulated attempts, whichever came first. During training, participants received 1-on-1 proctoring by a trainer and received feedback tailored to their performance after each attempt. All participants randomized to the curriculum achieved mastery at a mean ($\pm$ standard deviation) training time of 64 ± 40 minutes. As expected, the greater the previous experience with the TEP repair or the level of training, the less time required to achieve mastery of the curriculum. After training, participants were reassessed by both video recordings and observer scorings in the OR during all subsequent TEP repairs performed under supervision. Study results showed that when compared with their control counterparts, residents who trained under simulation-based conditions were on average 13 minutes faster (when corrected for any direct participation by the staff surgeon), were allowed by the staff surgeon to complete 15% more of the procedural time as the active surgeon, and were judged to be superior performers as demonstrated by an average 3.7 greater global ratings of performance on a 6 to 30 scale. But more importantly, patients in the simulation-based training group were 85% and 87% less likely to develop intraoperative and postoperative complications, respectively, and were 63% less likely to require an overnight stay after outpatient laparoscopic inguinal hernia surgery [5,26].

Simulation versus simulation studies

Hamilton and colleagues [27] compared residents who practiced a series of laparoscopic skills either on a video trainer or on a VR-type simulator. Transfer to the OR was assessed in the context of a laparoscopic cholecystectomy. Their results showed that although both groups improved, the performance as measured by a global rating scale and, hence, transfer was slightly superior for residents who trained with the VR-type simulator.

Gauger and colleagues [25] compared residents who underwent training with a structured curriculum consisting of repeated practice of laparoscopic tasks on a video trainer and on a VR simulator, either with or without proficiency targets. Their study suggested that during a laparoscopic cholecystectomy, residents who trained with proficiency targets were judged to be superior (better global ratings of performance and less errors) to those who had trained without proficiency targets.

SUMMARY OF CURRENT EVIDENCE AND IMPLICATIONS

Strong evidence supports the use of technology-enhanced simulation for the training of health professionals [4]. Independent of simulator fidelity and trainee level, improvements in the outcomes of laparoscopic procedures have been documented in the form of decreases in operative time, intraoperative errors and complications, improvements in residents' performance and participation, and clinically relevant patient outcomes in the form of decreases in postoperative complications and duration of the hospital stay. A key denominator to studies that have demonstrated such positive transfer of skills to the OR is purposeful repetition with appropriate feedback, termed deliberate practice, a key component of mastery learning or proficiency-based training. The authors, thus, return to the opening statement: repetition is the mother of learning, be it on a pig, cadaver, or simulator, it works and it is safer than practicing on patients.

With strong evidence to support the notion that when compared with no intervention, simulation works [4], the authors question the need for further studies attempting to *justify* the use of simulation-based education by addressing questions, such as *does it work?* Instead, questions should be aimed at trying to *clarify* when, how, to whom, under what circumstances, and in what combination is technology-enhanced simulation more efficient and cost-effective to train laparoscopic surgeons [4,28]. Theory-based head-to-head comparisons between different simulation modalities with one-at-a-time variations in the features of the instructional design will advance our understanding of the science of research in simulation-based education.

Acknowledgments

The authors would like to thank Dr Michael G. Sarr and Mrs Linda Haigh for their critical review of this article. The authors would also like to acknowledge Drs David A. Cook, Stan J. Hamstra, Rose Hatala, Ryan Brydges, Amy T. Wang, Jason H. Szostek and Ms Patricia J. Erwin for their respective contributions to the systematic review from which the data used in this work emerged [4].

References

[1] Fletcher DR, Hobbs MS, Tan P, et al. Complications of cholecystectomy: risks of the laparoscopic approach and protective effects of operative cholangiography: a population-based study. Ann Surg 1999;229(4):449–57.

[2] Kohn LT, Corrigan JM, Donaldson MS, editors. Committee on Quality of Health Care in America, Institute of Medicine. To err is human: building a safer health system. Washington, DC: The National Academies Press; 2000.

[3] Bridges M, Diamond DL. The financial impact of teaching surgical residents in the operating room. Am J Surg 1999;177(1):28–32.

[4] Cook DA, Hatala R, Brydges R, et al. Technology-enhanced simulation for health professions education: a systematic review and meta-analysis. JAMA 2011;306(9):978–88.

[5] Zendejas B, Cook DA, Bingener J, et al. Simulation-based mastery learning improves patient outcomes in laparoscopic inguinal hernia repair. A randomized controlled trial. Ann Surg 2011;254(3):502–11.

[6] Tsuda S, Scott D, Doyle J, et al. Surgical skills training and simulation. Curr Probl Surg 2009;46(4):271–370.

[7] Stefanidis D, Scerbo MW, Montero PN, et al. Simulator training to automaticity leads to improved skill transfer compared with traditional proficiency-based training: a randomized controlled trial. Ann Surg 2012;255(1):30–7.

[8] Kirkpatrick D. Great ideas revisited. Techniques for evaluating training programs. Revisiting Kirkpatrick's four-level model. Train Dev 1996;50(1):54–9.

[9] Cohen J. Statistical power analysis for the behavioral sciences. 2nd edition. Hillsdale (NJ): L Erlbaum Associates; 1988.

[10] Cook DA, Brydges R, Hamstra SJ, et al. Comparative effectiveness of technology-enhanced simulation vs other instructional methods: a systematic review and meta-analysis. Simul Healthc, in press.

[11] Hogle NJ, Chang L, Strong VE, et al. Validation of laparoscopic surgical skills training outside the operating room: a long road. Surg Endosc 2009;23(7):1476–82.

[12] Scott DJ, Bergen PC, Rege RV, et al. Laparoscopic training on bench models: better and more cost effective than operating room experience? J Am Coll Surg 2000;191(3):272–83.

[13] Hamilton EC, Scott DJ, Kapoor A, et al. Improving operative performance using a laparoscopic hernia simulator. Am J Surg 2001;182(6):725–8.

[14] Seymour NE, Gallagher AG, Roman SA, et al. Virtual reality training improves operating room performance: results of a randomized, double-blinded study. Ann Surg 2002;236(4):458–64.

[15] Sroka G, Feldman LS, Vassiliou MC, et al. Fundamentals of laparoscopic surgery simulator training to proficiency improves laparoscopic performance in the operating room-a randomized controlled trial. Am J Surg 2010;199(1):115–20.

[16] Calatayud D, Arora S, Aggarwal R, et al. Warm-up in a virtual reality environment improves performance in the operating room. Ann Surg 2010;251(6):1181–5.

[17] Ahlberg G, Enochsson L, Gallagher AG, et al. Proficiency-based virtual reality training significantly reduces the error rate for residents during their first 10 laparoscopic cholecystectomies. Am J Surg 2007;193(6):797–804.

[18] Cosman PH, Hugh TJ, Shearer CJ, et al. Skills acquired on virtual reality laparoscopic simulators transfer into the operating room in a blinded, randomised, controlled trial. Stud Health Technol Inform 2007;125:76–81.

[19] Mohan PVR, Chaudhry R. Laparoscopic simulators: are they useful! Med J Armed Forces India 2009;65(2):113–7.

[20] Grantcharov TP, Kristiansen VB, Bendix J, et al. Randomized clinical trial of virtual reality simulation for laparoscopic skills training. Br J Surg 2004;91(2):146–50.

[21] Banks EH, Chudnoff S, Karmin I, et al. Does a surgical simulator improve resident operative performance of laparoscopic tubal ligation? Am J Obstet Gynecol 2007;197(5):541.e1–5.

[22] Larsen CR, Soerensen JL, Grantcharov TP, et al. Effect of virtual reality training on laparoscopic surgery: randomised controlled trial. BMJ 2009;338:b1802.

[23] Van Sickle KR, Ritter EM, Baghai M, et al. Prospective, randomized, double-blind trial of curriculum-based training for intracorporeal suturing and knot tying. J Am Coll Surg 2008;207(4):560–8.

[24] Yang B, Zhang ZS, Xiao L, et al. A novel training model for retroperitoneal laparoscopic dismembered pyeloplasty. J Endourol 2010;24(8):1345–9.

[25] Gauger PG, Hauge LS, Andreatta PB, et al. Laparoscopic simulation training with proficiency targets improves practice and performance of novice surgeons. Am J Surg 2010;199(1): 72–80.

[26] Zendejas B, Cook DA, Hernandez-Irizarry R, et al. Mastery learning simulation-based curriculum for laparoscopic TEP inguinal hernia repair. J Surg Educ 2012;69(2):208–14.

[27] Hamilton EC, Scott DJ, Fleming JB, et al. Comparison of video trainer and virtual reality training systems on acquisition of laparoscopic skills. Surg Endosc 2002;16(3):406–11.

[28] Cook DA, Bordage G, Schmidt HG. Description, justification and clarification: a framework for classifying the purposes of research in medical education. Med Educ 2008;42(2): 128–33.

Hypertonic Resuscitation After Severe Injury: Is it of Benefit?

Eileen M. Bulger, MD[a],*, David B. Hoyt, MD[b]

[a]Department of Surgery, Harborview Medical Center, University of Washington, Box 359796, 325 9th Avenue, Seattle, WA 98104, USA; [b]American College of Surgeons, 633 North Saint Clair Street, Chicago, IL 60611, USA

Keywords
• Hypertonic saline • Hypovolemic shock resuscitation • Traumatic brain injury

Key Points
• Preclinical data suggests several potential benefits for resuscitation of hemorrhagic shock with hypertonic solutions including: improved tissue perfusion, improved microcirculatory flow, and modulation of the inflammatory response.
• Preclinical data also supports potential benefit for patients with traumatic brain injury with improved cerebral perfusion and reduced intracranial pressure.
• Despite these potential advantages, clinical trials have failed to demonstrate significant benefit from the early administration of these fluids to severely injured patients.

INTRODUCTION

Hypertonic fluids have been of interest for the resuscitation of severely injured patients for more than 30 years. Initial resuscitation of injured patients currently involves the administration of normal saline (0.9% NaCl) or lactated Ringer solution, followed by blood products as needed. Hypertonic fluids include a spectrum of solutions with increased NaCl concentrations with or without a colloid component. Reports in the literature regarding the administration of hypertonic fluids to patients range from a concentration of 1.5% to 23.4% [1,2]. Concentrations of 3% or less are usually administered as a continuous infusion, whereas higher concentrations are given as bolus therapy. The most widely studied solution is 7.5% saline (2400 mOsm/L) with or without 6% dextran-70. Indications for hypertonic resuscitation after injury have focused on resuscitation of patients with hemorrhagic shock or management of intracranial hypertension in patients with severe traumatic brain injury (TBI). The objective of this review is to discuss the mechanism of action of hypertonic fluids for these 2 indications and to summarize the experience in clinical trials with these fluids.

*Corresponding author. E-mail address: ebulger@u.washington.edu

0065-3411/12/$ – see front matter
doi:10.1016/j.yasu.2012.03.001

MECHANISM OF ACTION

Physiologic mechanism

Administration of hypertonic solutions results in an increase serum oncotic pressure, which can draw fluid from the interstitial space into the intravascular space. Thus a relatively small volume of fluid administered can result in significant volume expansion. It is estimated that administration of 250 mL of a 7.5% saline solution results in an equivalent volume expansion to 3 L of normal saline [3]. As a result, administration of these fluids for a hypovolemic patient can result in increased mean arterial pressure and improved cardiac output. Animal models of hemorrhagic shock have demonstrated rapid restoration of mean arterial pressure, improved tissue perfusion, improved cardiac contractility, and increased urinary output following resuscitation with hypertonic solutions [3]. A bolus of 4 mL/kg of 7.5% saline transiently increases serum osmolality by 30 to 50 mOsm, depending on the rate of infusion. This increase results in a total osmotic pressure of 500 to 1000 mm Hg, and rapid volume expansion begins during the infusion. Various colloids have been added to hypertonic saline, including 6% dextran-70 and hydroxyethyl starch, in an effort to increase the duration of these effects [3]. Studies by Velasco and colleagues [3,4] demonstrated that the addition of dextran to 7.5% saline increased the duration of volume expansion to greater than 3 hours.

One concern with this resuscitation approach has been that a transient increase in blood pressure could lead to increased blood loss in the setting of uncontrolled hemorrhage [5]. Animal studies have had conflicting results in this regard, with some showing evidence of increased hemorrhage with hypertonic fluids and others showing no such evidence [6–16]. In one study, although resuscitation with 7.5% saline/6% dextran-70 (hypertonic saline-dextran; HSD) led to increased hemorrhage, the degree of hemorrhage was less than that seen with conventional resuscitation with lactated Ringer [6]. In another study where the fluid was started 30 minutes after the injury and administered at a rate consistent with clinical intravenous infusion, there was no evidence of increased hemorrhage [7].

Microcirculatory effects

In addition to the macrocirculatory effects on blood pressure, several studies have demonstrated that resuscitation with hypertonic solutions can affect the microcirculation [17–24]. Impaired flow through the microcirculation following shock or TBI is thought to contribute to the progression of organ failure. Hypertonic fluids have been shown to result in improved capillary patency and arteriolar flow in several animal models [17]. The mechanisms of this effect include reduced endothelial cell swelling, reduced interactions between leukocytes and the endothelium, and constriction of capacitance vessels (for a review, see Pascual and colleagues [20]). Improvements in microcirculatory flow should result in decreased organ ischemia. In addition, the increased capillary permeability seen after severe injury, which results in a clinical capillary leak, is reduced. Some studies have suggested that the addition of the colloid to hypertonic solutions, especially dextran-70, results in further improvements in microcirculatory flow [21,22].

Immunologic effects

In addition to the physiologic and circulatory effects of hypertonic solutions, an extensive body of literature has demonstrated that these solutions have dramatic effects on the innate and cellular immune response. A fact only recently appreciated is that changes in volume affect a wide variety of cellular functions. Early on, it was determined that to migrate, polymorphonuclear neutrophils (PMN) have to undergo obligatory cell swelling [25,26]. Under hypertonic conditions PMN cell shrinkage suppresses cellular migration [25,27]. These effects on PMN motility were later explained by Rizoli and colleagues [26], who reported a major increase in actin polymerization under hypertonic conditions that resulted in impaired PMN motility, exocytosis, chemotaxis, adhesion, transmigration, and generation of reactive oxygen species. Hampton and colleagues [28] were the first to describe that PMN shrinkage, induced by exposure to hypertonicity, reduced PMN-mediated bacterial killing, generation of reactive oxygen species, and degranulation. The inability of PMN exposed to hypertonicity to mount an oxidative response has been extensively documented [26,29,30].

Hypertonicity also causes major changes in PMN expression of adhesion molecules, further incapacitating the PMN from adhering to the endothelium and becoming activated by interfering with the biochemical pathways triggered by these molecules. Hypertonicity causes an extensive shedding of CD62L from the cell surface while preventing the upregulation of CD11b/CD18 [31,32], which renders these cells unable to roll or adhere. In summary, exposure of isolated human neutrophils to hypertonicity results in a profound inhibition of most, if not all, PMN functions. These effects are transient and largely restored when the neutrophils are returned to an isotonic environment and are allowed to regain their original volume [33].

These in vitro findings have been confirmed in animal models of lung injury. Resuscitation by hypertonic saline has been shown to significantly attenuate inflammatory lung injury in a 2-hit animal model consisting of hemorrhagic shock with reperfusion followed by and intratracheal endotoxin challenge [31]. Lung injury was also attenuated by hypertonic resuscitation in a hemorrhagic-shock model by reducing hemorrhage-induced activation of neutrophil oxidative burst [30]. The timing of hypertonic saline administration seems to be crucial, as lung injury was attenuated by administration at the time of reperfusion, but was enhanced in animals given hypertonic saline after partial resuscitation with crystalloid [34].

Recent human studies have suggested that similar changes in PMN function are seen in injured patients receiving HSD in the prehospital setting [35,36]. However, injured patients have also been shown to have enhanced expression of the PMN adenosine A3 receptor, which may mitigate the anti-inflammatory effects of hypertonic saline [37].

The effect of hypertonic saline on monocyte/macrophage activation is less well defined. One study suggests that similar to the PMN effect, hypertonic preconditioning inhibits the macrophage responsiveness to inflammatory stimuli, such as endotoxin [38]. These studies demonstrated a significant reduction in production and activity of tumor necrosis factor α in response to endotoxin following hypertonic saline pretreatment. In addition, recent studies suggest that hypertonic treatment results in a shift in macrophage morphology from a proinflammatory to an anti-inflammatory phenotype [35]. Similar to the neutrophil data, these effects are transient with restoration of normal macrophage responsiveness, 20 hours following initial hypertonic conditioning.

The innate immune response after injury relies primarily on T-cell activation. Junger and colleagues [39] have demonstrated that increases in extracellular hypertonicity dramatically enhance T-cell proliferation. This effect was not restricted to NaCl, but was also observed when the extracellular tonicity was increased with other compounds, including KCl, sucrose, and choline chloride, indicating that hypertonicity, rather than NaCl per se, was responsible for the enhancing effects of hypertonic saline on T-cell function [39]. Further investigation of T-cell function in vivo revealed that hypertonic saline infusion in healthy animals increased cell-mediated immune function, as assessed by delayed-type hypersensitivity testing. Hypertonic saline, at clinically relevant levels, prevented the suppression of mouse T cells by prostaglandin E_2 in vitro [40], and hypertonic resuscitation reduced T-cell suppression and mortality in vivo in a mouse model of hemorrhagic shock followed by experimental sepsis [40–42]. In addition, hypertonic saline restored the function of human T cells that were exposed to anti-inflammatory mediators known to suppress T-cell function in trauma patients [43].

Impact on physiology after traumatic brain injury

Cerebral edema following TBI results from extravasation into areas of microvascular injury, vasoregulatory dysfunction, and the interstitial accumulation of osmotically active substances [44]. The injured brain loses its ability to autoregulate the vasculature in response to changes in blood flow, thus increasing its sensitivity to hypotension [45]. Thus the physiologic effects of hypertonic saline in improving mean arterial pressure and the osmotic effects leading to reduced brain swelling could both contribute to improved cerebral perfusion.

Hypertonic solutions have been shown to lower intracranial pressure (ICP) in several clinical trials and animal models [46–56]. The effect of hypertonic saline on ICP is thought to be due primarily to reduction of cerebral edema caused by increased osmotic load in the intravascular space. During cerebral injury, organic solutes that function as osmolytes are extruded into the extracellular space by several mechanisms thus contributing to the increase in ICP [44]. Increasing extracellular sodium levels by administration of hypertonic saline restores the active cellular sodium-osmolyte cotransporters, which restore the osmolytes to the intracellular space and thus restore normal cell polarity. This fact may explain the prolonged effects on ICP seen in human trials in which a 10- to 15-mEq/L increase in serum sodium lowered ICP for 72 hours [57].

In addition to its favorable effects on ICP, hypertonic saline has also been shown to have vasoregulatory, immunomodulatory, and neurochemical effects on the injured brain that may be beneficial [44]. Hypertonic saline counteracts hypoperfusion and vasospasm by increasing vessel diameter via volume expansion. In addition, hypertonic solutions may have direct effects on the vascular endothelium in the injured brain. Hypertonic saline infusion has also been associated with the release of nitric oxide, endothelins, and eicosanoids that alter vasomotor tone [58–60]. The systemic immunomodulatory effects of hypertonic saline (described in detail earlier) may also be beneficial in reducing the migration and activation of cerebral leukocytes that exacerbate acute cerebral injury. Much research has focused on inhibiting the effects of excitatory amino acids, such as glutamate, released as a result of brain injury and ischemia. HSD may be beneficial in this regard, as increasing extracellular sodium reestablishes the normal direction of the sodium/glutamate transporters, which restore intracellular glutamate levels [61].

A recent study of early resuscitation with HSD in humans with TBI has demonstrated significant reductions in biomarkers of brain injury including S100B, neuron-specific enolase, and myelin basic protein [62]. These findings suggest mitigation of brain injury.

CLINICAL TRIAL RESULTS

Before the year 2000 there were 8 clinical trials of HSD for the acute resuscitation of hypovolemic patients (Table 1) [63–70]. In 6 of these trials HSD was administered in the prehospital environment, while in 2 it was administered on arrival to the emergency department. In all trials there were no significant adverse events, attesting to the safety of this therapy. The 6 prehospital trials all demonstrated a survival benefit for patients treated with HSD versus conventional isotonic resuscitation, but did not reach statistical significance. The 2 emergency room trials showed no difference in survival, suggesting that the administration of this fluid at the time of initial reperfusion may be critical. In all prehospital trials, a 250-mL bolus of 7.5% saline (HS) with or without 6% dextran-70 versus a standard crystalloid solution (lactated Ringer or normal saline) was administered in a blinded fashion, followed by additional resuscitation with the standard crystalloid solution as required.

The largest of these early trials was a multicenter trial by Mattox and colleagues in 1991 [65]. This trial involved prehospital administration of HSD in 3 cities in the United States. Although designed to be representative of the entire trauma population, this trial had a much higher percentage of penetrating trauma victims (72%) than seen in most studies. As a result, the investigators were unable to evaluate any effect on TBI, although they did report a trend toward a decrease in the incidence of acute respiratory distress syndrome (ARDS). However, only 2 patients in the cohort developed ARDS, which is a much lower incidence than seen in the average blunt-trauma population.

There were 3 subsequent meta-analyses of these data by Wade and colleagues [71–73]. The first was a traditional meta-analysis of all the trials using HSD or HS published as of 1997, which concluded that HSD offers a survival benefit for the treatment of traumatic hypotension whereas there was no benefit from HS alone. These investigators acknowledged the limitations of including studies with significant differences in design, and so went on to perform 2 individual patient cohort analyses. The first, which included 1395 patients from previous trials,

Table 1
Clinical trials of hypertonic resuscitation after severe injury

Reference, year	Population	Design	N	Hypertonic fluid	Outcome
Holcroft et al [64], 1987	Prehospital trauma patients	Prospective, randomized	49	3% NaCl & 7.5% NaCl/6% dextran-70	Improved SBP
Holcroft et al [63], 1989	Hypovolemic shock (Emergency Dept SBP <80 mm Hg)	Prospective, randomized	32	7.5% NaCl/6% dextran-70	No difference in survival
Vassar et al [67], 1991	Hypovolemic shock (prehospital SBP <100 mm Hg)	Prospective, randomized	166	7.5% NaCl/6% dextran-70	Improved SBP and trend toward improved survival for TBI patients
Mattox et al [65], 1991	Hypovolemic shock (prehospital SBP <90 mm Hg)	Prospective, randomized	359	7.5% NaCl/6% dextran-70	Improved SBP, trend toward improved survival, decrease in ARDS
Younes et al [69], 1992	Hypovolemic shock (Emergency Dept SBP <80 mm Hg)	Prospective, randomized	105	7.5% NaCl & 7.5% NaCl/6% dextran-70	Improved SBP, no difference in survival
Vassar et al [66], 1993	Hypovolemic shock (prehospital SBP <90 mm Hg) Ground transport	Prospective, randomized	258	7.5% NaCl & 7.5% NaCl/6% dextran-70	Improved survival vs predicted survival based on Major Trauma Outcome Study
Vassar et al [68], 1993	Hypovolemic shock (prehospital SBP <90 mm Hg) Air transport	Prospective, randomized	194	7.5% NaCl & 7.5% NaCl/6% dextran-70	Improved survival vs predicted survival based on TRISS

Younes et al [70], 1997	Hypovolemic shock (Emergency Dept SBP <80 mm Hg)	Prospective, randomized	212	7.5% NaCl/6% dextran-70	Improved survival for subgroup with SBP <70 mm Hg
Cooper et al [74], 2004	Traumatic brain injury and shock (prehospital GCS <9 and SBP <100 mm Hg)	Prospective, randomized	229	7.5% NaCl	No difference in 6-month extended Glasgow Outcome Score
Bulger et al [76], 2008	Hypovolemic shock, blunt injury only (prehospital SBP <90 mm Hg)	Prospective, randomized	209	7.5% NaCl/6% dextran-70	No difference in 28-day ARDS-free survival, improvement in massive transfusion subgroup
Bulger et al [78], 2010	Hypovolemic shock (prehospital SBP <70 mm Hg or 70–90 mm Hg with HR >108 beats/min)	Prospective, randomized	894	7.5% NaCl & 7.5% NaCl/6% dextran-70	No difference in 28-day survival, higher mortality in a postrandomization subgroup
Bulger et al [78], 2010	Traumatic brain injury (prehospital GCS <9)	Prospective, randomized	1327	7.5% NaCl & 7.5% NaCl/6% dextran-70	No difference in 6-month extended Glasgow Outcome Score
Morrison et al [75], 2011	Traumatic brain injury (prehospital GCS <9)	Prospective, randomized	109	7.5% NaCl/6% dextran-70	No difference in outcome but limited neurologic follow-up

Abbreviations: ARDS, acute respiratory distress syndrome; GCS, Glasgow Coma Scale; HR, heart rate; SBP, systolic blood pressure; TBI, traumatic brain injury; TRISS, Trauma and Injury Severity Score.

demonstrated an improvement in overall survival to discharge in the HSD group (odds ratio [OR] 1.47, 95% confidence interval [CI] 1.04–2.08). Furthermore, patients who required blood transfusion or immediate surgical intervention for bleeding showed an even greater survival benefit from HSD. The second analysis focused on 223 patients with hypotension and TBI. The investigators concluded that HSD treatment in these patients resulted in a 2-fold increase in survival compared with conventional resuscitation.

A recent study assessed the effect of hypertonic resuscitation on outcome for patients with both hypotension and severe TBI [74]. This study enrolled 229 patients, randomized to 250 mL 7.5% saline without dextran versus lactated Ringer as the initial prehospital resuscitation fluid, and assessed neurologic outcome using the extended Glasgow Outcome Score 6 months after injury. This trial failed to identify any difference in neurologic outcome; however, there were significant limitations. Based on the authors' estimates the trial was severely underpowered to detect a meaningful difference in outcome. In addition, as this trial was confined to TBI patients with prehospital hypotension, there was very high mortality (50%), thus limiting the number of subjects available for follow-up evaluation. Although not statistically significant, a trend was observed toward improved survival at 6 months in the HS group (OR 1.17, 95% CI .9–1.5; $P = .23$). Of the patients who survived to the Emergency Department, the long-term survival was 67% for those receiving HS versus 55% for the lactated Ringer group (OR 1.72, 95% CI 0.95–3.1; $P = .073$). Another recent study that focused specifically on the TBI population enrolled 109 patients with a prehospital Glasgow Coma Scale (GCS) score of less than 9 randomized to HSD versus normal saline [75]. This study failed to draw any significant conclusions, owing to the insufficient 6-month follow-up.

The major limitations of the early studies of hypertonic resuscitation were either the insufficient patient number to enable detection of significant clinical differences in outcome, or the lack of focus on the specific patient population most likely to benefit. These studies were also conducted before the evolution of the basic science literature demonstrating the effects of hypertonicity on the immunoinflammatory response.

In 2005 a trial of HSD versus lactated Ringer following blunt traumatic injury with hypovolemic shock was closed for reasons of futility [76]. The primary end point for this trial was ARDS-free survival at 28 days. Twenty-eight-day survival, which was a secondary end point for this trial, was assessed by using Cox proportional hazards methods. There was no overall benefit to HSD resuscitation, with an unadjusted hazard ratio (HR) of 0.75 (95% CI 0.44–1.3). After adjusting for differences in baseline characteristics, the HR was 0.98 (95% CI 0.53–1.80) There was evidence of improved outcome for patients who were in severe shock, as manifested by the need for 10 units or more of packed red blood cells in the first 24 hours after injury. This finding was further evaluated using Cox proportional hazards methods with an interaction term to assess the effect of treatment in relation to amount of red cells transfused. The HR for 28-day survival was 2.49 (95% CI 1.1–5.6). The lack of an overall improvement in outcome in this study was attributed to the enrollment of a significant number of patients who were transiently hypotensive in the prehospital setting, but not truly in hemorrhagic shock, manifested by the fact that 45% of the patients enrolled did not receive any blood transfusions in the first 24 hours.

These data were used in the design of 2 subsequent trials conducted by the Resuscitation Outcomes Consortium from 2006 to 2009 [77–79]. These trials were randomized controlled trials of 250 mL 7.5% saline (HS), 7.5% saline/6% dextran-70 (HSD), or 0.9% saline (NS) as the initial resuscitation fluid administered in the prehospital setting following severe traumatic injury with evidence of either hypovolemic shock or severe TBI. The shock cohort was based on initial vital signs of systolic blood pressure of less than 70 mm Hg or 70 to 90 mm Hg, with a heart rate of 108 beats/min or greater. The TBI cohort was based on a prehospital GCS score of 8 or less. Patients meeting both entry criteria were analyzed in the shock cohort.

Enrollment in the shock cohort was suspended by the Data Safety Monitoring Board in August 2008, secondary to futility and a potential safety concern in the hypertonic groups (N = 894) [77]. There was no difference in 28-day survival: HSD 74.5%, HS 73.0%, and NS 74.4% ($P = .91$). There was a higher mortality for the postrandomization subgroup of patients who did not receive blood transfusions in the first 24 hours and who received hypertonic fluids compared with normal saline (28-day mortality: HSD 10%, HS 12.2%, NS 4.8%; $P < .01$) This result was attributed to a shift toward earlier mortality in the hypertonic groups. Enrollment in the TBI cohort was suspended in 2009 secondary to futility (N = 1327) [78]. There was no difference in 6-month neurologic outcome: extended Glasgow Outcome Score of 4 or less (death or severe disability) HSD 53.7%, HS 54.3%, NS 51.5% ($P = .67$). There was no statistically significant difference in 28-day survival or in the distribution of the extended Glasgow Outcome Score or disability rating score by treatment group.

SUMMARY

There is a wealth of preclinical data suggesting potential benefit from the administration of hypertonic solutions after severe injury with hypovolemic shock, including improved tissue perfusion, improved flow through the microcirculation, and modulation of the inflammatory response, which may mitigate subsequent organ failure. However, despite these potential advantages, clinical trials of hypertonic resuscitation early after injury have failed to demonstrate significant benefit for resuscitation of hemorrhagic shock, and although there is no difference in overall mortality, there appears to be a trend toward earlier mortality among those receiving hypertonic fluids.

Likewise, for TBI there are data suggesting that hypertonic fluids should support cerebral perfusion and mitigate intracranial hypertension, yet the clinical trials of early administration to these patients have also failed to show benefit. Further study is warranted in this patient population, as a longer period of hypertonicity may be required to show a clinical effect. Assessment of long-term neurologic outcome in this patient population remains the gold standard in determining benefit.

References

[1] Shackford SR, Bourguignon PR, Wald SL, et al. Hypertonic saline resuscitation of patients with head injury: a prospective, randomized clinical trial. J Trauma 1998;44(1):50–8.
[2] Kerwin AJ, Schinco MA, Tepas JJ 3rd, et al. The use of 23.4% hypertonic saline for the management of elevated intracranial pressure in patients with severe traumatic brain injury: a pilot study. J Trauma 2009;67(2):277–82.
[3] Kramer GC. Hypertonic resuscitation: physiologic mechanisms and recommendations for trauma care. J Trauma 2003;54(Suppl 5):S89–99.
[4] Velasco IT, Rocha e Silva M, Oliveira MA, et al. Hypertonic and hyperoncotic resuscitation from severe hemorrhagic shock in dogs: a comparative study. Crit Care Med 1989;17(3): 261–4.
[5] Dubick MA, Bruttig SP, Wade CE. Issues of concern regarding the use of hypertonic/hyperoncotic fluid resuscitation of hemorrhagic hypotension. Shock 2006;25(4):321–8.
[6] Bickell WH, Bruttig SP, Millnamow GA, et al. Use of hypertonic saline/dextran versus lactated Ringer's solution as a resuscitation fluid after uncontrolled aortic hemorrhage in anesthetized swine. Ann Emerg Med 1992;21(9):1077–85.
[7] Bruttig SP, O'Benar JD, Wade CE, et al. Benefit of slow infusion of hypertonic saline/dextran in swine with uncontrolled aortotomy hemorrhage. Shock 2005;24(1):92–6.
[8] Doucet JJ, Hall RI. Limited resuscitation with hypertonic saline, hypertonic sodium acetate, and lactated Ringer's solution in a model of uncontrolled hemorrhage from a vascular injury. J Trauma 1999;47(5):956–63.
[9] Elgjo GI, Knardahl S. Low-dose hypertonic saline (NaCl 8.0%) treatment of uncontrolled abdominal hemorrhage: effects on arterial versus venous injury. Shock 1996;5(1): 52–8.
[10] Gross D, Landau EH, Assalia A, et al. Is hypertonic saline resuscitation safe in 'uncontrolled' hemorrhagic shock? J Trauma 1988;28(6):751–6.
[11] Kentner R, Safar P, Prueckner S, et al. Titrated hypertonic/hyperoncotic solution for hypotensive fluid resuscitation during uncontrolled hemorrhagic shock in rats. Resuscitation 2005;65(1):87–95.
[12] Krausz MM, Landau EH, Klin B, et al. Hypertonic saline treatment of uncontrolled hemorrhagic shock at different periods from bleeding. Arch Surg 1992;127(1):93–6.
[13] Matsuoka T, Hildreth J, Wisner DH. Liver injury as a model of uncontrolled hemorrhagic shock: resuscitation with different hypertonic regimens. J Trauma 1995;39(4):674–80.
[14] Riddez L, Drobin D, Sjostrand F, et al. Lower dose of hypertonic saline dextran reduces the risk of lethal rebleeding in uncontrolled hemorrhage. Shock 2002;17(5):377–82.
[15] Stern SA, Jwayyed S, Dronen SC, et al. Resuscitation of severe uncontrolled hemorrhage: 7.5% sodium chloride/6% dextran 70 vs 0.9% sodium chloride. Acad Emerg Med 2000;7(8):847–56.
[16] Stern SA, Kowalenko T, Younger J, et al. Comparison of the effects of bolus vs. slow infusion of 7.5% NaCl/6% dextran-70 in a model of near-lethal uncontrolled hemorrhage. Shock 2000;14(6):616–22.
[17] Bauer M, Marzi I, Ziegenfuss T, et al. Comparative effects of crystalloid and small volume hypertonic hyperoncotic fluid resuscitation on hepatic microcirculation after hemorrhagic shock. Circ Shock 1993;40(3):187–93.
[18] Hartl R, Medary MB, Ruge M, et al. Hypertonic/hyperoncotic saline attenuates microcirculatory disturbances after traumatic brain injury. J Trauma 1997;42(Suppl 5):S41–7.
[19] Mittlmeier T, Vollmar B, Menger MD, et al. Small volume hypertonic hydroxyethyl starch reduces acute microvascular dysfunction after closed soft-tissue trauma. J Bone Joint Surg Br 2003;85(1):126–32.

[20] Pascual JL, Khwaja KA, Chaudhury P, et al. Hypertonic saline and the microcirculation. J Trauma 2003;54(Suppl 5):S133–40.

[21] Strecker U, Dick W, Madjidi A, et al. The effect of the type of colloid on the efficacy of hypertonic saline colloid mixtures in hemorrhagic shock: dextran versus hydroxyethyl starch. Resuscitation 1993;25(1):41–57.

[22] Victorino GP, Newton CR, Curran B. Dextran modulates microvascular permeability: effect in isotonic and hypertonic solutions. Shock 2003;19(2):183–6.

[23] Zakaria el R, Tsakadze NL, Garrison RN. Hypertonic saline resuscitation improves intestinal microcirculation in a rat model of hemorrhagic shock. Surgery 2006;140(4):579–87 [discussion: 587–8].

[24] Zhao L, Wang B, You G, et al. Effects of different resuscitation fluids on the rheologic behavior of red blood cells, blood viscosity and plasma viscosity in experimental hemorrhagic shock. Resuscitation 2009;80(2):253–8.

[25] Worthen GS, Henson PM, Rosengren S, et al. Neutrophils increase volume during migration in vivo and in vitro. Am J Respir Cell Mol Biol 1994;10(1):1–7.

[26] Rizoli SB, Rotstein OD, Parodo J, et al. Hypertonic inhibition of exocytosis in neutrophils: central role for osmotic actin skeleton remodeling. Am J Physiol Cell Physiol 2000;279(3): C619–33.

[27] Rosengren S, Henson PM, Worthen GS. Migration-associated volume changes in neutrophils facilitate the migratory process in vitro. Am J Physiol 1994;267(6 Pt 1):C1623–32.

[28] Hampton MB, Chambers ST, Vissers MC, et al. Bacterial killing by neutrophils in hypertonic environments. J Infect Dis 1994;169(4):839–46.

[29] Junger WG, Hoyt DB, Davis RE, et al. Hypertonicity regulates the function of human neutrophils by modulating chemoattractant receptor signaling and activating mitogen-activated protein kinase p38. J Clin Invest 1998;101(12):2768–79.

[30] Angle N, Hoyt DB, Coimbra R, et al. Hypertonic saline resuscitation diminishes lung injury by suppressing neutrophil activation after hemorrhagic shock. Shock 1998;9(3): 164–70.

[31] Rizoli SB, Kapus A, Fan J, et al. Immunomodulatory effects of hypertonic resuscitation on the development of lung inflammation following hemorrhagic shock. J Immunol 1998;161(11): 6288–96.

[32] Thiel M, Buessecker F, Eberhardt K, et al. Effects of hypertonic saline on expression of human polymorphonuclear leukocyte adhesion molecules. J Leukoc Biol 2001;70(2): 261–73.

[33] Rizoli SB, Kapus A, Parodo J, et al. Hypertonic immunomodulation is reversible and accompanied by changes in CD11b expression. J Surg Res 1999;83(2):130–5.

[34] Murao Y, Hoyt DB, Loomis W, et al. Does the timing of hypertonic saline resuscitation affect its potential to prevent lung damage? Shock 2000;14(1):18–23.

[35] Rizoli SB, Rhind SG, Shek PN, et al. The immunomodulatory effects of hypertonic saline resuscitation in patients sustaining traumatic hemorrhagic shock: a randomized, controlled, double-blinded trial. Ann Surg 2006;243(1):47–57.

[36] Bulger EM, Cuschieri J, Warner K, et al. Hypertonic resuscitation modulates the inflammatory response in patients with traumatic hemorrhagic shock. Ann Surg 2006;245(4): 635–41.

[37] Bulger EM, Tower CM, Warner KJ, et al. Increased neutrophil adenosine A3 receptor expression is associated with hemorrhagic shock and injury severity in trauma patients. Shock 2011;36(5):435–9.

[38] Cuschieri J, Gourlay D, Garcia I, et al. Hypertonic preconditioning inhibits macrophage responsiveness to endotoxin. J Immunol 2002;168:1389–96.

[39] Junger WG, Liu FC, Loomis WH, et al. Hypertonic saline enhances cellular immune function. Circ Shock 1994;42(4):190–6.

[40] Coimbra R, Junger WG, Liu FC, et al. Hypertonic/hyperoncotic fluids reverse prostaglandin E2 (PGE2)-induced T-cell suppression. Shock 1995;4(1):45–9.

[41] Coimbra R, Junger WG, Hoyt DB, et al. Hypertonic saline resuscitation restores hemorrhage-induced immunosuppression by decreasing prostaglandin E2 and interleukin-4 production. J Surg Res 1996;64(2):203–9.

[42] Coimbra R, Hoyt DB, Junger WG, et al. Hypertonic saline resuscitation decreases susceptibility to sepsis after hemorrhagic shock. J Trauma 1997;42(4):602–6 [discussion: 606–7].

[43] Loomis WH, Namiki S, Hoyt DB, et al. Hypertonicity rescues T cells from suppression by trauma-induced anti- inflammatory mediators. Am J Physiol Cell Physiol 2001;281(3): C840–8.

[44] Doyle JA, Davis DP, Hoyt DB. The use of hypertonic saline in the treatment of traumatic brain injury. J Trauma 2001;50(2):367–83.

[45] Rosner MJ, Rosner SD, Johnson AH. Cerebral perfusion pressure: management protocol and clinical results. J Neurosurg 1995;83(6):949–62.

[46] Sheikh AA, Matsuoka T, Wisner DH. Cerebral effects of resuscitation with hypertonic saline and a new low- sodium hypertonic fluid in hemorrhagic shock and head injury. Crit Care Med 1996;24(7):1226–32.

[47] Battistella FD, Wisner DH. Combined hemorrhagic shock and head injury: effects of hypertonic saline (7.5%) resuscitation. J Trauma 1991;31(2):182–8.

[48] Berger S, Schurer L, Hartl R, et al. 7.2% NaCl/10% dextran 60 versus 20% mannitol for treatment of intracranial hypertension. Acta Neurochir Suppl 1994;60:494–8.

[49] Berger S, Schurer L, Hartl R, et al. Reduction of post-traumatic intracranial hypertension by hypertonic/hyperoncotic saline/dextran and hypertonic mannitol. Neurosurgery 1995;37(1): 98–107 [discussion: 107–8].

[50] Ducey JP, Mozingo DW, Lamiell JM, et al. A comparison of the cerebral and cardiovascular effects of complete resuscitation with isotonic and hypertonic saline, hetastarch, and whole blood following hemorrhage. J Trauma 1989;29(11):1510–8.

[51] Prough DS, Johnson JC, Poole GV Jr, et al. Effects on intracranial pressure of resuscitation from hemorrhagic shock with hypertonic saline versus lactated Ringer's solution. Crit Care Med 1985;13(5):407–11.

[52] Zornow MH, Scheller MS, Shackford SR. Effect of a hypertonic lactated Ringer's solution on intracranial pressure and cerebral water content in a model of traumatic brain injury. J Trauma 1989;29(4):484–8.

[53] Freshman SP, Battistella FD, Matteucci M, et al. Hypertonic saline (7.5%) versus mannitol: a comparison for treatment of acute head injuries. J Trauma 1993;35(3):344–8.

[54] Qureshi AI, Suarez JI. Use of hypertonic saline solutions in treatment of cerebral edema and intracranial hypertension. Crit Care Med 2000;28(9):3301–13.

[55] Simma B, Burger R, Falk M, et al. A prospective, randomized, and controlled study of fluid management in children with severe head injury: lactated Ringer's solution versus hypertonic saline. Crit Care Med 1998;26(7):1265–70.

[56] Schatzmann C, Heissler HE, Konig K, et al. Treatment of elevated intracranial pressure by infusions of 10% saline in severely head injured patients. Acta Neurochir Suppl 1998;71:31–3.

[57] Qureshi AI, Suarez JI, Bhardwaj A, et al. Use of hypertonic (3%) saline/acetate infusion in the treatment of cerebral edema: effect on intracranial pressure and lateral displacement of the brain. Crit Care Med 1998;26(3):440–6.

[58] Kraus GE, Bucholz RD, Yoon KW, et al. Cerebrospinal fluid endothelin-1 and endothelin-3 levels in normal and neurosurgical patients: a clinical study and literature review. Surg Neurol 1991;35(1):20–9.

[59] Steenbergen JM, Bohlen HG. Sodium hyperosmolarity of intestinal lymph causes arteriolar vasodilation in part mediated by EDRF. Am J Physiol 1993;265(1 Pt 2):H323–8.

[60] Hariri RJ, Ghajar JB, Pomerantz KB, et al. Human glial cell production of lipoxygenase-generated eicosanoids: a potential role in the pathophysiology of vascular changes following traumatic brain injury. J Trauma 1989;29(9):1203–10.

[61] Phillis JW, Song D, O'Regan MH. Effects of hyperosmolarity and ion substitutions on amino acid efflux from the ischemic rat cerebral cortex. Brain Res 1999;828(1–2):1–11.

[62] Baker AJ, Rhind SG, Morrison LJ, et al. Resuscitation with hypertonic saline-dextran reduces serum biomarker levels and correlates with outcome in severe traumatic brain injury patients. J Neurotrauma 2009;26(8):1227–40.

[63] Holcroft JW, Vassar MJ, Perry CA, et al. Use of a 7.5% NaCl/6% dextran 70 solution in the resuscitation of injured patients in the emergency room. Prog Clin Biol Res 1989;299: 331–8.

[64] Holcroft JW, Vassar MJ, Turner JE, et al. 3% NaCl and 7.5% NaCl/dextran 70 in the resuscitation of severely injured patients. Ann Surg 1987;206(3):279–88.

[65] Mattox KL, Maningas PA, Moore EE, et al. Prehospital hypertonic saline/dextran infusion for post-traumatic hypotension. The U.S.A. Multicenter Trial. Ann Surg 1991;213(5): 482–91.

[66] Vassar MJ, Fischer RP, O'Brien PE, et al. A multicenter trial for resuscitation of injured patients with 7.5% sodium chloride. The effect of added dextran 70. The Multicenter Group for the Study of Hypertonic Saline in Trauma Patients. Arch Surg 1993;128(9):1003–11 [discussion: 1011–3].

[67] Vassar MJ, Perry CA, Gannaway WL, et al. 7.5% sodium chloride/dextran for resuscitation of trauma patients undergoing helicopter transport. Arch Surg 1991;126(9):1065–72.

[68] Vassar MJ, Perry CA, Holcroft JW. Prehospital resuscitation of hypotensive trauma patients with 7.5% NaCl versus 7.5% NaCl with added dextran: a controlled trial. J Trauma 1993;34(5):622–32 [discussion: 632–3].

[69] Younes RN, Aun F, Accioly CQ, et al. Hypertonic solutions in the treatment of hypovolemic shock: a prospective, randomized study in patients admitted to the emergency room. Surgery 1992;111(4):380–5.

[70] Younes RN, Aun F, Ching CT, et al. Prognostic factors to predict outcome following the administration of hypertonic/hyperoncotic solution in hypovolemic patients. Shock 1997;7(2):79–83.

[71] Wade CE, Grady JJ, Kramer GC. Efficacy of hypertonic saline dextran (HSD) in patients with traumatic hypotension: meta-analysis of individual patient data. Acta Anaesthesiol Scand Suppl 1997;110:77–9.

[72] Wade CE, Grady JJ, Kramer GC, et al. Individual patient cohort analysis of the efficacy of hypertonic saline/dextran in patients with traumatic brain injury and hypotension. J Trauma 1997;42(Suppl 5):S61–5.

[73] Wade CE, Kramer GC, Grady JJ, et al. Efficacy of hypertonic 7.5% saline and 6% dextran-70 in treating trauma: a meta-analysis of controlled clinical studies. Surgery 1997;122(3): 609–16.

[74] Cooper DJ, Myles PS, McDermott FT, et al. Prehospital hypertonic saline resuscitation of patients with hypotension and severe traumatic brain injury: a randomized controlled trial. JAMA 2004;291(11):1350–7.

[75] Morrison LJ, Baker AJ, Rhind SG, et al. The Toronto prehospital hypertonic resuscitation–head injury and multiorgan dysfunction trial: feasibility study of a randomized controlled trial. J Crit Care 2011;26(4):363–72.

[76] Bulger E, Jurkovich G, Nathens A, et al. Hypertonic resuscitation of hypovolemic shock after blunt trauma: a randomized controlled trial. Arch Surg 2008;143:139–48.

[77] Bulger EM, May S, Kerby J, et al; the ROC Investigators. Prehospital hypertonic resuscitation following traumatic hypovolemic shock: a randomized, placebo controlled trial. Ann Surg 2011;23:431–41.

[78] Bulger EM, May S, Brasel KJ, et al. Out-of-hospital hypertonic resuscitation following severe traumatic brain injury: a randomized controlled trial. JAMA 2010;304(13):1455–64.

[79] Brasel K, Bulger E, Cook A, et al. Hypertonic resuscitation: design and implementation of a prehospital intervention trial. J Am Coll Surg 2008;206(2):220–32.

What is the Prognosis After Retransplantation of the Liver?

Ali Zarrinpar, MD, PhD, Johnny C. Hong, MD*

Division of Liver and Pancreas Transplantation, Department of Surgery, David Geffen School of Medicine at University of California, Los Angeles, 650 C.E. Young Drive South, 77-120 CHS, Box 957054, Los Angeles, CA 90095, USA

Keywords
- Retransplantation of the liver • Prognostic index
- Patient survival after liver retransplantation • Risk stratification

Key Points
- Hepatic retransplantation (ReLT) in patients with failing liver grafts cannot be abandoned.
- Risk stratification of retransplant candidates is essential to optimize patient survival.
- Long-term patient and graft survival outcomes after ReLT are excellent and acceptable for the low and intermediate groups, respectively.
- ReLT in transplant candidates in high-risk patients cannot be recommended.
- ReLT should be reserved for centers equipped to manage the difficulties of the process.

INTRODUCTION

Long-term patient survival outcomes after primary (first time) orthotopic liver transplantation (OLT) are excellent largely because of the surgical innovations and advances in perioperative and intraoperative management and immunosuppression regimens. After primary OLT, 10% to 22% of recipients will require retransplantation of the liver (ReLT) for various reasons [1,2]. For patients with failing hepatic grafts, ReLT is the only option for survival. In numerous studies, ReLT has been associated with lower survival rates than the first transplantation [1] and is considered a high-risk procedure because of the technical demands of the operation and the severity of the illness of the ReLT candidates.

---

*Corresponding author. UCLA-Pfleger Liver Institute, Dumont-UCLA Transplant and Liver Cancer Centers, Division of Liver and Pancreas Transplantation, Department of Surgery, David Geffen School of Medicine at University of California, Los Angeles, 650 C.E. Young Drive South, 77-120 CHS, Box 957054, Los Angeles, CA 90095-7054. *E-mail address:* Johnnyhong@mednet.ucla.edu

0065-3411/12/$ – see front matter
doi:10.1016/j.yasu.2012.03.005

With the dramatic success of OLT, patients awaiting OLT continue to outnumber the available organs leading to a heated debate about organ allocation prioritization (Fig. 1) (based on Organ Procurement and Transplantation Network [OPTN] data as of October 21, 2011). Not only are there attendant medical and surgical problems but these are also accompanied by financial and ethical issues because of the increased resource use of ReLT and the idea of denying patients awaiting their first transplant access to grafts. Nevertheless, good long-term survival has been demonstrated in select groups of re-transplant recipients [1–3]. A trend toward improved 1-year survival is also reflected in OPTN data (Fig. 2; from Scientific Registry of Transplant Recipients [SRTR]). Objectively, the decision of whether to retransplant a patient should involve the same considerations as the first time: the operative risk and the chances of long-term survival. As such, it is important for clinicians to have tools to risk stratify ReLT candidates so that they can have an accurate predictor of survival after ReLT.

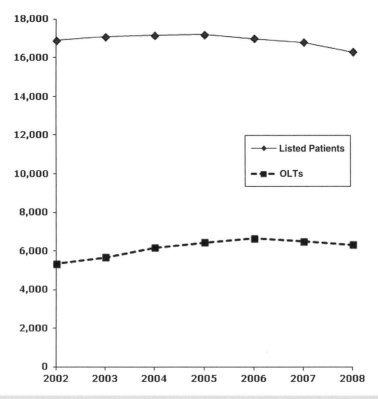

Fig. 1. Number of liver transplant candidates on the waiting list at the end of the calendar year and the number of liver transplant operations during that calendar year. (*Data from* SRTR analysis, data as of May 2009.)

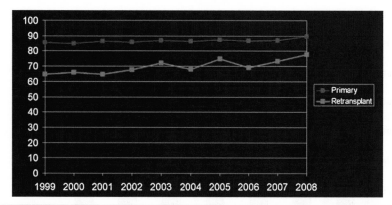

Fig. 2. One-year patient survival for primary and retransplantation by year of transplantation. (*Data from* SRTR analysis, data as of May 2009.)

INCIDENCE/EPIDEMIOLOGY

Although the long-term patient survival outcomes after OLT are steadily improving, with more than 74% of transplant recipients surviving more than 5 years, the primary liver disease can recur for almost all indications for primary OLT [4]. Most of these recipients will ultimately develop end-stage liver failure again and, thus, require additional grafts. The expectation is that the number of patients requiring ReLT will continue to grow to a proportion similar to those awaiting primary transplantation [5].

The reported rates of ReLT have not remained constant over time, probably reflecting changes in clinical practice with new discoveries in immunosuppression and antiviral agents as well as modification of surgical techniques (Fig. 3; from SRTR) [1,6]. Pediatric patients have a higher retransplantation rate largely because smaller grafts (whether partial or whole) are associated with an increased risk for vascular complications that predispose to graft failure. Although microsurgical techniques have decreased the incidence of hepatic artery thrombosis (HAT) in pediatric patients [4], vascular complications are still the most common indication for ReLT (35%). Graft failure caused by primary graft dysfunction and chronic rejection composes up to 19% and 15% of ReLT in children, respectively [7]. In adults, the 2 most common causes of hepatic graft failure are chronic rejection and recurrence of liver disease.

INDICATIONS FOR RETRANSPLANTATION

The causes of hepatic graft failure can be divided into early and late (Table 1; data from Thuluvath and colleagues [8]). These causes can be compared with the causes for the primary liver failure in first-time recipients (Table 2; data from Hong and colleagues [9]). Currently, the most common causes of graft failure leading to ReLT are the early causes: primary nonfunction (PNF), delayed nonfunction, or initial poor function. This occurrence will likely increase as more

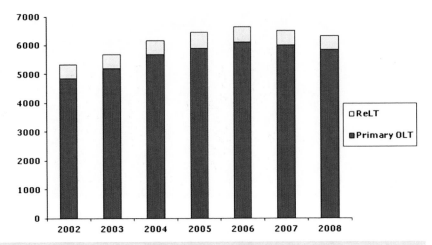

Fig. 3. Number of liver transplant operations during that calendar year, primary and retransplantation. (*Data from* SRTR analysis, data as of May 2009.)

grafts are obtained from marginal or extended criteria donors (those at higher risk based on demographic, clinical, laboratory, and histologic data) [10,11]. HAT and other vascular complications are other common early causes of graft failure [12,13]. The incidence of HAT has not significantly increased even with the use of partial grafts from deceased and living donors [14].

The most common late cause of graft failure is chronic rejection. Chronic rejection remains a major problem despite the improvement in immunosuppression therapy. The immunologic injury to the liver usually results from severe, uncontrolled, or recurrent acute rejection episodes, leading to the progressive destruction of the bile ducts, the development of perivenular and portal fibrosis, and arterial narrowing. Its occurrence is exacerbated by

Table 1
Causes of hepatic graft failure

Cause of graft failure	Early (<7 mo) (%)	Late (>7 mo) (%)	Percent of total
Primary graft failure	82	18	40
Vascular thrombosis	78	22	19
Biliary tract complication	44	56	3
Recurrent hepatitis	11	89	11
Recurrent disease	4	96	5
Acute rejection	60	40	—
Chronic rejection	8	92	18
Infection	56	44	—

Data from Thuluvath PJ, Guidinger MK, Fung JJ, et al. Liver transplantation in the United States, 1999–2008. Am J Transplant 2010;10(4 Pt 2):1003–19; and Hong JC, Kaldas FM, Kositamongkol P, et al. Predictive index for long-term survival after retransplantation of the liver in adult recipients: analysis of a 26-year experience in a single center. Ann Surg 2011;254(3):444–9.

Table 2
Causes of liver failure

Cause of liver failure	All recipients (%)	Primary liver disease in ReLT recipients (%)
Malignancy	21	12
Alcohol-induced	21	12
Hepatitis C	20	31
Cholestatic	10	15
Cryptogenic	9	8
Acute liver failure	7	8
Hepatitis B	5	5
Other	7	7

Data from Hong JC, Kosari K, Benjamin E, et al. Does race influence outcomes after primary liver transplantation? A 23-year experience with 2700 patients. J Am Coll Surg 2008;206(5):1009–16 [discussion: 1016–8]; and Hong JC, Kaldas FM, Kositamongkol P, et al. Predictive index for long-term survival after retransplantation of the liver in adult recipients: analysis of a 26-year experience in a single center. Ann Surg 2011;254(3):444–9.

reperfusion injury, viral infections, diabetes, hypertension, hyperlipidemia, and episodes of acute rejection [7,8,15].

Another indication for retransplantation is complex biliary strictures related to a variety of causes [9,16]. Nonanastomotic ischemic-type biliary strictures are characterized by a complex series of strictures and dilations involving only the biliary tree of the graft and are often associated with stone or sludge formation leading to episodes of cholangitis [17]. Ischemia, whether caused by prolonged warm or cold ischemic times or as a result of hepatic artery thrombosis or immunologically induced injury and cytotoxic injury induced by bile salts, increases the incidence of biliary strictures, which is reported to be between 5% and 15%. Ischemic-type cholangiopathy is also a major complication after OLT using donation after cardiac death grafts [18,19], although the use of tissue plasminogen activator has been reported to be protective [20].

The recurrence of the primary disease is the next most common late cause and is becoming increasingly prevalent, especially as hepatitis C virus (HCV) cirrhosis continues to be the leading indication for primary OLT. The inexorable recurrence of HCV leads to variable outcomes in the recipients and there are a host of interrelated viral, donor, and recipient factors that determine the development and progression of hepatic fibrosis [21,22]. Berenguer and colleagues [23] found that a high Child-Turcotte-Pugh score, low albumin level at the time of diagnosis of graft cirrhosis, and a short interval between OLT and the development of graft cirrhosis predicted clinical decompensation and mortality. They also found that the rate of decompensation and mortality were much higher with recurrence than the first time, thus suggesting that ReLT should be performed before decompensation. Because of these caveats, the approach to retransplantation for recurrent HCV varies widely among centers, with some choosing not to perform the procedure. Although most studies show that individuals undergoing retransplantation for HCV have worse outcomes than those undergoing primary transplantations, their outcomes do not seem to be worse than those after retransplantation for other causes. However, individuals with early aggressive recurrence and graft failure within the first year, referred to as fibrosing cholestatic hepatitis, have very poor outcomes after retransplantation and many recommend against ReLT in these patients except under highly selected conditions [21].

Other causes of liver failure have lower rates of recurrence. Alcoholic liver disease, the second most common cause of liver failure in the United States, also has high recidivism rates (up to 34%) [24]. Although hepatic graft failure from primary toxicity does occur in a small subset of these patients, more grafts fail because of the associated lack of adherence to the immunosuppression regimen. Primary biliary cirrhosis and primary sclerosing cholangitis were initially thought not to lead to recurrent disease. However, several studies have found that not to be the case. A group from the Mayo Clinic found evidence of primary sclerosing cholangitis (PSC) recurrence in 20% of liver transplant recipients [25] and another group found the recurrence of primary biliary cirrhosis (PBC) in more than 15% of their patients [26]. However, less than 5% of those patients ultimately required ReLT for graft failure from recurrent disease. Recurrent autoimmune hepatitis, however, has led to graft failure; in one study, 23% of the patients have required ReLT [27]. Previously, hepatitis B virus was plagued by a very high recurrence after OLT, especially in patients with active viral replication pre-OLT. This recurrence resulted in low enthusiasm for transplantation of these patients and even denial of coverage by some third-party payers, such as Medicare. This situation is now moot, however, with the development of effective antiviral therapies that have dropped the recurrence of hepatitis B to less than 2% [28].

SURGICAL/TECHNICAL DIFFICULTIES

The key to successful recipient hepatectomy for ReLT is to shorten the duration of total hepatectomy and to avoid significant intraoperative blood loss. The difficulty of the recipient hepatectomy will vary greatly depending on the interval between the primary operation and the subsequent transplant and cause of hepatic graft failure. On the one hand, early reoperation caused by primary graft nonfunction requires significantly less dissection, and the degree of portal hypertension is much less than the typical liver transplantation. However, in a late retransplantation caused by graft failure secondary to the recurrence of HCV cirrhosis or biliary strictures with repeated biliary infection and instrumentation, the presence of dense adhesions and scar tissue can make the recipient total hepatectomy challenging because most blood loss comes from raw surface areas of the liver parenchyma and abdominal wall, which underscores the need for expeditious control of vascular inflow to minimize blood loss.

In the presence of severe scarring or collateral vessel formation, venovenous bypass becomes essential for the decompression of the portal-mesenteric venous system and to minimize the hemodynamic fluctuations associated with the hepatectomy for patients with tenuous hemodynamic status. Portal-mesenteric venous decompression can be achieved with cannulation of either the recipient portal vein or inferior mesenteric vein. The use of the piggyback technique allows venous blood return to the heart without the need for venovenous bypass; however, this technique does not decompress the portal-mesenteric venous system. For this reason, others have advocated a creation of a temporary portacaval shunt to reduce splanchnic circulation congestion when the piggyback technique is used [29].

During excision of the liver graft, leaving the previous vena cava anastomosis intact is critical in allowing enough length for the new anastomosis. In cases when the length of the suprahepatic vena cuff is inadequate for the placement of the vascular clamp before excision of the liver graft, vascular control of the suprahepatic vena cava can be achieved in the pericardium [4]. An incision is made on the diaphragm a few centimeters anterior to the suprahepatic vena cava to permit the application of a vascular clamp on the intrapericardial IVC.

Although retaining the previous suprahepatic vena cava is usually necessary to facilitate the implantation of the new liver graft, the infrahepatic vena cava and the portal vein anastomoses will only occasionally require portions of the previous graft vessels. The reuse of the graft hepatic artery is not advisable because of the risk of necrosis of the vessel that may lead to arterial thrombosis or rupture. This fact, along with the frequent presence of HAT in the recipient, may require an alternative method of arterial reconstruction: either the use of the recipient splenic artery or the creation of an aortic conduit for hepatic graft arterialization. Similarly, the graft bile duct should not be reused and the viability of the recipient bile duct should be closely scrutinized. A Roux-en-Y choledochojejunostomy is mandatory in the presence of questionable recipient duct quality or anastomotic tension [4,30].

TIMING OF RETRANSPLANTATION

The timing of retransplantation plays an important role in both patient and graft outcome because it reflects the acuity of illness of the ReLT candidate and the severity of intra-abdominal adhesions [2,6,31]. Receiving a transplant more than 30 days after the initial OLT has been better than those who got ReLT between 8 and 30 days after OLT. Survival in patients after ReLT in the first week was nearly equivalent to the chronic group, emphasizing the need for early recognition of patients who require retransplantation, especially for PNF or HAT.

CAUSES OF DEATH

The development of sepsis and multiorgan failure accounts for most of the deaths in patients with ReLT, with the largest proportion of deaths occurring in the first 4 weeks after ReLT [32]; among those who died of sepsis, nearly 50% in the University of California, Los Angeles series died of a fungal infection [2]. This finding may reflect the higher cumulative immunosuppression and severity of illness in the ReLT group. As such, it is imperative to establish a dynamic goal in immunosuppression, titrating the level of immunosuppression based on the acuity of the illness without increasing the risk for acute rejection. However, a validated method of immune monitoring is not currently available [33–35]. In addition to the tailoring of immunosuppression after ReLT, an extended period of antimicrobial prophylaxis that includes antifungal agents is equally important in reducing the risk for serious post-ReLT infections.

PROGNOSIS/MODELS

Although ReLT continues to be controversial because of inferior survival outcomes compared with primary OLT and the consequent perceived injustice of using a scarce resource for these inferior outcomes [31,36], good long-term survival has been demonstrated when appropriate retransplant recipients have been identified [1,3]. With properly matched recipients and graft types, the 10-year survival rates for the retransplantation of both adults and children approach 50% or higher [2].

The issue, therefore, becomes patient selection. Independent predictors of diminished survival from previous studies have included recipient age greater than 18 years, need for mechanical ventilation at the time of ReLT, total bilirubin greater than 13 mg/dL, serum creatinine greater than 1.6 mg/dL, and graft ischemia time greater than 12 hours [2,37]. The clinical practice of liver transplantation has dramatically changed since these first analyses. Most importantly, the implementation in the United States of the Model for End-Stage Liver Disease (MELD) system of liver organ allocation in 2002 [38] has led to liver grafts being allocated to transplant candidates with the highest acuity of illness, therefore, limiting any recipient-to-graft matching. Oftentimes in these cases, the quality of the allocated graft may not be adequate for ReLT candidates who are usually sicker than patients undergoing primary OLT. Furthermore, with increase experience, the clinical practice today has allowed a more liberal acceptance policy for transplant candidates. The addition of many sicker patients has further widened the gap between donor organ supply and demand [8,11,39].

Several clinical models have been proposed to guide patient and donor selection for ReLT and to aid in the optimal use of a scarce resource. Rosen and colleagues [40] initially developed a model to predict survival following retransplantation and their findings were later validated using an international database [41,42]. Using registry data, the risk scores for individual patients were calculated by combining the values of 5 prognostic factors (recipient age, serum bilirubin, serum creatinine, cause of graft failure of prior transplant, and United Network for Organ Sharing [UNOS] status). The 5-year patient survival was 68% for the low-risk, 62% for the intermediate, and 38% for the high-risk groups. This model, although somewhat impractical because of its reliance on a cumbersome mathematical calculation, is no longer relevant because of its use of the UNOS status, which is a variable no longer used in the allocation of grafts. Furthermore, donor and operative factors were not included. Another group [43] evaluated donor and recipient variables to devise a risk-score point system using a multivariate model for determining long-term survival among patients after ReLT. Their model provided a good retrospective prediction of patient outcome using the recipient's age, creatinine, urgency of retransplantation, and whether the first graft failed early or late. In this model, the 5-year patient survival was 77% for the low-risk, 61% for the intermediate, and 16% for the high-risk groups. One drawback of this study is its use of data from transplants from more than a decade ago, which may not accurately reflect clinical practice in liver transplantation today. Also, the use of the urgency status for ReLT (elective vs urgent vs emergency) was based on a subjective evaluation and may not be universally applicable or reproducible.

A recent study defines a predictive model based on available preoperative clinical information for the risk stratification of patients undergoing ReLT [44]. In their analysis, Hong and colleagues [44] identified independent predictors for graft failure after ReLT (Table 3). These predictors included 5 recipient risk factors (age >55 years, prior OLT >1, MELD score >27, and the requirement of mechanical ventilator and serum albumin <2.5 g/dL at the time of ReLT), 2 operative risk factors (the time interval from the prior OLT to ReLT and the requirement for intraoperative packed red blood cells (Prbc) transfusion >30 units), and 1 donor factor (donor age >45 years). Each predictor was assigned a risk score point (RS) proportional to the log hazard ratio for tte graft failure. These points are then added together to place patients in 1 of 4 risk categories, with the 5-year graft failure–free survival rates (Table 4) of 65% for the low-risk (Predictive Index Risk Category I, RS = 0), 53% for low-intermediate, (Predictive Index Risk Category II, RS = 1–2), 43% for intermediate (Predictive Index Risk Category III, RS = 3–4), and 20% for the high-risk groups (Predictive Index Risk Category IV, RS = 5–12). Fig. 4 shows that patient survival rates were excellent and acceptable for the low, low-intermediate, and intermediate groups. This prognostic model allows for the risk stratification of candidates for retransplantation preoperatively (without the intraoperative blood use information). It also provides

Table 3
Independent predictors and assigned risk score points

Variables	Risk score points
Intraoperative Prbc >30 units	2
Prior OLT >1	2
Requirement for ventilator at time of ReLT	2
Interval of prior OLT to ReLT	
15–30 d	2
31–180 d	1
Donor age >45 y	1
MELD score >27	1
Serum albumin <2.5 g/dL at time of ReLT	1
Recipient age >55 y	1

Data from Hong JC, Kaldas FM, Kositamongkol P, et al. Predictive index for long-term survival after retransplantation of the liver in adult recipients: analysis of a 26-year experience in a single center. Ann Surg 2011;254(3):444–9.

Table 4
Collected series of liver retransplantation

Author	Year	Category	Risk factors (if applicable)	Patient survival (%) 1 y	3 y	5 y
Markmann et al [2]	1997	Adults		50	45	42
		Children		65	65	55
Rosen et al [40]	1999	Low risk	Recipient age	72	70	68
		Intermediate risk	Serum bilirubin	65	62	62
		High risk	Serum creatinine	42	38	38
			Cause of graft failure			
			UNOS status at ReLT			
Facciuto et al [32]	2000	Adults		60		42
Azoulay et al [1]	2002	Adults		61		50
Yao et al [46]	2004	Adults		70	68	65
Linhares et al [43]	2006	Low risk	Urgency of ReLT	85	82	77
		Intermediate risk	Recipient age	69	66	61
		High risk	Serum creatinine	21	19	16
			Timing of first graft failure			
Marudanayagam et al [47]	2010	Adults		66	61	57
Hong et al [44]	2011	Low risk	Intraoperative blood loss	84	79	79
		Low-intermediate risk	Number of prior OLTs	75	67	59
			Ventilator requirement			
		Intermediate risk	preoperative	63	57	49
		High risk	Interval from prior OLT to ReLT	33	26	22
			Donor age >45 y			
			MELD score >27			
			Serum albumin <2.5			
			Recipient age >55 y			

Data from Hong JC, Kaldas FM, Kositamongkol P, et al. Predictive index for long-term survival after retransplantation of the liver in adult recipients: analysis of a 26-year experience in a single center. Ann Surg 2011;254(3):444–9.

prognostic information about the expected survival after ReLT postoperatively, by revising the risk category, adding 2 points to the preoperative score for any patient who experienced extensive intraoperative blood loss (>30 units). Another recipient risk factor was hypoalbuminemia. Hypoalbuminemia closely correlates with malnutrition and hepatocellular deficiency in patients with end-stage liver disease; not surprisingly, it is an independent risk factor for mortality in these patients [45]. Several studies [3,16,44] have also found that high acuity of illness as measured by MELD, number of prior transplants, and respiratory failure were independent predictors for graft failure after ReLT.

As a measure of the level of technical challenge of this demanding procedure, and the role the timing of the operation played in the outcome, intraoperative blood loss is a predictive factor. The complexity of the procedure, compounded

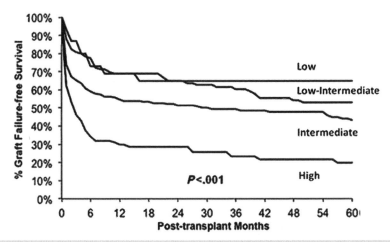

Fig. 4. Five-year graft failure–free survival after retransplantation of the liver. (*From* Hong JC, Kaldas FM, Kositamongkol P, et al. Predictive index for long-term survival after retransplantation of the liver in adult recipients: analysis of a 26-year experience in a single center. Ann Surg 2011;254(3):444–9; with permission.)

by dense postoperative vascular adhesions from prior operations, the frequent need for complex vascular reconstructions because of HAT or portal vein thrombosis (PVT), and the tenuous hemodynamic status of the patients can lead to prodigious amounts of blood loss. Two studies demonstrated a strong correlation between intraoperative blood product use and posttransplant survival [32,44].

Many groups' results suggest the existence of clearly different outcomes for elective and emergency retransplantation patients. In many studies, the elective group of retransplantation patients had survival curves similar to the primary transplant recipients [1], with perhaps a trend toward a longer hospital stay and higher costs. However, patients needing urgent retransplantation have very different outcomes, much worse than urgent primary transplant patients. These patients, often critically ill with worsening multiorgan failure and at increased risk for infection from the failing transplanted graft, are the ones who require ReLT between 15 to 180 days [44]. These patients are different from those with lower acuity of illness undergoing ReLT more than 2 years after the prior OLT or those suffering from PNF and needing an emergent ReLT within 2 weeks of the primary operation.

SUMMARY

In patients with failing liver grafts, hepatic retransplantation cannot be abandoned for the ethical and practical reasons that have been detailed previously. The current recommendations involve a strategy for risk stratification of re-transplant candidates. The long-term patient and graft survival outcomes after ReLT are excellent and acceptable for the low and intermediate groups, respectively. However, pursuing ReLT in transplant candidates in the high-risk category cannot be recommended. Furthermore, ReLT should be reserved for centers equipped to manage the difficulties of the endeavor because it is a technically demanding operation that requires surgical expertise and excellent anesthesiology and critical care support both before and after transplantation.

References

[1] Azoulay D, Linhares MM, Huguet E, et al. Decision for retransplantation of the liver: an experience- and cost-based analysis. Ann Surg 2002;236(6):713–21 [discussion: 721].

[2] Markmann JF, Markowitz JS, Yersiz H, et al. Long-term survival after retransplantation of the liver. Ann Surg 1997;226(4):408–18 [discussion: 418–20].

[3] Uemura T, Randall HB, Sanchez EQ, et al. Liver retransplantation for primary nonfunction: analysis of a 20-year single-center experience. Liver Transpl 2007;13(2):227–33.

[4] Lerner SM, Markmann JF, Jurim O, et al. Retransplantation. In: Busuttil RW, Klintmalm GB, editors. Transplantation of the liver, vol. 1. 2nd edition. Elsevier Saunders; 2005. p. 767–75.

[5] Wall WJ. Recurrent disease after liver transplantation: implications for the future. Liver Transpl Surg 1997;3(5 Suppl 1):S62–7.

[6] Powelson JA, Cosimi AB, Lewis WD, et al. Hepatic retransplantation in New England– a regional experience and survival model. Transplantation 1993;55(4):802–6.

[7] Ng V, Anand R, Martz K, et al. Liver retransplantation in children: a SPLIT database analysis of outcome and predictive factors for survival. Am J Transplant 2008;8(2):386–95.

[8] Thuluvath PJ, Guidinger MK, Fung JJ, et al. Liver transplantation in the United States, 1999-2008. Am J Transplant 2010;10(4 Pt 2):1003–19.

[9] Hong JC, Kosari K, Benjamin E, et al. Does race influence outcomes after primary liver transplantation? A 23-year experience with 2,700 patients. J Am Coll Surg 2008;206(5): 1009–16 [discussion: 1016–8].

[10] Melendez HV, Heaton ND. Understanding "marginal" liver grafts. Transplantation 1999;68(4):469–71.

[11] Cameron AM, Ghobrial RM, Yersiz H, et al. Optimal utilization of donor grafts with extended criteria: a single-center experience in over 1000 liver transplants. Ann Surg 2006;243(6):748–53 [discussion: 753–5].

[12] Busuttil RW, Farmer DG, Yersiz H, et al. Analysis of long-term outcomes of 3200 liver transplantations over two decades: a single-center experience. Ann Surg 2005;241(6):905–16 [discussion: 916–8].

[13] Duffy JP, Hong JC, Farmer DG, et al. Vascular complications of orthotopic liver transplantation: experience in more than 4,200 patients. J Am Coll Surg 2009;208(5):896–903 [discussion: 903–5].

[14] Hong JC, Yersiz H, Farmer DG, et al. Longterm outcomes for whole and segmental liver grafts in adult and pediatric liver transplant recipients: a 10-year comparative analysis of 2,988 cases. J Am Coll Surg 2009;208(5):682–9 [discussion: 689–91].

[15] Blakolmer K, Jain A, Ruppert K, et al. Chronic liver allograft rejection in a population treated primarily with tacrolimus as baseline immunosuppression: long-term follow-up and evaluation of features for histopathological staging. Transplantation 2000;69(11): 2330–6.

[16] Jain A, Reyes J, Kashyap R, et al. Long-term survival after liver transplantation in 4,000 consecutive patients at a single center. Ann Surg 2000;232(4):490–500.

[17] Buis CI, Hoekstra H, Verdonk RC, et al. Causes and consequences of ischemic-type biliary lesions after liver transplantation. J Hepatobiliary Pancreat Surg 2006;13(6):517–24.

[18] Maheshwari A, Maley W, Li Z, et al. Biliary complications and outcomes of liver transplantation from donors after cardiac death. Liver Transpl 2007;13(12):1645–53.

[19] Reich DJ, Hong JC. Current status of donation after cardiac death liver transplantation. Curr Opin Organ Transplant 2010;15(3):316–21.
[20] Hashimoto K, Eghtesad B, Gunasekaran G, et al. Use of tissue plasminogen activator in liver transplantation from donation after cardiac death donors. Am J Transplant 2010;10(12): 2665–72.
[21] Brown RS. Hepatitis C and liver transplantation. Nature 2005;436(7053):973–8.
[22] Cameron AM, Ghobrial RM, Hiatt JR, et al. Effect of nonviral factors on hepatitis C recurrence after liver transplantation. Ann Surg 2006;244(4):563–71.
[23] Berenguer M, Prieto M, Rayon JM, et al. Natural history of clinically compensated hepatitis C virus-related graft cirrhosis after liver transplantation. Hepatology 2000;32(4 Pt 1):852–8.
[24] Lucey MR. Management of alcoholic liver disease. Clin Liver Dis 2009;13(2):267–75.
[25] Graziadei IW, Wiesner RH, Batts KP, et al. Recurrence of primary sclerosing cholangitis following liver transplantation. Hepatology 1999;29(4):1050–6.
[26] Hubscher SG, Elias E, Buckels JA, et al. Primary biliary cirrhosis. Histological evidence of disease recurrence after liver transplantation. J Hepatol 1993;18(2):173–84.
[27] Devlin J, Donaldson P, Portmann B, et al. Recurrence of autoimmune hepatitis following liver transplantation. Liver Transpl Surg 1995;1(3):162–5.
[28] Saab S, Desai S, Tsaoi D, et al. Posttransplantation hepatitis B prophylaxis with combination oral nucleoside and nucleotide analog therapy. Am J Transplant 2011;11(3):511–7.
[29] Belghiti J, Noun R, Sauvanet A. Temporary portocaval anastomosis with preservation of caval flow during orthotopic liver transplantation. Am J Surg 1995;169(2):277–9.
[30] Lerut JP, Bourlier P, de Ville de Goyet J, et al. Improvement of technique for adult orthotopic liver retransplantation. J Am Coll Surg 1995;180(6):729–32.
[31] Doyle HR, Morelli F, McMichael J, et al. Hepatic retransplantation—an analysis of risk factors associated with outcome. Transplantation 1996;61(10):1499–505.
[32] Facciuto M, Heidt D, Guarrera J, et al. Retransplantation for late liver graft failure: predictors of mortality. Liver Transpl 2000;6(2):174–9.
[33] Kowalski RJ, Post DR, Mannon RB, et al. Assessing relative risks of infection and rejection: a meta-analysis using an immune function assay. Transplantation 2006;82(5):663–8.
[34] Huskey J, Gralla J, Wiseman AC. Single time point immune function assay (ImmuKnow) testing does not aid in the prediction of future opportunistic infections or acute rejection. Clin J Am Soc Nephrol 2011;6(2):423–9.
[35] Torio A, Fernandez EJ, Montes-Ares O, et al. Lack of association of immune cell function test with rejection in kidney transplantation. Transplant Proc 2011;43(6):2168–70.
[36] Pelletier SJ, Schaubel DE, Punch JD, et al. Hepatitis C is a risk factor for death after liver retransplantation. Liver Transpl 2005;11(4):434–40.
[37] Markmann JF, Gornbein J, Markowitz JS, et al. A simple model to estimate survival after retransplantation of the liver. Transplantation 1999;67(3):422–30.
[38] Wiesner RH, McDiarmid SV, Kamath PS, et al. MELD and PELD: application of survival models to liver allocation. Liver Transpl 2001;7(7):567–80.
[39] Klein AS, Messersmith EE, Ratner LE, et al. Organ donation and utilization in the United States, 1999-2008. Am J Transplant 2010;10(4 Pt 2):973–86.
[40] Rosen HR, Madden JP, Martin P. A model to predict survival following liver retransplantation. Hepatology 1999;29(2):365–70.
[41] Marti J, Charco R, Ferrer J, et al. Optimization of liver grafts in liver retransplantation: a European single-center experience. Surgery 2008;144(5):762–9.
[42] Rosen HR, Prieto M, Casanovas-Taltavull T, et al. Validation and refinement of survival models for liver retransplantation. Hepatology 2003;38(2):460–9.
[43] Linhares MM, Azoulay D, Matos D, et al. Liver retransplantation: a model for determining long-term survival. Transplantation 2006;81(7):1016–21.
[44] Hong JC, Kaldas FM, Kositamongkol P, et al. Predictive index for long-term survival after retransplantation of the liver in adult recipients: analysis of a 26-year experience in a single center. Ann Surg 2011;254(3):444–9.

[45] Filloux B, Chagneau-Derrode C, Ragot S, et al. Short-term and long-term vital outcomes of cirrhotic patients admitted to an intensive care unit. Eur J Gastroenterol Hepatol 2010;22(12):1474–80.

[46] Yao FY, Saab S, Bass NM, et al. Prediction of survival after liver retransplantation for late graft failure based on preoperative prognostic scores. Hepatology 2004;39(1):230–8.

[47] Marudanayagam R, Shanmugam V, Sandhu B, et al. Liver retransplantation in adults: a single-centre, 25-year experience. HPB (Oxford) 2010;12(3):217–24.

Screening for Abdominal Aortic Aneurysms

Joseph L. Bobadilla, MD, K. Craig Kent, MD*

Department of Surgery, University of Wisconsin–Madison, Clinical Science Center H4/710, 600 Highland Avenue, Madison, WI 53792-7375, USA

Keywords
• Abdominal aortic aneurysm • Screening • Guidelines

Key Points
• AAA screening programs have been shown to decrease the incidence of aneurysm rupture and reduce aneurysm related deaths.
• Tobacco use, age, and gender are the most significant risk factors related to abdominal aneurysm formation.
• A scoring system to assist in identifying patients at risk for aneurysm development has been devised to guide in patient screening selection.

OVERVIEW

Aneurysmal dilatation of the abdominal aorta is defined as an aortic diameter that is 50% greater than the immediately adjacent aorta, or a diameter of greater than 3.0 cm in the average person [1]. It is estimated that more than 1 million persons in the United States population have an abdominal aortic aneurysm (AAA), with more than 200,000 newly diagnosed each year. Large aneurysms (>5.5 cm maximal diameter) are responsible for roughly 30,000 deaths each year in the United States, and significantly more worldwide [2]. The Veterans Affairs Cooperative Study Group found the prevalence of large aneurysms to be 0.5% in men aged 50 to 79 years [3]. Significant and well-established risk factors for the development of AAA include age, male gender, history of smoking, and a first-degree relative with AAA [4–7]. Maximal aneurysm diameter continues to be the strongest predictor of risk of rupture, although a host of other factors including rapid expansion (>1 cm/y) as well as aneurysm type and configuration should also be considered [8–10].

Despite increases in the frequency of abdominal imaging, the incidence of ruptured AAA has only modestly diminished over time. Moreover, the overall mortality associated with ruptured AAA is approximately 85%. Most individuals

*Corresponding author. E-mail address: kent@surgery.wisc.edu

0065-3411/12/$ – see front matter
doi:10.1016/j.yasu.2012.03.006

with ruptured AAA do not survive long enough to access medical care or undergo intervention. For those who are surgically treated for rupture, the mortality approaches 50%. In addition, the morbidity and cost associated with aneurysm rupture are significantly greater than those of elective repair. The costs of renal replacement therapy, prolonged ventilator support, treatment of congestive heart failure, and other such interventions following ruptured AAA have been well documented [11]. It has been suggested that there would be a potential $50 million annual cost saving if treatment of ruptured aneurysms was replaced by screening and elective aneurysm repair [12]. The clear-cut benefit of avoiding rupture repair in terms of saving lives and cost has fueled the argument for widespread initiation of screening protocols in the United States and elsewhere around the world. The efficacy of aneurysm screening has been evaluated in a number studies [13–20]. Most notable is the Oxford Multicentre Aneurysm Screening Study (MASS), in which 67,800 men aged 65 to 74 years were randomized to screening or not screening. These investigators found a 53% reduction in aneurysm-related mortality in those who attended ultrasound screening [20]. However, the identity of the cohort of individuals that should be subjected to screening is still controversial.

SCREENING PRINCIPLES

Medical screening is defined as a test applied to a defined high-risk population to detect a disease in individuals before the development of signs or symptoms. The goal of medical screening is to reduce the morbidity and mortality associated with delayed diagnosis of a disease. In general, screening protocols are most useful when a disease has a defined latency period, and when an intervention during this latency period can reduce the long-term risk and morbidity. With regard to AAA, the goal of screening is to reduce death caused by rupture and also to reduce the frequency of emergent aneurysm repair and the associated cost and morbidity. When determining the efficacy of screening for a disease, there are many important factors. These factors include the cost, ease, and acceptance of the screening test; the prevalence of disease in the population chosen for screening; the cost and effectiveness of early treatment of the disease; and the long-term outcome for patients whose disease is not detected by screening. An important factor is patient acceptance of the screening test. If patients are not receptive to being screened, the test is useless. Patients with significant risk factors for vascular disease are often the least compliant. Many of the forgoing issues are included in the World Health Organization's guiding principles of medical screening, summarized in Table 1. Screening for AAA with a quick-screen ultrasound meets each of these requirements [21].

SCREENING TECHNIQUES

The first step in screening is a routine history and physical. Patients should be asked whether they smoke and about other risk factors such as a personal or family history of AAA. Some aneurysms can be identified on physical examination, which should include slow, firm, and deep palpation of the epigastrium

Table 1
Screening guidelines

World Health Organization screening criteria (1968)	AAA-specific screening (2010)
The condition should be an important health problem	Approximately 30,000 people in the United States die of ruptured AAA each year
There should be a treatment for the condition	Open and endovascular options for elective repair exist
Facilities for diagnosis and treatment should be available	Thousands of established diagnostic vascular laboratories
There should be a latent stage of the disease	Small, and even large, aneurysms that have not yet ruptured
There should be a test or examination for the condition	Quick-screen abdominal ultrasound
The test should be acceptable to the population	Test is noninvasive and quick
The natural history of the disease should be adequately understood	Annual growth rates 2–4 mm/y
There should be an agreed policy on whom to treat	Symptomatic aneurysms and aneurysms greater than 5.5 cm
The total cost of finding a case should be economically balanced in relation to medical expenditures as a whole	Refs. [13–20]
Case finding should be continuous process, not just a once-and-for-all project	Screening could be incorporated into yearly history and physical

with the thumbs paramidline and the hands wrapped toward the flank. However, physical examination alone is, at best, moderately reliable, with approximately a 20% rate of detection when applied to a broad population [22]. Sensitivity is likely increased in the hands of a vascular specialist, which is not relevant when considering large-population screening. Consequently, effective screening for AAA requires imaging. Imaging techniques include ultrasound, computed tomography (CT), and/or magnetic resonance. Although each of these modalities has its unique features, because of cost and convenience, ultrasound is the imaging modality of choice.

Abdominal B-mode ultrasonography is a 30-minute to 45 minute test that allows imaging of the aorta as well as other important abdominal vessels and organs. It does not produce radiation or require intravenous contrast. Although a traditional abdominal ultrasound provides highly detailed information about the aorta, its branches, the kidneys, and adjacent organs, for purposes of AAA screening, only 1 question needs to be answered: is the aorta greater than 3 cm in diameter? With this in mind, a quick screen for AAA was devised. The goal of this study is to measure the infrarenal aorta at its largest diameter and determine whether or not the size is greater than 3 cm. A quick screen can be performed in most vascular laboratories within 5 minutes with a high accuracy. To that end, some have advocated the use of handheld ultrasound in a primary care physician's office as an adjunct to physical examination [23]. However, ultrasound imaging is not always straightforward, particularly in patients with an increased body mass index (BMI) or if there is overlying bowel gas [24–26]. Nevertheless, in the hands of an appropriately trained technologist, a quick-screen ultrasound is a safe and convenient test for aneurysmal disease. If a AAA is identified by ultrasound, particularly if repair is being contemplated, a CT angiogram will eventually be required to help with planning for either open surgery or endovascular repair.

Once aneurysms have been identified through screening, those that are not repaired should be followed through surveillance. A recent consensus statement from the Society for Vascular Surgery, the American Association of Vascular Surgery, and the Society for Vascular Medicine and Biology provided the following guidelines for surveillance intervals [27]: (1) aneurysms less than 4.0 cm can be monitored on an annual basis unless they show evidence for rapid expansion [27–29]; (2) aneurysms greater than or equal to 4 cm should be monitored at 6-month intervals. Patients who are not deemed candidates for repair should not be further evaluated. These recommended surveillance intervals are summarized in Table 2.

SCREENING TRIALS

To date, there have been 3 large-scale prospective, randomized trials of AAA screening: the MASS, Chichester United Kingdom, and Viborg County Denmark studies [19,20,30,31]. In MASS, 70,495 men aged 65 to 74 years were followed; 33,839 were randomized to screening. Of these, 80% of those invited accepted the invitation and were screened. The incidence of AAA in this population was 5%. At 4 years' follow-up, there were 113 aneurysm-related deaths in the control group and 65 in screened patients, with an overall and statistically significant 42% risk reduction in AAA death [20]. In the Chichester United Kingdom study, a total of 6058 men aged 65 to 80 years were followed, 74% of whom accepted a screening invitation. The rate of AAA detection was 7.6%. In this study, the AAA-related rate of death was reduced by 41% at 5 years and 21% at 10 years [30]. In the Viborg study 12,658 men age 65 to 73 years were randomized. Of these, 76% accepted an

| Table 2 | |
| Recommended surveillance intervals | |
Maximal AAA diameter (cm)	Recommendations
<3.0	No further surveillance
3.0–4.0	Image every 12 mo
4.0–4.5	Image every 6 mo
4.5–5.5	Referral to vascular specialist
>5.5	Consider elective repair

Data from Brewster DC, Cronenwett JL, Hallett JW Jr, et al. Guidelines for the treatment of abdominal aortic aneurysms. Report of a subcommittee of the Joint Council of the American Association for Vascular Surgery and Society for Vascular Surgery. J Vasc Surg 2003;37:1106–17.

invitation for screening and the rate of detection of AAAs was 4%. Over a mean follow-up period of 5.13 years, there was an in-hospital mortality reduction of 68%, with a total number of deaths of 6 in the screening cohort and 19 in the unscreened cohort [19]. The frequency of emergency operation in the screened group was reduced by 74% (95% confidence interval [CI] 54%–89%) over the same period of time [19]. Taken together, these studies imply that, given a rate of screening of 74% to 80% of those invited, quick-screen AAA ultrasound in men aged 65 years or older results in a measurable and significant reduction in aneurysm-related deaths. Furthermore, this benefit seems to be sustained over time. In the MASS, cost-effectiveness was evaluated. The findings were favorable with regard to the cost-effectiveness of AAA screening, with an incremental cost per quality life year saved of $12,000 at 10 years [32–35]. Moreover, the MASS data suggest that those patients with an initially negative screening study need no further evaluation [32].

CURRENT SCREENING RECOMMENDATIONS IN THE UNITED STATES

The current recommendation for AAA screening comes from the United States Preventive Services Task Force (USPSTF) and is for a one-time ultrasound screening for aneurysm in ever-smoking men aged 65 to 75 years [36]. In addition, the USPSTF recommended against routine screening for AAA in women, regardless of smoking status. As a consequence of this recommendation, the United States SAAAVE (Screening Abdominal Aortic Aneurysm Very Efficiently) Act was passed on January 1, 2007. The SAAAVE Act provides a free, one-time, ultrasound AAA screening benefit for individuals turning 65 years that is included as part of a Welcome-to-Medicare physical. Inclusion criteria are age greater than 65 years but less than 75 years, and either men who have smoked at least 100 cigarettes during their life or men/women with a family history of AAA. Patients must visit their primary care physician for a Welcome-to-Medicare physical within 6 months of enrollment to qualify for the aneurysm screening. The Medicare AAA screening benefit became law on February 8, 2006 (effective January 1, 2007) as part of the Deficit Reduction Act of 2005, provision S.1932.

NEW DIRECTIONS IN SCREENING

Despite a law now mandating screening for aneurysms, the Welcome-to-Medicare physical has been grossly undersubscribed. Only a few individuals turning 65 years have been screened using this mechanism. Moreover, at the time of passage of the bill, no provision was made to screen the large number of Medicare patients already more than 65 years of age. In addition, the USPSTF recommendations exclude from screening 4 significant populations: women, nonsmokers, and patients less than 65 years or greater than 75 years of age. These 4 populations account for greater than one-third of reported aneurysms in historical series [37–39].

Although the incidence of rupture in men seems to be declining, the rate of rupture in women is increasing. It seems likely that this, at least in part, is related to the exclusion of women from screening protocols. Because of these concerns,

Table 3
Multivariate AAA risk score

Variable	Odds ratio	95% CI	Risk score
Male (vs female)	5.71	5.57–5.85	18
Age (vs <55 y)			
55–59	2.76	2.55–3.00	11
60–64	5.35	4.97–5.76	17
65–69	9.41	8.76–10.12	23
70–74	14.46	13.45–15.55	28
75–79	20.43	18.99–21.99	31
80–84	28.37	26.31–30.59	35
Race/Ethnicity (vs White)			
Hispanic	0.69	0.62–0.77	−4
African American	0.72	0.66–0.78	−3
Asian	0.72	0.59–0.75	−4
High blood pressure	1.25	1.21–1.28	2
Coronary artery disease	1.72	1.69–1.76	6
Family history of AAA	3.80	3.66–3.95	14
High cholesterol	1.34	1.31–1.37	3
Diabetes	0.75	0.73–0.77	−3
Peripheral arterial disease	1.59	1.54–1.65	5
Carotid disease	1.51	1.46–1.56	4
Cerebrovascular history	1.18	1.14–1.21	2
Smoking (packs/d)			
≤10 y			
<0.5	2.61	2.47–2.74	10
0.5–1	3.19	2.93–3.46	12
>1	3.20	2.88–3.56	12
11–20 y			
<0.5	4.87	4.63–5.12	16
0.5–1	5.79	5.48–6.12	18
>1	6.00	5.66–6.35	19
21–35 y			
<0.5	7.29	6.97–7.64	21
0.5–1	7.99	7.62–8.38	22
>1	8.41	8.57–9.36	22
>35 y			
<0.5	8.96	8.57–9.36	23
0.5–1	11.19	10.76–11.64	25
>1	12.13	11.66–12.61	26
Quit Smoking			
<5 y ago	0.87	0.84–0.912	−1
5–10 y ago	0.68	0.65–0.71	−4
>10 y ago	0.42	0.41–0.43	−9
Fruit and vegetables >3 times/wk	0.91	0.88–0.92	−1
Nuts >3 times/wk	0.90	0.89–0.93	−1
Exercise ≥1 time/wk	0.86	0.85–0.88	−2
BMI≥25 kg/m^2	1.20	1.17–1.22	2

The model was developed on 50% of the Life Line Screening cohort and validated on the remaining 50%. The area under the receiver operator curve of the model (C statistic) was 0.893. The overall accuracy of the scoring system as measured by the C statistic was 0.842.

Data from Kent KC, Zwolak RM, Egorova NN, et al. Analysis of risk factors for abdominal aortic aneurysm in a cohort of more than 3 million individuals. J Vasc Surg 2010;52:539–48.

our group has recently attempted to more inclusively define the cohort of patients that should be screened. For this analysis, we used data from 3.1 million patients derived from Life Line Screening, which is a for-profit screening program in which, in addition to a quick screen, more than 30 pieces of data are collected from each patient evaluated [40,41]. These data represent the largest ever analysis of both men and women screened for aneurysmal disease. Moreover, included in the populace screened were men, women, smokers, nonsmokers, and a range of ages from young to elderly. Patient data and risk factors were evaluated using a multivariate logistic regression model, and a clinical risk score was developed. In addition to the previous well-defined risk factors including smoking, age, gender, and family history, we found a plethora of additional risk factors that, to a lesser extent, predicted AAA. These risk factors included coronary artery disease and increased cholesterol and hypertension. New risk factors for AAA that had not previously been identified included ethnic status as well as diet and exercise. Patients with diabetes were less likely to develop AAA. The correlation with smoking was strong. Risk of AAA closely correlated with length of smoking as well as number of packs smoked per day. There was also a significant reduction in the incidence of AAA associated with smoking cessation. We devised a scoring system that correlated well with incidence of AAA and thus might be used to determine an inclusive subset of patients that might benefit from screening. It is necessary to choose a threshold score for individuals to be referred for screening. If this threshold score is high, a smaller subset of patients is screened with lower cost; however, the total number of AAAs identified is small. If the threshold score is low, more individuals are screened at a higher cost, but the total number of AAAs identified is increased. The threshold that is chosen depends on what Medicare and/or society is willing to pay for AAA screening. Again, a lower threshold is associated with a greater number of aneurysms identified. We then compared our newly devised screening model with the status quo recommendations by the USPSTF (ever-smoking man aged 65–75 years). We found that our model identified a substantially larger number of aneurysms for the same number of individuals screened compared with the USPSTF criteria. We were able to identify women with aneurysms in individuals with multiple risk factors. In addition, our model identified younger individuals with AAA as well as aneurysms in men who did not smoke. The complete scoring model is outlined in Table 3. In sum, this model allows the selection for screening of a larger and more diverse group of individuals with AAA.

SUMMARY

Ruptured AAA ranks as the 15th leading cause of death overall in the United States, and the 10th leading cause of death in men older than 55 years. Early identification of AAA can save lives and diminish cost. Screening programs have been implemented and studied in other countries and have shown a measurable and significant reduction in overall rate of aneurysm-related death. Currently, screening is not widely used in the United States and Medicare, at best, provides one-time screening of a small number of ever-smoking men when they turn 65 years old. Because more than 30,000 individuals in the United States die each year of ruptured AAA, a great deal of progress must be made to eradicate rupture from aneurysmal disease. A more comprehensive system of screening is required and this should be uniformly applied to the US population. It is hoped that scoring systems such as the one outlined in this article, if widely adopted, can greatly enhance screening for aneurysmal disease and prevent the high mortality that stems from this serious vascular disease.

References

[1] Johnston KW, Rutherford RB, Tilson MD, et al. Suggested standards for reporting on arterial aneurysms. Subcommittee on Reporting Standards for Arterial Aneurysms, Ad Hoc Committee on Reporting Standards, Society for Vascular Surgery and North American Chapter, International Society for Cardiovascular Surgery. J Vasc Surg 1991;13:452–8.
[2] Gillum RF. Epidemiology of aortic aneurysm in the United States. J Clin Epidemiol 1995;48: 1289–98.
[3] Lederle FA, Johnson GR, Wilson SE, et al. Prevalence and associations of abdominal aortic aneurysm detected through screening. Aneurysm Detection and Management (ADAM) Veterans Affairs Cooperative Study Group. Ann Intern Med 1997;126:441–9.
[4] Brown LC, Powell JT. Risk factors for aneurysm rupture in patients kept under ultrasound surveillance. UK Small Aneurysm Trial Participants. Ann Surg 1999;230:289–96 [discussion: 96–7].
[5] Cronenwett JL, Sargent SK, Wall MH, et al. Variables that affect the expansion rate and outcome of small abdominal aortic aneurysms. J Vasc Surg 1990;11:260–8 [discussion: 268–9].
[6] Sterpetti AV, Cavallaro A, Cavallari N, et al. Factors influencing the rupture of abdominal aortic aneurysms. Surg Gynecol Obstet 1991;173:175–8.
[7] Strachan DP. Predictors of death from aortic aneurysm among middle-aged men: the White-hall Study. Br J Surg 1991;78:401–4.
[8] Nevitt MP, Ballard DJ, Hallett JW Jr. Prognosis of abdominal aortic aneurysms. A population-based study. N Engl J Med 1989;321:1009–14.
[9] Glimaker H, Holmberg L, Elvin A, et al. Natural history of patients with abdominal aortic aneurysm. Eur J Vasc Surg 1991;5:125–30.
[10] Wilmink AB, Quick CR. Epidemiology and potential for prevention of abdominal aortic aneurysm. Br J Surg 1998;85:155–62.
[11] Patel ST, Korn P, Haser PB, et al. The cost-effectiveness of repairing ruptured abdominal aortic aneurysms. J Vasc Surg 2000;32:247–57.
[12] Pasch AR, Ricotta JJ, May AG, et al. Abdominal aortic aneurysm: the case for elective resection. Circulation 1984;70:II-4.
[13] Bengtsson H, Bergqvist D, Ekberg O, et al. A population based screening of abdominal aortic aneurysms (AAA). Eur J Vasc Surg 1991;5:53–7.
[14] Morris GE, Hubbard CS, Quick CR. An abdominal aortic aneurysm screening programme for all males over the age of 50 years. Eur J Vasc Surg 1994;8:156–60.
[15] Scott RA, Ashton HA, Kay DN. Abdominal aortic aneurysm in 4237 screened patients: prevalence, development and management over 6 years. Br J Surg 1991;78:1122–5.
[16] Heather BP, Poskitt KR, Earnshaw JJ, et al. Population screening reduces mortality rate from aortic aneurysm in men. Br J Surg 2000;87:750–3.
[17] Vardulaki KA, Walker NM, Couto E, et al. Late results concerning feasibility and compliance from a randomized trial of ultrasonographic screening for abdominal aortic aneurysm. Br J Surg 2002;89:861–4.
[18] Scott RA, Bridgewater SG, Ashton HA. Randomized clinical trial of screening for abdominal aortic aneurysm in women. Br J Surg 2002;89:283–5.

[19] Lindholt JS, Juul S, Fasting H, et al. Hospital costs and benefits of screening for abdominal aortic aneurysms. Results from a randomised population screening trial. Eur J Vasc Endovasc Surg 2002;23:55–60.

[20] Ashton HA, Buxton MJ, Day NE, et al. The Multicentre Aneurysm Screening Study (MASS) into the effect of abdominal aortic aneurysm screening on mortality in men: a randomised controlled trial. Lancet 2002;360:1531–9.

[21] Lee TY, Korn P, Heller JA, et al. The cost-effectiveness of a "quick-screen" program for abdominal aortic aneurysms. Surgery 2002;132:399–407.

[22] Pleumeekers HJ, Hoes AW, Hofman A, et al. Selecting subjects for ultrasonographic screening for aneurysms of the abdominal aorta: four different strategies. Int J Epidemiol 1999;28:682–6.

[23] Lin PH, Bush RL, McCoy SA, et al. A prospective study of a hand-held ultrasound device in abdominal aortic aneurysm evaluation. Am J Surg 2003;186:455–9.

[24] Quill DS, Colgan MP, Sumner DS. Ultrasonic screening for the detection of abdominal aortic aneurysms. Surg Clin North Am 1989;69:713–20.

[25] Graeve AH, Carpenter CM, Wicks JD, et al. Discordance in the sizing of abdominal aortic aneurysm and its significance. Am J Surg 1982;144:627–34.

[26] Gomes MN, Schellinger D, Hufnagel CA. Abdominal aortic aneurysms: diagnostic review and new technique. Ann Thorac Surg 1979;27:479–88.

[27] Kent KC, Zwolak RM, Jaff MR, et al. Screening for abdominal aortic aneurysm: a consensus statement. J Vasc Surg 2004;39:267–9.

[28] Brewster DC, Cronenwett JL, Hallett JW Jr, et al. Guidelines for the treatment of abdominal aortic aneurysms. Report of a subcommittee of the Joint Council of the American Association for Vascular Surgery and Society for Vascular Surgery. J Vasc Surg 2003;37:1106–17.

[29] Gadowski GR, Pilcher DB, Ricci MA. Abdominal aortic aneurysm expansion rate: effect of size and beta-adrenergic blockade. J Vasc Surg 1994;19:727–31.

[30] Scott RA, Wilson NM, Ashton HA, et al. Influence of screening on the incidence of ruptured abdominal aortic aneurysm: 5-year results of a randomized controlled study. Br J Surg 1995;82:1066–70.

[31] Multicentre Aneurysm Screening Study Group. Multicentre aneurysm screening study (MASS): cost effectiveness analysis of screening for abdominal aortic aneurysms based on four year results from randomised controlled trial. BMJ 2002;325:1135.

[32] Thompson SG, Ashton HA, Gao L, et al. Screening men for abdominal aortic aneurysm: 10 year mortality and cost effectiveness results from the randomised Multicentre Aneurysm Screening Study. BMJ 2009;338:b2307.

[33] Crow P, Shaw E, Earnshaw JJ, et al. A single normal ultrasonographic scan at age 65 years rules out significant aneurysm disease for life in men. Br J Surg 2001;88:941–4.

[34] Scott RA, Vardulaki KA, Walker NM, et al. The long-term benefits of a single scan for abdominal aortic aneurysm (AAA) at age 65. Eur J Vasc Endovasc Surg 2001;21:535–40.

[35] Lederle FA, Johnson GR, Wilson SE, et al. Yield of repeated screening for abdominal aortic aneurysm after a 4-year interval. Aneurysm Detection and Management Veterans Affairs Cooperative Study Investigators. Arch Intern Med 2000;160:1117–21.

[36] U.S. Preventive Services Task Force. Screening for abdominal aortic aneurysm: recommendation statement. Ann Intern Med 2005;142:198–202.

[37] Mureebe L, Egorova N, Giacovelli JK, et al. National trends in the repair of ruptured abdominal aortic aneurysms. J Vasc Surg 2008;48:1101–7.

[38] Kung HC, Hoyert DL, Xu J, et al. Deaths: final data for 2005. Natl Vital Stat Rep 2008;56:1–120.

[39] Longo C, Upchurch GR Jr. Abdominal aortic aneurysm screening: recommendations and controversies. Vasc Endovascular Surg 2005;39:213–9.

[40] Greco G, Egorova NN, Gelijns AC, et al. Development of a novel scoring tool for the identification of large ≥5 cm abdominal aortic aneurysms. Ann Surg 2010;252:675–82.

[41] Kent KC, Zwolak RM, Egorova NN, et al. Analysis of risk factors for abdominal aortic aneurysm in a cohort of more than 3 million individuals. J Vasc Surg 2010;52:539–48.

Novel Management Strategies in the Treatment of Severe *Clostridium difficile* Infection

Ibrahim Nassour, MD[a], Evie H. Carchman, MD[a],
Richard L. Simmons, MD[a], Brian S. Zuckerbraun, MD[a,b,*]

[a]Department of Surgery, University of Pittsburgh, 200 Lothrop Street, F1200 PUH, Pittsburgh, PA 15213, USA; [b]Surgical Service Line, VA Pittsburgh Healthcare System, University Drive, Pittsburgh, PA 15240, USA

Keywords
• Vancomycin • Colectomy • Ileostomy • Colonic lavage

Key Points
• In the setting of the clinical syndrome of CDI and risk factors, do not delay empiric therapy for laboratory confirmation of CDI.
• Adequate fluid and electrolyte resuscitation.
• Vancomycin 125 mg PO four times per day *PLUS* metronidazole 500 mg IV three times per day for severe, complicated disease.
• If ileus is suspected or patient is immunocompromised add vancomycin enemas (500 mg in 500 mL saline four times a day).
• Surgical consultation early.
• Surgical therapy prior to decompensation.
• Consider colon preserving surgery (loop ileostomy/colonic lavage).

The epidemiology of *Clostridium difficile* infection (CDI) has evolved significantly during the past decade, with a major increase in incidence, severity, and mortality. According to the US Department of Health and Human Services through data retrieved from the Healthcare Cost and Utilization Project, the total number of hospitalizations related to CDI increased from 133,151 in 1999 to 336,565 in 2009, with a respective increase in the national bill from 0.4 to 3.7 billion dollars [1,2]. Since 2001, outbreaks of CDI secondary to a more virulent strain, which likely results in more severe disease and worse outcomes, has been reported in the United States, Canada, and Europe [3–8].

As a result, several newer tactics for prevention and treatment have been implemented. Standardized and more intense hospital infection control strategies

*Corresponding author. F1200 PUH, 200 Lothrop Street, Pittsburgh, PA 15213. E-mail address: zuckerbraunbs@upmc.edu

0065-3411/12/$ – see front matter
doi:10.1016/j.yasu.2012.03.009
Published by Elsevier Inc.

are essential to prevent disease transmission; there is no known substitute. But earlier recognition and newer treatments must be developed to reduce morbidity and mortality. A multidisciplinary approach to treatment is going to be necessary in patients with the more severe stages of disease. Early surgical consultation should be obtained in patients who are failing to improve with standard medical therapy, in those with significant comorbidities or who are immunosuppressed, or in patients who require intensive care support. This review proposes management guidelines for CDI, with a focus on patients with severe, complicated disease, in whom surgical therapy should be considered.

PATHOPHYSIOLOGY

Clostridium difficile is a gram-positive, spore-forming anaerobic bacillus that can colonize the large intestines of humans. *Clostridium difficile* is acquired after oral ingestion of either the vegetative form of the bacteria or spores (which can live in the environment for years). Typically, *Clostridium difficile* colonization follows disruption of normal gut microflora by antibiotic therapy or other host factors. Although this organism typically can be cultured in the stool of 1% to 6% of the general population [9,10], colonization rates increase with the use of antibiotics and the duration of hospitalization. The use of antibiotics disrupts the normal colonic microbiome, allowing *Clostridium difficile* to proliferate. Studies have shown that a single dose of perioperative antibiotics can increase the colonization rate to more than 20% [11].

    Clostridium difficile was recognized as the causative agent of pseudomembranous colitis in 1978; it had been previously described as clindamycin-associated colitis [12]. CDI occurs when bacteria numbers increase and toxins are produced. The vegetative form colonizes the colonic epithelium by producing microtubule-based cellular protrusions that increase surface adhesion [13]. The bacteria then release toxins, leading to the disease state. *Clostridium difficile* has a 19Kb pathogenic locus in its genome that includes tcdA and tcdB genes encoding for the major toxins responsible for its pathogenicity [14]. Toxin A and toxin B share 74% of their amino acid sequences, particularly in the enzymatic and substrate binding regions [15]. Both toxins are internalized by endocytosis into the epithelial cell, where they extrude their enzymatic domains into the cytoplasm by forming pores in the endosomes in a pH-dependent manner [16]. Once in the cytoplasm, the enzymes become activated and glycosylate and inactivate Rho and Ras family guanosine triphosphatases, which, in turn, leads to disruption of cytoskeletal integrity and intercellular junctional complexes; a secretory diarrhea is the result [14,17]. Although it was once believed that toxin A was the major virulence factor, animal studies have shown that toxin A-only producing bacteria are nonpathogenic, whereas toxin B-only secreting organisms can produce the disease [14,18]. Most toxigenic strains produce both toxins [19].

    The inflammatory response marked by invasion of leukocytes and the release of cytokines contributes significantly to the injury of the colonic epithelium. An inflammatory exudate on the colonic epithelium can form the classic pseudomembrane appearance.

THE EPIDEMIOLOGY OF CDI

Over the past decade, several epidemics of CDI in the United States, Canada, and Europe have led to the recognition of a more virulent strain of *Clostridium difficile*. The strain of *Clostridium difficile* leading to the initial outbreaks in the United States and Canada was identical, and has been given the classification of the BI/NAP1/027 strain [3,6], referring to pulsed field gel electrophoresis (PFGE) pattern (NAP1; North America PFGE type 1), its restriction endonuclease analysis pattern (B1), and its polymerase chain reaction (PCR) ribotype designation (027). This strain was retrieved from 82% of stool samples of patients in Quebec and 51% of isolates during the US outbreak [3]. This strain was responsible for only 0.002% of the cases in the past [20]. The emergence of this new strain may be related to widespread usage of fluoroquinolones during this period to which the new strain is resistant [3], and it implies that the transmission of this strain is more effective than others [21]. BI/NAP1 has spread beyond the United States and Canada [22] and has reached England [23], The Netherlands [24], other parts of Europe [25], and Asia [26].

Not only has the incidence of CDI increased over the last decade but the apparent morbidity and mortality associated with this infection have also increased. The percentage of patients developing severe, complicated disease (defined by the presence of perforation, ileus, megacolon, need for surgery, or cardiopulmonary deterioration) increased from 7.1% to 18.2% with an overall 30-day mortality increase from 4.7% to 13.8% during the period of 1991 to 2003 [2,27]. According to a 12-year follow-up study performed at the University of Pittsburgh Medical Center, the incidence of death or colectomy had increased from 0% in 1990 to 3.2% in 2000 [8].

The dramatic increase in disease-specific mortality in patients with *Clostridium difficile* in the recent outbreaks was because of a higher incidence of severe, complicated (fulminant) disease that was linked to the appearance of the BI/NAP1 strain [28]. The high virulence of this strain is partly attributed to a mutation in the tcdC gene [23]. This gene is located within the pathogenicity locus (PaLoc) and encodes a regulatory protein that inhibits the production of toxin A and B [29]. BI/NAP1 has an 18 base pair deletion in the tcdC gene, leading to an increased production of toxins A and B [30,31], and hypothetically increased virulence. Warny and colleagues [23] measured the in vitro production of toxins A and B by BI/NAP1 and control isolates using an enzyme-linked immunoassay, and found that BI/NAP1 produced 16 and 23 times higher concentrations of toxins A and B, respectively. In addition, these strains produce a binary toxin know as *Clostridium difficile* transferase (CDT), which is made of 2 proteins (Cdta and Cdtb) encoded by the transferase locus located downstream from the pathogenicity locus [27]. The role of this toxin is not clear because strains that produce it alone are not pathogenic in animal models [32]. On the molecular level, this toxin causes adenosine diphosphate (ADP)-ribosylation of G-actin, inhibiting actin polymerization. It also causes rearrangement of microtubules, leading to formation of long protrusions on the cell surface, increasing the adherence of *Clostridium difficile* [13]. This toxin may contribute to the virulence of this strain.

RISK FACTORS FOR THE DEVELOPMENT OF CDI

The most important risk factor for the development of CDI is antibiotic use, and any antibiotic has the potential to cause CDI. Kelly and LaMont [33] reported that 96% of patients who developed CDI had been treated with an antibiotic within the previous 2 months. Antibiotics disrupt the normal colonic microbiome, which then allows relatively resistant *Clostridium difficile* to proliferate. It was shown that longer duration of antibiotic use, as well as the use of multiple antibiotics, increase the risk of developing CDI [34].

Several antibiotics have an increased association with the development of CDI. Clindamycin was the original antibiotic that was implicated in the pathogenesis of this disease. Cephalosporins and fluoroquinolones have also been shown to increase the incidence of CDI [6,34–37]. During the last decade, because of widespread use of fluoroquinolones, this class of antibiotic has become a major cause of CDI, leading to an increase up to 3-fold of the incidence in hospitalized patients [36].

Hospitalization is a further risk factor for the development of CDI. This factor is clearly related to increased risk of exposure in this environment, as well as associated use of antibiotics in hospitalized patients. The duration of hospitalization directly correlates with risk for the development of CDI [38]. Increasing age is a substantial risk factor for the development of CDI [39]. This factor is in part secondary to increased exposure to highly contaminated environments, including hospitals and nursing homes, plus the fact that comorbid medical conditions are associated with the development of CDI [40].

Suppression of gastric acid by proton pump inhibitors or histamine receptor 2 blockers are also found to be associated with a doubling of CDI risk [10,41–43]. The suppression of acid hypothetically decreases the innoculum of either ingested vegetative bacteria or spores required to result in colonization with *Clostridium difficile*. It may also be secondary to relative changes in gut microflora as a result of gastric acid suppression [27].

Immunosuppression [21,39], chemotherapy [44,45], gastrointestinal (GI) surgery [46], intensive care unit (ICU) stay, and inflammatory bowel disease [47,48] are also associated with CDI.

CLINICAL MANIFESTATIONS

According to the Society for Healthcare Epidemiology of America (SHEA), CDI is defined as the presence of diarrhea with one of the following laboratory findings: a positive stool test for toxigenic *Clostridium difficile* or its toxin, or alternatively, the documentation of pseudomembranous colitis on colonoscopy [21].

In clinical practice, the use of antibiotics is usually considered one of the diagnostic criteria, based on the fact the most patients with CDI have received antibiotics within the 2 weeks of their disease [49]. However, it is appropriately not included in the definition because of the increasing incidence of community-acquired CDI that occurs in the absence of previous antibiotic use [50].

Patients with mild to moderate disease present with uncomplicated diarrhea that may be slightly mucoid or bloody. The diarrhea has a characteristic foul-smelling odor that is associated with production of the volatile short-chain fatty acids butyrate and succinate, as well as aromatic amines [51]. There may also be associated abdominal crampy pain with distention and fever. These symptoms most often begin within 4 to 9 days after antibiotic intake [28], but may be associated with antibiotic use up to 3 months previously.

A common laboratory finding is an unusually high serum white blood cell count with or without an increased band count. It is not unusual to see a white blood cell count in the 20,000 to 30,000 range.

The spectrum of disease ranges from relatively mild diarrhea to the development of life-threatening sepsis syndrome with organ failure. In more severe disease, the abrupt resolution of diarrhea in the setting of continued clinical symptoms including pain, abdominal distention, or cardiopulmonary deterioration is an ominous sign. This symptom represents the development of an ileus or a clinical picture similar to toxic megacolon seen in inflammatory bowel disease, and should prompt an escalation of care and surgical consultation.

Although patients with advanced disease may, on rare occasions, even go on to develop colonic necrosis and perforation, we do not believe that these complications are inherently part of the syndrome of CDI. The colon does not die or perforate as a result of the pathophysiology. Rather, when colonic necrosis or perforation is encountered in CDI, this is as a result of either hypoperfusion secondary to the development of shock and vasopressor usage or as a result of vascular compromise because of colonic distension or the abdominal compartment syndrome with resultant malperfusion of the colon. In our experience, colonic perforation or necrosis is found in only 1% to 2% of patients taken to the operating room for severe complicated CDI.

The Infectious Diseases Society of America (IDSA) and SHEA have devised a severity scoring system based on a combination of laboratory and clinical criteria [21] (Table 1). This system includes mild to moderate disease, which

Table 1
Classification schema for CDI and recommended antibiotic treatment strategy as outlined in SHEA/IDSA treatment guidelines

Category	Criteria	Treatment
Mild or moderate	Diarrhea	Metronidazole 500 mg orally 3 times a day
Severe	White blood cell count >15,000 cells/µL or creatinine increased 1.5 fold > baseline	Vancomycin 125 mg orally 4 times a day
Severe, complicated	Ileus, megacolon, hypotension, or shock	Metronidazole 500 mg intravenously 3 times a day + vancomycin 500 mg orally 4 times a day (+ vancomycin enemas in ileus)

This scoring system is not yet validated.
Data from Cohen SH, Gerding DN, Johnson S, et al. Clinical practice guidelines for *Clostridium difficile* infection in adults: 2010 update by the Society for Healthcare Epidemiology of America (SHEA) and the Infectious Diseases Society of America (IDSA). Infect Control Hosp Epidemiol 2010;31(5):431–55.

is characterized by diarrhea. Patients are classified as having severe disease when the white blood cell count is greater than 15,000 or serum creatinine level is increased 50% greater than baseline. These criteria are relatively nonspecific but suggest a progression of disease and have been shown to be signs associated with increased morbidity. Severe, complicated disease (inclusive of what is sometimes referred to as fulminant disease) is characterized by CDI with ileus/megacolon, hypotension, or systemic shock.

The percentage of patients with CDI who progress to severe or severe, complicated disease using this classification schema is relatively unknown. Several case series have reported overall mortality in patients with CDI from 4% to 10% [52]. However, mortality in patients who develop signs of shock requiring vasopressors as a result of CDI is estimated to be greater than 50% [8,53,54].

We use the classification schema of SHEA/IDSA throughout, but believe that this scoring system fails to adequately identify and guide the management of patients who have a mortality risk from this disease. Additional scoring and prognostic criteria have been identified and are highlighted in the next section.

SEVERITY AND PROGNOSTIC SCORING CRITERIA

A particular challenge for clinicians has been the management and treatment of patients with severe, complicated CDI. One reason has been the lack of ability to identify patients who fail medical therapy and go on to deteriorate. Another reason is that the main therapy in the management of patients who have failed antibiotic therapy and are clinically deteriorating has been total abdominal colectomy. Clinicians have been reluctant to execute this therapy except as a salvage procedure, offered only once patients are critically ill and have signs of cardiopulmonary compromise.

Several scoring systems and prognostic criteria have been developed [52–58]. In general, these scoring criteria have an excellent negative predictive value, but a relatively poor positive predictive value concerning failure of medical therapy or mortality. In the absence of these criteria or a higher score, most patients have a good prognosis; however, the presence of these criteria or a higher score have not been able to adequately stratify which of these sicker patients go on to fail. Nevertheless, at this point, these evolving prognostic scoring systems can help clinicians to understand the severity of disease and overall chances of mortality associated with CDI.

Most scoring and prognostic systems have used a combination of similar clinical and laboratory criteria that have been shown to be associated with poorer outcomes (Box 1). These criteria include increasing age, history of organ transplantation or malignancy, ileus, cardiopulmonary compromise, increased serum white blood cell counts, increased serum band counts, increased serum creatinine, increased lactate, decreased albumin, or increased American Association of Anaesthetists (ASA) class or APACHE (Acute Physiology and Chronic Health Evaluation) scores. In addition, some scoring systems use the abdominal computed tomography (CT) scan findings as part of the criteria.

Box 1: Factors that have been associated with a poor prognosis from CDI

Nonmodifiable patient factors:
- Age older than 65 years
- Preexisting renal or pulmonary disease
- Immunosuppression
- High ASA class

Physical examination/clinical findings:
- Fever
- Hypotension/shock requiring vasopressors
- Need for intubation/mechanical ventilation
- Mental status changes
- Ileus/distention

Laboratory values:
- High white blood cell count (>20,000 cells/μL)
- Increased creatinine/renal dysfunction
- Increasing lactate
- Low albumin

CT scan findings:
- Pancolitis/ascites

A broad interpretation of all of these studies is that patients who are likely to have a poor prognosis are those with more comorbidities, increasing age, and critical illness and shock. We currently use several of these components as thresholds for both recommendations for surgical consultation and inclusion criteria for those to be offered surgical therapy, as opposed to achieving a definitive score. This subject is discussed further in the next section.

ESTABLISHED MANAGEMENT STRATEGIES

The most important aspect any health care provider can undertake in the treatment of CDI is infection control measures to prevent the disease in the first place. These measures include: (1) basic hygiene in the interaction with all patients; (2) adequate environmental cleaning in hospitals and nursing homes using bleach-based solutions to kill *Clostridium difficile* spores; (3) isolation of patients with CDI; (4) use of proper barrier precautions; and (5) hand-washing with soap and water when making contact patients with known or suspected CDI. The spores are not susceptible to alcohol-based antiseptic solutions and gels.

Several initial steps are generally recommended in the treatment of any patient with CDI. Resuscitation with intravenous fluids and correction of electrolytes is often necessary given the volume of diarrhea. This aspect must not be overlooked.

In addition, treatment with the inciting antimicrobial(s) should be stopped if it is still ongoing. This strategy is not always possible given the need to treat an active infection. Thus, if antibiotics need to be continued, then the recommendation is to change to an antibiotic that is less likely to promote CDI. These antibiotics include sulfamethoxazole, macrolides, aminoglycosides, tigecycline, and intravenous vancomycin. There are no randomized data to support this approach. Avoidance of antibiotics that have a higher association of CDI is recommended (these include cephalosporins, fluoroquinolones, and clindamycin). At one time, discontinuation of inciting antibiotics was considered to be the only initial treatment in cases of mild or moderate CDI [59]. However, this strategy is no longer considered prudent given the evolving epidemiology and prevalence of the more virulent BI/NAP1 strain. Avoidance of antiperistaltic agents and minimalization of opioid analgesics is generally recommended despite the diarrhea [21].

Established antibiotic management

Several antibiotics with known activity against *Clostridium difficile* have been shown to be effective in treating CDI. These antibiotics include metronidazole, vancomycin, teicoplanin, fusidic acid, bacitracin, nitazoxanide, tolevamer, and fidaxomicin. The mainstay of medical treatment of CDI involves the use of either metronidazole or enteral vancomycin. Both enteral and intravenous metronidazole can achieve concentrations in the lumen of the colon under diarrheal conditions to effectively treat CDI, but metronidazole is not therapeutic in formed stool [60]. Intravenous vancomycin does not enter the lumen of the GI tract and is never a treatment of CDI. All references to vancomycin therapy in this article refer to direct enteral delivery, either via the oral route, enteric tubes, or enemas.

The choice of antibiotic (metronidazole or vancomycin) depends on the severity of disease and other considerations, such as the presence of an ileus [21]. The greatest experience with dosing regimens has been with metronidazole 500 mg 3 times per day for 10 to 14 days (current recommended regimen) or 250 mg 4 times a day for 10 to 14 days. Vancomycin dosing has been 125 mg orally 4 times per day for 10 to 14 days. Vancomycin was approved by the US Food and Drug Administration (FDA) in 1978 for the treatment of CDI [61], and up until recently was the only approved drug with this indication.

Traditionally, metronidazole has been first-line therapy based on its significantly lower cost and initial small, prospective randomized trials that showed metronidazole or vancomycin to be equally effective [59,62]. Metronidazole was also recommended as first-line therapy by a Cochrane review [63]. More recent observational studies have suggested that metronidazole is not as effective as previously suggested [64,65]. This finding may be because of the changes in the microbe and the altered epidemiology of this disease. The most recent prospective, double-blind, randomized study showed that the clinical cure rate in patients with severe CDI was significantly better with vancomycin than with metronidazole (97% vs 76%) [66]. Thus, the current recommendations of SHEA and IDSA are the use of metronidazole for mild or moderate disease at an oral dose of 500 mg 3 times per day for 10 to 14 days. In severe disease, oral vancomycin is recommended at a dose of 125 mg 4 times per day for 10 to 14 days [21]. Severe is defined as a patient with a leukocytosis of more than 15,000 cells/μL or a creatinine level more than 1.5 times the baseline (see Table 1).

Antibiotic management for severe, complicated disease

The data, and thus the specific recommendations, for the treatment of severe, complicated disease are based on small case series and expert opinion. Severe, complicated CDI has been defined as patients with ileus, megacolon, hypotension, or shock. We believe the definition should also encompass patients with extreme white blood cell counts (>30,000 cells/μL or <2000 cells/μL), high serum band percentages (>50%), mental status changes, worsening examinations or white blood cell counts on CDI directed antibiotic treatment, patients requiring intubation/mechanical ventilation because of CDI, and patients with acute kidney injury because of CDI. We believe that this category should be explicitly more inclusive to ensure the escalation of care in more patients, with the goal of improving outcomes. The treatment recommendations from SHEA and IDSA include vancomycin 500 mg 4 times per day orally or via nasogastric tube plus the addition of metronidazole 500 mg intravenously 3 times per day. Our experience has been that patients with more advanced disease often do not respond to more intense antibiotic therapy, especially if the effective delivery of antibiotic to the colon may be substantially reduced by the presence of an ileus. The SHEA/IDSA recommended increased dose of vancomycin is not based on strong data, but rather on the logic that in the setting of impaired GI motility, doubling the dose may increase the levels that reach the colon. The recommended use of intravenous metronidazole avoids the need for oral intake, but delivery to the colon is still dependent on biliary excretion of the metronidazole to the small bowel and subsequent GI motility to reach the colon. The SHEA/IDSA recommendations also include the adjunctive use of vancomycin enemas to ensure delivery to the colon. Several small studies lend support to this recommendation [49,67]. We support the use of vancomycin enemas, but stress that the volume of the enema must be sufficient to reflux into the right colon. Former recommendations of vancomycin enemas have been for 500 mg in 100 mL of saline 4 times per day. We believe the vancomycin volume should be at least 500 mL.

The role of surgery for severe, complicated CDI

The recommendations from SHEA and IDSA have also been more nebulous for surgical therapies. Subtotal colectomy is most commonly recommended when severe complicated CDI fails to respond to antibiotic use. There is no consensus on the indications or timing of surgery. The rare perforation is 1 clear indication. The vague term clinical deterioration in already critically ill patients failing medical therapy is frequently mentioned. These strategies rely on surgery as a salvage therapy, which may account for the poor outcomes associated with subtotal colectomy in severe, complicated CDI, with mortality ranging from 35% to 85% [8,53,54,68,69].

We join others in advocating earlier surgical consultation as soon as the diagnosis of severe or severe complicated CDI is considered [28,70]. This strategy would likely help to identify patients earlier in the course of the disease process, before decompensation. At our institution, we advocate surgical consultation in all patients prescribed vancomycin for an acute episode of CDI. This approach may be too inclusive and cumbersome. Other strategies may be less stringent but should at least include any patient in the ICU because of CDI, patients with ileus or abdominal distention, or who fail to improve or have worsening white blood cell counts on medical therapy. Patients who are immunosuppressed or those with extreme white blood cell counts (>30,000 cells/μL or <2000 cells/μL) often fit the definition of severe complicated CDI. In addition, we advocate the use of CT scanning of the abdomen and pelvis in this patient population if there is no immediate indication for operative intervention. CT scanning may aid in the diagnosis and help clinicians to recognize the severity of disease by identifying findings such as pancolitis, colonic thickening, ascites, ileus, and megacolon. Although this strategy is not supported by data, it has been shown that patients treated in surgical departments have a higher rate of operation with a lower rate of mortality compared with those treated in a nonsurgical department [53]. This finding suggests a benefit of early surgical consultation.

The timing of surgical therapy needs to be better defined. We put forth the following recommendations for indications for surgery (Box 2). A diagnosis of CDI should be made based on one of the following: (1) laboratory confirmation of a diagnosis; (2) endoscopic findings of pseudomembranes; or (3) CT scan consistent with CDI in the setting of an appropriate history. These 3 characteristics plus any one of the following findings might complete a set of indications: (1) peritonitis; (2) worsening abdominal distention/pain; (3) sepsis;

Box 2: Indications for operative management in patients with CDI

A diagnosis of CDI as determined by one of the following:

1. Laboratory confirmation of *Clostridium difficile*
2. Endoscopic findings
3. CT scan findings consistent with CDI (pancolitis ± ascites)

Plus any one of the following criteria:

1. Peritonitis
2. Worsening abdominal distention/pain
3. Sepsis
4. Intubation secondary to CDI
5. Vasopressor requirement secondary to CDI
6. Mental status changes
7. Unexplained clinical deterioration
8. Failure to improve with standard therapy within 96 hours as determined by resolving symptoms and physical examination, resolving white blood cell/band count

(4) intubation as a result of CDI; (5) vasopressor requirement as a result of CDI; (6) mental status changes; (7) unexplained clinical deterioration; or (8) failure to improve with standard therapy within 96 hours. Clinical judgment must be applied to these indications.

The choice of surgical therapy for these patients has, in the absence of an alternative, traditionally been exploratory laparotomy with total abdominal colectomy and end ileostomy. Total abdominal colectomy has been more successful than segmental colectomy in several series [28,54,71]. One particular challenge for surgeons has been the deceptive findings at the time of laparotomy. In most patients, the serosal surface of the colon, although boggy and edematous, is usually intact, viable, and without evidence of necrosis. Thus, inexperienced surgeons are tempted to perform segmental colectomy, thereby removing only segments that seem to be nonviable or seriously diseased; however, outcomes have been worse with this strategy, seemingly because the extent of the disease is not obvious from the serosal aspect. Although it is patchy, patients with severe/complicated CDI have extensive mucosal damage throughout the colon. However, the finding that the colon is usually viable and nonnecrotic has implications for evolving surgical therapies, which are believed to have advantages when compared with subtotal colectomy and are discussed later.

The treatment algorithm that we currently use is highlighted in Fig. 1. This algorithm uses the SHEA/IDSA guidelines for antimicrobial management for mild, moderate, and severe disease. It differs in severe, complicated CDI. For these patients, the recommendation is for operative therapy if they meet the criteria described earlier (ie, that the patient has cardiopulmonary compromise, sepsis syndrome, end organ dysfunction, mental status changes, peritonitis, or is clinically deteriorating). In the absence of these findings, this group is at high risk for ileus and delayed GI motility. The recommended antimicrobial strategy uses vancomycin enemas (500 mg rectally 4 times a day; same dose as the SHEA/IDSA guidelines) in a volume of 500 mL. This dose is higher than the 100-mL volume that has been recommended, but the increased volume is necessary to have the enema reach the proximal part of the colon (right and proximal transverse colon). This group also receives metronidazole intravenously and vancomycin orally or via nasogastric tube. We use a dose of 125 mg orally 4 times a day, as opposed to 500 mg orally 4 times a day, because all of these patients are receiving the additional rectal vancomycin. Daily assessment is necessary to determine response, and further care adjusted based on clinical assessments.

Recurrent CDI

One aspect of the medical management of CDI that has been challenging has been the high recurrence rates. Recurrence rates are lower with vancomycin than metronidazole, but still approach 25% [64,66,72,73]. In general, second episodes should be treated with an antibiotic strategy that is the same as a first episode based on severity. Recurrent CDI occurs in 33% to 65% of patients who have had more than 2 previous episodes [64,74–77]. The antibiotic strategy most used in these patients has been a vancomycin pulse (10–14 days' standard

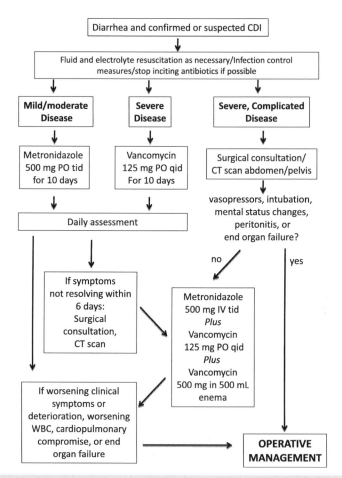

Fig. 1. This treatment algorithm uses the SHEA/IDSA guidelines for antimicrobial management for mild, moderate, and severe disease.

therapy) and taper strategy (dose frequency tapered over an additional 4–6 weeks). Adjunctive therapies to prevent recurrences, including probiotics and fecal bacteriotherapy, are highlighted later.

Recurrences are generally not attributed to the development of resistance to metronidazole or vancomycin [78]. It is believed that reinfection occurs either as a result of continued environmental exposure or from spores in the GI tract as an endogenous source. One prevailing hypothesis relates more to an impaired humoral host immune response [79], which has implications for developing therapies.

ADVANCES IN MEDICAL MANAGEMENT

Poor outcomes, high recurrence rates, and increasing incidence and severity continue to drive interest in novel therapeutic strategies in the management of CDI. These advances in care have been in areas of diagnosis, active and passive immunization to treat or prevent CDI, novel antibiotics, the use of fecal bacteriotherapy or probiotics, delivery strategies of vancomycin and other antibiotics. Several of these advances are highlighted later and in Box 3.

Advances in diagnosis

A summary of diagnostic tests is given in Table 2. The gold standard for diagnosis of CDI is stool culture under anaerobic conditions. However, this test is cumbersome and is often not diagnostic for up to 96 hours. Therefore it has less use in the clinical setting, but is essential for epidemiologic studies. Most diagnostic tests rely on detection of toxin. Toxin has been detected by cell cytotoxin culture, which uses coculture of cells with stool supernatants looking for cytotoxic effects, or by enzyme immunoassay. Some advocate an initial screen for the *Clostridium difficile* antigen glutamate dehydrogenase (GDH), followed by a toxin assay to increase sensitivity, but results vary depending on methods used for GDH detection [80,81].

PCR testing is relatively new and is increasing in use in clinical laboratories. In 2009, several PCR assays were approved by the US FDA. This approach has the advantage of being rapid, sensitive, and specific [82,83]. One study compared PCR and enzyme immunoassay techniques with gold standard anaerobic culture. Sensitivity and specificity were better for PCR than enzyme immunoassay (93% and 97% vs 73% and 97%, respectively) [83]. In a recent study comparing the Cepheid Xpert *Clostridium difficile* PCR assay (Sunnyvale, CA, USA) with cell cytotoxicity assays for diagnosis of CDI, the sensitivity and specificity of the PCR assay were 97 and 93%, respectively [82].

Box 3: Novel medical treatment strategies for CDI

Antibiotics:
- Fidaxomicin (FDA approved)
- Rifaximin
- Nitazoxanide
- Teicoplanin
- Ramoplanin

Immunization therapy:
- Toxoid vaccines
- Anti-*Clostridium difficile* toxin antibodies
- Intravenous immunoglobulin (IVIG)

Biotherapy:
- Fecal bacteriotherapy
- Nontoxigenic *Clostridium difficile* strains
- Probiotics

Table 2
Diagnostic tests available for CDI

Test	Advantages	Disadvantages
Anaerobic stool culture	Gold standard	72–96-h turnaround
	Typing of strain possible	Labor intensive
Cytotoxin assay	Sensitivity (76%–90%)	48-h turnaround
	Specificity (99%–100%)	Requires tissue culture
Enzyme immunoassay for toxin A or toxins A and B	Specificity (95%–100%)	Reduced sensitivity
	Rapid turnaround time	(65%–85%)
	Technically less demanding	
Glutamate dehydrogenase followed by enzyme immunoassay	Increased sensitivity compared with enzyme immunoassay alone	Sensitivity limited by glutamate dehydrogenase kit used
	Same-day turnaround time	
PCR for toxin genes	Sensitivity (93%–97%)	Increased skill required
	Specificity (93%–97%)	
	Rapid turnaround time	

In general, testing should be done only on unformed stools and in patients with the clinical syndrome of CDI.

Two important aspects should always be considered when ordering diagnostic tests for CDI. The first is that only unformed stools should be tested. Only patients with the clinical syndrome of CDI should be tested for CDI. The second is that repeat stool testing during the same diarrhea episode is generally not indicated. It had become adopted practice at many centers to send at least 3 specimens; however, with increasing sensitivity and sensitivity of clinical diagnostic tests, this is not necessary.

Immunization strategies against *Clostridium difficile*
The use of both passive and active immunization strategies in the treatment of CDI is appealing, especially considering findings that progression to severe disease or disease recurrence may be related to impaired host immune responses [79]. One of the most encouraging studies has been in the area of passive immunization. In a prospective, randomized, double-blind, placebo-controlled trial, Lowy and colleagues [72] showed that the use of monoclonal antibodies against toxin A and B in conjunction with vancomycin decreased the recurrence rate from 25% to 7% compared with vancomycin alone. This strategy was even effective in patients with the epidemic BI/NAP1 strain and patients with previous episodes. These monoclonal antibodies are not yet available for clinical use.

Passive immunization has also been attempted with pooled IVIG. IVIG is from pooled human serum and has been documented to contain antibodies against *Clostridium difficile* toxins. IVIG has been used in recurrent disease and in severe, complicated disease. This approach has not been well studied, but several case series or retrospective studies do not suggest a significant benefit [84–86].

Active immunization strategies are currently under clinical trial. Preliminary trials with vaccines containing toxoids have proved to be safe and can effectively result in an antitoxin response in healthy adults [87,88]. Sougioultzis and colleagues [89] showed that 3 patients with recurrent CDI requiring continuous treatment with vancomycin were successfully weaned off after vaccination.

Novel antibiotics for CDI

Antimicrobial drug development for CDI is an obvious area for development. Several established antibiotics are being investigated for activity and effectiveness in CDI, whereas others are being developed. These drugs include nitazoxanide, rifamixin, ramoplanin, teicoplanin, and most notably fidaxomicin.

Fidaxomicin was recently approved by the FDA for the treatment of CDI. This is a macrocyclic antibiotic with narrow therapeutic spectrum. Its bactericidal effect is caused by its ability to inhibit bacterial RNA polymerase [90]. In a prospective, randomized trial, Louie and colleagues [73] showed that the clinical cure rate of fidaxomicin was noninferior compared with vancomycin. The main advantage of this drug was the lower overall recurrence rate compared with vancomycin (15.4% vs 25.3%, respectively). However, no significant difference was seen in recurrence rate in patients with the BI/NAP1 strain.

Vancomycin and fidaxomicin have a similar safety profile [91]. The lower recurrence rate of fidaxomicin may be explained by the narrower spectrum of fidaxomicin compared with vancomycin, leading to less disruption of the intestinal microflora. It has been shown that fidaxomicin was associated with less disruption of the anaerobe *Bacteroides* in the colon compared with vancomycin and that there may be less of an associated risk for the development of selecting out for vancomycin-resistant *Enterococci* [92].

At this point, fidaxomicin is not being used as a first-line therapy at most centers. There is no major cost advantage over vancomycin, many large centers have a high prevalence of BI/NAP1 strain, and concerns about the development of resistance have limited its use. Fidaxomicin may be an appropriate therapy in patients with CDI or perhaps as initial therapy in patients deemed a high risk for developing recurrent disease; however, the integration of this drug into treatment algorithms is still being developed.

Rifaximin is a semisynthetic, rifamycin derivative that is highly active against *Clostridium difficile* in vitro. It is not absorbed by the intestinal mucosal, leading to a high intraluminal concentration, which may be beneficial in treating and preventing CDI. Johnson and colleagues [93] used rifaximin immediately after vancomycin treatment in patients with high recurrence and found that 67% of patients were cured. Although results were initially encouraging, the major drawback of this antimicrobial is the emergence of resistance, and it is unlikely to be a significant advancement in the treatment of this disease. Rifalazil is a new benzoxazinorifamycin that has been studied in hamsters and was shown to be superior to vancomycin in the treatment and prevention of recurrent CDI [94]. However, resistance to this drug is also highly likely.

Nitazoxanide is a thiazolide antibiotic marketed in the United States for the treatment of intestinal parasites. Nitazoxanide has a potent effect on *Clostridium difficile* in vitro by affecting the pyruvate ferredoxin oxidoreductase pathway, which is necessary for the anaerobic metabolism [95,96]. Musher and colleagues [97] compared 27 patients receiving vancomycin and 23 receiving nitazoxanide in a randomized trial; response rates were 87% in the vancomycin group and 94% in the nitazoxanide group. There was a similar interval of time for resolution of symptoms. This study was too underpowered to draw any significant conclusions.

Ramoplanin, a glycolipodepsipeptide antibiotic, exerts its bactericidal effect by inhibiting cell wall biosynthesis. Freeman and colleagues [98] used in vitro gut and hamster models and showed that ramoplanin is as effective as vancomycin in reducing toxin production in vitro and in achieving clinical cure in the hamster model. Ramoplanin was also more effective than vancomycin in preventing disease recurrence in this animal model.

Teicoplanin, a glycopeptide antibiotic, inhibits bacterial cell wall synthesis and has a similar spectrum of activity to vancomycin. Wenisch and colleagues [62] showed in a randomized clinical trial that teicoplanin was as effective as metronidazole and vancomycin in achieving clinical cure of CDI, was equivalent in the rapidity of response and was more effective than metronidazole in achieving fecal cytotoxicity resolution. Teicoplanin has a high cost and is associated with an increased resistance rate [99].

Biotherapeutic strategies

Biotherapeutic approaches to restore the microflora of the GI system to prevent or treat CDI are of great interest. These approaches include probiotics, fecal bacteriotherapy, and the use of nontoxigenic strains of *Clostridium difficile.*

Probiotics refers to the biotherapeutic strategy of delivering viable microorganisms with the goal of maintaining or restoring normal gut microbiome. Common species that have been investigated include *Saccharomyces boulardii, Lactobacillus rhamnosus,* and *Lactobacillus acidophilus* [100]. A Cochrane review to evaluate the use of probiotics alone or in conjunction with conventional antibiotics for the treatment of CDI was performed. Four studies were included and the review suggested that probiotics are likely effective, but because of study heterogeneity, the evidence was inconclusive in supporting the use of probiotic therapy [101]. Of all probiotics used in CDI, *S boulardii* is the best studied. In a prospective, randomized, controlled trial studying recurrent CDI, treatment with a high-dose vancomycin plus *S boulardii* showed a significant trend toward reduced recurrences [102]. Several cases of bacteremia or fungemia have been reported after treatment with *Lactobacillus* species or *S boulardii,* respectively, in immunocompromised hosts [103–105], and therefore should be used with caution in these populations.

Fecal bacteriotherapy or stool transplants have obvious aesthetic concerns but holds great promise. Typically fresh feces from a household donor, which has previously been tested for *Clostridium difficile* and other infectious diseases, is blended and particulate matter is removed. The mixture is then delivered via colonoscopy, enema, or nasogastric tube. It is believed that the stool must be fresh to ensure that the anaerobic population remains viable. This approach has mainly been studied in the setting of relapsing recurrences or in mild or moderate disease. In a review, Bakken reported the results of 100 patients with CDI recurrences who failed conventional therapies and showed that fecal bacteriotherapy was successful in treating 89% of the recurrent cases of CDI [106]. Case reports have shown fecal bacteriotherapy to be effective in cases of severe, complicated CDI [107]. The use of bacteria mixtures that mimic stool flora has also been investigated [108]. This simple and inexpensive procedure will likely increase in popularity over time given that the strategy is the most natural way to restore normal colonic microbiome.

The use of nontoxigenic *Clostridium difficile* strain has also been postulated for the management of CDI. It was found in an animal model that the administration of nonpathogenic strain during or after antimicrobial management successfully led to GI colonization and prevention of further CDI recurrence [109–111]. This approach has also been used in patients in case reports with some success [112].

ADVANCES IN SURGICAL MANAGEMENT

Subtotal or total abdominal colectomy with end ileostomy had become the gold standard in the surgical management of severe, complicated CDI. As mentioned earlier, this therapy improves outcomes in some patients who have advanced disease, yet the outcomes remain poor even with colectomy once the disease has advanced to the severe, complicated state. These outcomes are likely secondary to associated patient comorbidities, use of colectomy as a salvage therapy in deteriorating patients, and the stresses of total colectomy in this patient population under such conditions. Clinicians have been reluctant to consider early total colectomy because of the long-term effects of even a successful life-saving outcome. Few surviving patients undergo reconstruction of their GI tract after subtotal colectomy.

Our group has recently reported our experience with performing loop ileostomy and colonic lavage with a polyethylene glycol 3350/balanced electrolyte solution (Go-lytely, Braintree Labs) followed by postoperative antegrade vancomycin colonic flushes for the treatment of severe, complicated CDI [113]. Fig. 2 highlights the operative procedure. This case series reported mortality of 19% in 42 patients using this therapy compared with 50% from the previous 42 patients who underwent colectomy at the same center. There were no statistically significant differences in demographics of these critically ill patient populations with regards to age, sex, immunosuppression, and APACHE II scores. More than 80% of these operations were performed laparoscopically, and of the patients followed for at least 6 months postoperatively, 79% had reversal of their ileostomy performed and their GI tract continuity restored.

The success of this operative approach is likely multifactorial. The surgical insult is minimized compared with total abdominal colectomy. The combination of fecal diversion, high-volume washout, and antegrade colonic delivery of vancomycin achieves several goals. The washout with polyethylene glycol solution reduces resident colonic flora, including *Clostridium difficile* and toxins. This strategy

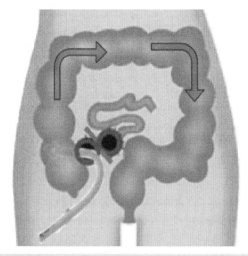

Fig. 2. Creation of diverting loop ileostomy. On-table colonic lavage with warm 8 L PEG3350/balanced electrolyte solution (collection of effluent via rectal tube). Postoperative antegrade vancomycin flushes via efferent limb of ileostomy (500 mg in 500 mL of lactated Ringer solution 3 times per day for 10 days).

has been used successfully in several patients with relapsing disease in the past via oral or nasogastric or colonoscopic delivery of polyethylene glycol solution [114,115]. A possible pharmacologic effect of polyethylene glycol is hypothesized but not proved [116,117]. The direct installation of vancomycin into the efferent limb of the ileostomy and antegrade into the colon has the obvious benefit of being directed antimicrobial therapy. Vancomycin delivery into the colon via cecostomy tube or colonoscopically has been shown to be effective [49,118]. Fecal diversion has the hypothetical advantage of colonic bowel rest of the inflamed colon, as well as possible changes in oxygen tension of the colon after diversion. Blowhole- type ostomies have been used in toxic megacolon for ulcerative colitis [119]. Future investigations may prove 1 or more of these steps unnecessary.

Additional potential advantages of this approach may be the willingness of clinicians to offer this surgical therapy earlier in the course of disease in patients with severe, complicated CDI.

The current surgical strategy that we recommend based on this experience is highlighted in Fig. 3. Once a decision to offer a patient surgical therapy is made, it is important to determine if the patient has abdominal compartment syndrome. From our experience, the rate of abdominal compartment syndrome found in patients managed operatively is around 5%. These patients require laparotomy and abdominal decompression. Although we have managed these patients via a staged approach with decompressive laparotomy, loop ileostomy and colonic lavage, and temporary management of an open abdomen with a negative pressure dressing followed by subsequent closure, we now favor a single-stage approach with colectomy and end ileostomy. The compartment syndrome

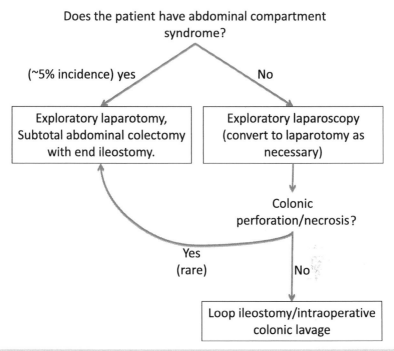

Fig. 3. Operative management strategy for CDI.

is usually resolved by colectomy and facilitates definitive management and closure. In most patients, one can proceed with laparoscopy (or laparotomy if necessary). If the patient does not have a necrotic colon or perforation (which is rare and usually occurs only in the setting of abdominal compartment syndrome or nonocclusive ischemia as a result of volume depletion and vasopressors), the loop ileostomy and intraoperative colonic lavage is performed. Clinical improvement is assessed and most often seen within 24 to 48 hours and should be seen within 5 days. This group of patients often has significant comorbidities or has been allowed to progress to organ failure before surgical consultation, both of which can delay clinical resolution. In addition, the inflamed colon is left in place and although the inciting CDI infection is treated, the resolution of the colonic inflammation and the systemic consequences of this can take several days to resolve. Furthermore, this operation does not preclude subsequent colectomy in the setting of deterioration. We have managed 3 patients (of 70 patients we have treated with loop ileostomy) who have developed abdominal compartment syndrome postoperatively requiring further surgery. Two were treated with decompressive laparotomy alone and one with colectomy. We have performed total abdominal colectomies on 3 additional patients for the indication of clinical deterioration after ileostomy and colonic lavage. These treatments were performed on postoperative days 4, 7, and 8 after the original procedure. No perforation or colonic ischemia was encountered and the pathology reports showed resolving colitis on all of these patients. Further experiences and a planned randomized controlled trial compared with colectomy will add to this experience.

SUMMARY

CDI is increasing in incidence and severity. Clinicians must have a low threshold to consider the diagnosis and to treat patients with the clinical syndrome and risk factors before laboratory confirmation of the diagnosis. In patients who have signs of advanced disease, escalation of care with antimicrobial strategies and multidisciplinary care including surgical consultation is necessary. Furthermore, lowering the threshold for surgery compared with traditional approaches likely results in improved survival. Novel surgical approaches may obviate total abdominal colectomy and the associated immediate and long-term morbidity in this often fragile patient population, thus allowing clinicians to embrace surgical therapy earlier in the course of severe, complicated disease.

References

[1] Song X, Bartlett JG, Speck K, et al. Rising economic impact of *Clostridium difficile*-associated disease in adult hospitalized patient population. Infect Control Hosp Epidemiol 2008;29(9):823–8.

[2] US Department of Health and Human Services. HCUPnet 2010. Available at: www.hcupnet. ahrq.gov. Accessed May 24, 2012.

[3] McDonald LC, Killgore GE, Thompson A, et al. An epidemic, toxin gene-variant strain of *Clostridium difficile*. N Engl J Med 2005;353(23):2433–41.

[4] Muto CA, Pokrywka M, Shutt K, et al. A large outbreak of *Clostridium difficile*-associated disease with an unexpected proportion of deaths and colectomies at a teaching hospital following increased fluoroquinolone use. Infect Control Hosp Epidemiol 2005;26(3): 273–80.

[5] Gaynes R, Rimland D, Killum E, et al. Outbreak of *Clostridium difficile* infection in a long-term care facility: association with gatifloxacin use. Clin Infect Dis 2004;38(5):640–5.

[6] Loo VG, Poirier L, Miller MA, et al. A predominantly clonal multi-institutional outbreak of *Clostridium difficile*-associated diarrhea with high morbidity and mortality. N Engl J Med 2005;353(23):2442–9.

[7] Pepin J, Valiquette L, Alary ME, et al. *Clostridium difficile*-associated diarrhea in a region of Quebec from 1991 to 2003: a changing pattern of disease severity. CMAJ 2004;171(5): 466–72.

[8] Dallal RM, Harbrecht BG, Boujoukas AJ, et al. Fulminant *Clostridium difficile*: an underappreciated and increasing cause of death and complications. Ann Surg 2002;235(3): 363–72.

[9] Ricciardi R, Rothenberger DA, Madoff RD, et al. Increasing prevalence and severity of *Clostridium difficile* colitis in hospitalized patients in the United States. Arch Surg 2007;142(7): 624–31 [discussion: 631].

[10] Loo VG, Bourgault AM, Poirier L, et al. Host and pathogen factors for *Clostridium difficile* infection and colonization. N Engl J Med 2011;365(18):1693–703.

[11] Privitera G, Scarpellini P, Ortisi G, et al. Prospective study of *Clostridium difficile* intestinal colonization and disease following single-dose antibiotic prophylaxis in surgery. Antimicrob Agents Chemother 1991;35(1):208–10.

[12] Heinlen L, Ballard JD. *Clostridium difficile* infection. Am J Med Sci 2010;340(3): 247–52.

[13] Schwan C, Stecher B, Tzivelekidis T, et al. *Clostridium difficile* toxin CDT induces formation of microtubule-based protrusions and increases adherence of bacteria. PLoS Pathog 2009;5(10):e1000626.

[14] Rupnik M, Wilcox MH, Gerding DN. *Clostridium difficile* infection: new developments in epidemiology and pathogenesis. Nat Rev Microbiol 2009;7(7):526–36.

[15] Reinert DJ, Jank T, Aktories K, et al. Structural basis for the function of *Clostridium difficile* toxin B. J Mol Biol 2005;351(5):973–81.

[16] Jank T, Giesemann T, Aktories K. Rho-glucosylating *Clostridium difficile* toxins A and B: new insights into structure and function. Glycobiology 2007;17(4):15R–22R.

[17] Giesemann T, Egerer M, Jank T, et al. Processing of *Clostridium difficile* toxins. J Med Microbiol 2008;57(Pt 6):690–6.

[18] Lyras D, O'Connor JR, Howarth PM, et al. Toxin B is essential for virulence of *Clostridium difficile*. Nature 2009;458(7242):1176–9.

[19] Drudy D, Harnedy N, Fanning S, et al. Isolation and characterisation of toxin A-negative, toxin B-positive *Clostridium difficile* in Dublin, Ireland. Clin Microbiol Infect 2007;13(3): 298–304.

[20] Bartlett JG. *Clostridium difficile*: progress and challenges. Ann N Y Acad Sci 2010;1213: 62–9.

[21] Cohen SH, Gerding DN, Johnson S, et al. Clinical practice guidelines for *Clostridium difficile* infection in adults: 2010 update by the Society for Healthcare Epidemiology of America (SHEA) and the Infectious Diseases Society of America (IDSA). Infect Control Hosp Epidemiol 2010;31(5):431–55.

[22] Eggertson L. Quebec strain of C. difficile in 7 provinces. CMAJ 2006;174(5):607–8.

[23] Warny M, Pepin J, Fang A, et al. Toxin production by an emerging strain of *Clostridium difficile* associated with outbreaks of severe disease in North America and Europe. Lancet 2005;366(9491):1079–84.

[24] Kuijper EJ, van den Berg RJ, Debast S, et al. *Clostridium difficile* ribotype 027, toxinotype III, the Netherlands. Emerg Infect Dis 2006;12(5):827–30.

[25] Kuijper EJ, Barbut F, Brazier JS, et al. Update of *Clostridium difficile* infection due to PCR ribotype 027 in Europe, 2008. Euro Surveill 2008;13(31):Article 5.

[26] Kato H, Ito Y, van den Berg RJ, et al. First isolation of *Clostridium difficile* 027 in Japan. Euro Surveill 2007;12(2):Article 3.

[27] Ananthakrishnan AN. *Clostridium difficile* infection: epidemiology, risk factors and management. Nat Rev Gastroenterol Hepatol 2011;8(1):17–26.

[28] Olivas AD, Umanskiy K, Zuckerbraun B, et al. Avoiding colectomy during surgical management of fulminant *Clostridium difficile* colitis. Surg Infect (Larchmt) 2010;11(3): 299–305.

[29] Halsey J. Current and future treatment modalities for *Clostridium difficile* -associated disease. Am J Health Syst Pharm 2008;65(8):705–15.

[30] Musher DM, Logan N, Mehendiratta V. Epidemic *Clostridium difficile*. N Engl J Med 2006;354(11):1199–203 [author reply: 1199–203].

[31] Akerlund T, Svenungsson B, Lagergren A, et al. Correlation of disease severity with fecal toxin levels in patients with *Clostridium difficile* -associated diarrhea and distribution of PCR ribotypes and toxin yields in vitro of corresponding isolates. J Clin Microbiol 2006;44(2):353–8.

[32] Geric B, Carman RJ, Rupnik M, et al. Binary toxin-producing, large clostridial toxin-negative *Clostridium difficile* strains are enterotoxic but do not cause disease in hamsters. J Infect Dis 2006;193(8):1143–50.

[33] Kelly CP, LaMont JT. *Clostridium difficile* infection. Annu Rev Med 1998;49:375–90.

[34] Owens RC Jr, Donskey CJ, Gaynes RP, et al. Antimicrobial-associated risk factors for *Clostridium difficile* infection. Clin Infect Dis 2008;46(Suppl 1):S19–31.

[35] Bartlett JG. Narrative review: the new epidemic of *Clostridium difficile*-associated enteric disease. Ann Intern Med 2006;145(10):758–64.

[36] Pepin J, Saheb N, Coulombe MA, et al. Emergence of fluoroquinolones as the predominant risk factor for *Clostridium difficile*-associated diarrhea: a cohort study during an epidemic in Quebec. Clin Infect Dis 2005;41(9):1254–60.

[37] Gerding DN. Clindamycin, cephalosporins, fluoroquinolones, and *Clostridium difficile*-associated diarrhea: this is an antimicrobial resistance problem. Clin Infect Dis 2004;38(5):646–8.

[38] McFarland LV, Mulligan ME, Kwok RY, et al. Nosocomial acquisition of *Clostridium difficile* infection. N Engl J Med 1989;320(4):204–10.

[39] Bartlett JG, Gerding DN. Clinical recognition and diagnosis of *Clostridium difficile* infection. Clin Infect Dis 2008;46(Suppl 1):S12–8.

[40] Diggs NG, Surawicz CM. Evolving concepts in *Clostridium difficile* colitis. Curr Gastroenterol Rep 2009;11(5):400–5.

[41] Dial S, Delaney JA, Barkun AN, et al. Use of gastric acid-suppressive agents and the risk of community-acquired *Clostridium difficile*-associated disease. JAMA 2005;294(23):2989–95.

[42] Cunningham R, Dale B, Undy B, et al. Proton pump inhibitors as a risk factor for *Clostridium difficile* diarrhoea. J Hosp Infect 2003;54(3):243–5.

[43] Dial S, Alrasadi K, Manoukian C, et al. Risk of *Clostridium difficile* diarrhea among hospital inpatients prescribed proton pump inhibitors: cohort and case-control studies. CMAJ 2004;171(1):33–8.

[44] Anand A, Glatt AE. *Clostridium difficile* infection associated with antineoplastic chemotherapy: a review. Clin Infect Dis 1993;17(1):109–13.

[45] Morales Chamorro R, Serrano Blanch R, Mendez Vidal MJ, et al. Pseudomembranous colitis associated with chemotherapy with 5-fluorouracil. Clin Transl Oncol 2005;7(6):258–61.

[46] Thibault A, Miller MA, Gaese C. Risk factors for the development of *Clostridium difficile*-associated diarrhea during a hospital outbreak. Infect Control Hosp Epidemiol 1991;12(6):345–8.

[47] Ingle M, Deshmukh A, Desai D, et al. Prevalence and clinical course of *Clostridium difficile* infection in a tertiary-care hospital: a retrospective analysis. Indian J Gastroenterol 2011;30(2):89–93.

[48] Sinh P, Barrett TA, Yun L. *Clostridium difficile* infection and inflammatory bowel disease: a review. Gastroenterol Res Pract 2011;2011:136064.

[49] Olson MM, Shanholtzer CJ, Lee JT Jr, et al. Ten years of prospective *Clostridium difficile*-associated disease surveillance and treatment at the Minneapolis VA Medical Center, 1982-1991. Infect Control Hosp Epidemiol 1994;15(6):371–81.

[50] Kyne L, Merry C, O'Connell B, et al. Community-acquired *Clostridium difficile* infection. J Infect 1998;36(3):287–8.

[51] Bartlett JG. Detection of *Clostridium difficile* infection. Infect Control Hosp Epidemiol 2010;31(Suppl 1):S35–7.

[52] Dudukgian H, Sie E, Gonzalez-Ruiz C, et al. C. difficile colitis–predictors of fatal outcome. J Gastrointest Surg 2010;14(2):315–22.

[53] Sailhamer EA, Carson K, Chang Y, et al. Fulminant *Clostridium difficile* colitis: patterns of care and predictors of mortality. Arch Surg 2009;144(5):433–9 [discussion: 439–40].

[54] Perera AD, Akbari RP, Cowher MS, et al. Colectomy for fulminant *Clostridium difficile* colitis: predictors of mortality. Am Surg 2010;76(4):418–21.

[55] Lungulescu OA, Cao W, Gatskevich E, et al. CSI: a severity index for *Clostridium difficile* infection at the time of admission. J Hosp Infect 2011;79(2):151–4.

[56] Greenstein AJ, Byrn JC, Zhang LP, et al. Risk factors for the development of fulminant *Clostridium difficile* colitis. Surgery 2008;143(5):623–9.

[57] Gujja D, Friedenberg FK. Predictors of serious complications due to *Clostridium difficile* infection. Aliment Pharmacol Ther 2009;29(6):635–42.

[58] Belmares J, Gerding DN, Parada JP, et al. Outcome of metronidazole therapy for Clostridium difficile disease and correlation with a scoring system. J Infect 2007;55(6): 495–501.

[59] Teasley DG, Gerding DN, Olson MM, et al. Prospective randomised trial of metronidazole versus vancomycin for Clostridium difficile-associated diarrhoea and colitis. Lancet 1983;2(8358):1043–6.

[60] Bolton RP, Culshaw MA. Faecal metronidazole concentrations during oral and intravenous therapy for antibiotic associated colitis due to Clostridium difficile. Gut 1986;27(10): 1169–72.

[61] Keighley MR, Burdon DW, Arabi Y, et al. Randomised controlled trial of vancomycin for pseudomembranous colitis and postoperative diarrhoea. Br Med J 1978;2(6153):1667–9.

[62] Wenisch C, Parschalk B, Hasenhundl M, et al. Comparison of vancomycin, teicoplanin, metronidazole, and fusidic acid for the treatment of Clostridium difficile -associated diarrhea. Clin Infect Dis 1996;22(5):813–8.

[63] Bricker E, Garg R, Nelson R, et al. Antibiotic treatment for Clostridium difficile -associated diarrhea in adults. Cochrane Database Syst Rev 2005;1:CD004610.

[64] Pepin J, Alary ME, Valiquette L, et al. Increasing risk of relapse after treatment of Clostridium difficile colitis in Quebec, Canada. Clin Infect Dis 2005;40(11):1591–7.

[65] Musher DM, Aslam S, Logan N, et al. Relatively poor outcome after treatment of Clostridium difficile colitis with metronidazole. Clin Infect Dis 2005;40(11):1586–90.

[66] Zar FA, Bakkanagari SR, Moorthi KM, et al. A comparison of vancomycin and metronidazole for the treatment of Clostridium difficile-associated diarrhea, stratified by disease severity. Clin Infect Dis 2007;45(3):302–7.

[67] Pasic M, Jost R, Carrel T, et al. Intracolonic vancomycin for pseudomembranous colitis. N Engl J Med 1993;329(8):583.

[68] Lamontagne F, Labbe AC, Haeck O, et al. Impact of emergency colectomy on survival of patients with fulminant Clostridium difficile colitis during an epidemic caused by a hypervirulent strain. Ann Surg 2007;245(2):267–72.

[69] Longo WE, Mazuski JE, Virgo KS, et al. Outcome after colectomy for Clostridium difficile colitis. Dis Colon Rectum 2004;47(10):1620–6.

[70] Butala P, Divino CM. Surgical aspects of fulminant Clostridium difficile colitis. Am J Surg 2010;200(1):131–5.

[71] Medich DS, Lee KK, Simmons RL, et al. Laparotomy for fulminant pseudomembranous colitis. Arch Surg 1992;127(7):847–52 [discussion: 852–3].

[72] Lowy I, Molrine DC, Leav BA, et al. Treatment with monoclonal antibodies against Clostridium difficile toxins. N Engl J Med 2010;362(3):197–205.

[73] Louie TJ, Miller MA, Mullane KM, et al. Fidaxomicin versus vancomycin for Clostridium difficile infection. N Engl J Med 2011;364(5):422–31.

[74] McFarland LV, Elmer GW, Surawicz CM. Breaking the cycle: treatment strategies for 163 cases of recurrent Clostridium difficile disease. Am J Gastroenterol 2002;97(7): 1769–75.

[75] McFarland LV. Alternative treatments for Clostridium difficile disease: what really works? J Med Microbiol 2005;54(Pt 2):101–11.

[76] McFarland LV, Surawicz CM, Rubin M, et al. Recurrent Clostridium difficile disease: epidemiology and clinical characteristics. Infect Control Hosp Epidemiol 1999;20(1): 43–50.

[77] Barbut F, Richard A, Hamadi K, et al. Epidemiology of recurrences or reinfections of Clostridium difficile -associated diarrhea. J Clin Microbiol 2000;38(6):2386–8.

[78] Johnson S, Sanchez JL, Gerding DN. Metronidazole resistance in Clostridium difficile. Clin Infect Dis 2000;31(2):625–6.

[79] Kyne L, Warny M, Qamar A, et al. Association between antibody response to toxin A and protection against recurrent Clostridium difficile diarrhoea. Lancet 2001;357(9251): 189–93.

[80] Snell H, Ramos M, Longo S, et al. Performance of the TechLab C. DIFF CHEK-60 enzyme immunoassay (EIA) in combination with the C. difficile Tox A/B II EIA kit, the Triage C. difficile panel immunoassay, and a cytotoxin assay for diagnosis of Clostridium difficile -associated diarrhea. J Clin Microbiol 2004;42(10):4863–5.

[81] Zheng L, Keller SF, Lyerly DM, et al. Multicenter evaluation of a new screening test that detects Clostridium difficile in fecal specimens. J Clin Microbiol 2004;42(8):3837–40.

[82] Huang H, Weintraub A, Fang H, et al. Comparison of a commercial multiplex real-time PCR to the cell cytotoxicity neutralization assay for diagnosis of Clostridium difficile infections. J Clin Microbiol 2009;47(11):3729–31.

[83] Peterson LR, Manson RU, Paule SM, et al. Detection of toxigenic Clostridium difficile in stool samples by real-time polymerase chain reaction for the diagnosis of C. difficile-associated diarrhea. Clin Infect Dis 2007;45(9):1152–60.

[84] Abougergi MS, Broor A, Cui W, et al. Intravenous immunoglobulin for the treatment of severe Clostridium difficile colitis: an observational study and review of the literature. J Hosp Med 2010;5(1):E1–9.

[85] Juang P, Skledar SJ, Zgheib NK, et al. Clinical outcomes of intravenous immune globulin in severe Clostridium difficile -associated diarrhea. Am J Infect Control 2007;35(2):131–7.

[86] Wilcox MH. Descriptive study of intravenous immunoglobulin for the treatment of recurrent Clostridium difficile diarrhoea. J Antimicrob Chemother 2004;53(5):882–4.

[87] Kotloff KL, Wasserman SS, Losonsky GA, et al. Safety and immunogenicity of increasing doses of a Clostridium difficile toxoid vaccine administered to healthy adults. Infect Immun 2001;69(2):988–95.

[88] Aboudola S, Kotloff KL, Kyne L, et al. Clostridium difficile vaccine and serum immunoglobulin G antibody response to toxin A. Infect Immun 2003;71(3):1608–10.

[89] Sougioultzis S, Kyne L, Drudy D, et al. Clostridium difficile toxoid vaccine in recurrent C. difficile-associated diarrhea. Gastroenterology 2005;128(3):764–70.

[90] Gerding DN, Johnson S. Management of Clostridium difficile infection: thinking inside and outside the box. Clin Infect Dis 2010;51(11):1306–13.

[91] Shue YK, Sears PS, Shangle S, et al. Safety, tolerance, and pharmacokinetic studies of OPT-80 in healthy volunteers following single and multiple oral doses. Antimicrob Agents Chemother 2008;52(4):1391–5.

[92] Louie TJ, Emery J, Krulicki W, et al. OPT-80 eliminates Clostridium difficile and is sparing of bacteroides species during treatment of C. difficile infection. Antimicrob Agents Chemother 2009;53(1):261–3.

[93] Johnson S, Schriever C, Patel U, et al. Rifaximin Redux: treatment of recurrent Clostridium difficile infections with rifaximin immediately post-vancomycin treatment. Anaerobe 2009;15(6):290–1.

[94] Anton PM, O'Brien M, Kokkotou E, et al. Rifalazil treats and prevents relapse of Clostridium difficile -associated diarrhea in hamsters. Antimicrob Agents Chemother 2004;48(10):3975–9.

[95] Freeman J, Baines SD, Todhunter SL, et al. Nitazoxanide is active against Clostridium difficile strains with reduced susceptibility to metronidazole. J Antimicrob Chemother 2011;66(6):1407–8.

[96] McVay CS, Rolfe RD. In vitro and in vivo activities of nitazoxanide against Clostridium difficile. Antimicrob Agents Chemother 2000;44(9):2254–8.

[97] Musher DM, Logan N, Hamill RJ, et al. Nitazoxanide for the treatment of Clostridium difficile colitis. Clin Infect Dis 2006;43(4):421–7.

[98] Freeman J, Baines SD, Jabes D, et al. Comparison of the efficacy of ramoplanin and vancomycin in both in vitro and in vivo models of clindamycin-induced Clostridium difficile infection. J Antimicrob Chemother 2005;56(4):717–25.

[99] Dworczynski A, Sokol B, Meisel-Mikolajczyk F. Antibiotic resistance of Clostridium difficile isolates. Cytobios 1991;65(262-263):149–53.

[100] Elmer GW. Probiotics: "living drugs". Am J Health Syst Pharm 2001;58(12):1101–9.

[101] Pillai A, Nelson R. Probiotics for treatment of Clostridium difficile -associated colitis in adults. Cochrane Database Syst Rev 2008;1:CD004611.
[102] Surawicz CM, McFarland LV, Greenberg RN, et al. The search for a better treatment for recurrent Clostridium difficile disease: use of high-dose vancomycin combined with Saccharomyces boulardii. Clin Infect Dis 2000;31(4):1012–7.
[103] Enache-Angoulvant A, Hennequin C. Invasive Saccharomyces infection: a comprehensive review. Clin Infect Dis 2005;41(11):1559–68.
[104] Lherm T, Monet C, Nougiere B, et al. Seven cases of fungemia with Saccharomyces boulardii in critically ill patients. Intensive Care Med 2002;28(6):797–801.
[105] Salminen MK, Rautelin H, Tynkkynen S, et al. Lactobacillus bacteremia, clinical significance, and patient outcome, with special focus on probiotic L. rhamnosus GG. Clin Infect Dis 2004;38(1):62–9.
[106] Bakken JS. Fecal bacteriotherapy for recurrent Clostridium difficile infection. Anaerobe 2009;15(6):285–9.
[107] You DM, Franzos MA, Holman RP. Successful treatment of fulminant Clostridium difficile infection with fecal bacteriotherapy. Ann Intern Med 2008;148(8):632–3.
[108] Tvede M, Rask-Madsen J. Bacteriotherapy for chronic relapsing Clostridium difficile diarrhoea in six patients. Lancet 1989;1(8648):1156–60.
[109] Borriello SP, Barclay FE. Protection of hamsters against Clostridium difficile ileocaecitis by prior colonisation with non-pathogenic strains. J Med Microbiol 1985;19(3):339–50.
[110] Wilson KH, Sheagren JN. Antagonism of toxigenic Clostridium difficile by nontoxigenic C. difficile. J Infect Dis 1983;147(4):733–6.
[111] Sambol SP, Merrigan MM, Tang JK, et al. Colonization for the prevention of Clostridium difficile disease in hamsters. J Infect Dis 2002;186(12):1781–9.
[112] Seal D, Borriello SP, Barclay F, et al. Treatment of relapsing Clostridium difficile diarrhoea by administration of a non-toxigenic strain. Eur J Clin Microbiol 1987;6(1):51–3.
[113] Neal MD, Alverdy JC, Hall DE, et al. Diverting loop ileostomy and colonic lavage: an alternative to total abdominal colectomy for the treatment of severe, complicated Clostridium difficile associated disease. Ann Surg 2011;254(3):423–7 [discussion: 427–9].
[114] Liacouras CA, Piccoli DA. Whole-bowel irrigation as an adjunct to the treatment of chronic, relapsing Clostridium difficile colitis. J Clin Gastroenterol 1996;22(3):186–9.
[115] Persky SE, Brandt LJ. Treatment of recurrent Clostridium difficile-associated diarrhea by administration of donated stool directly through a colonoscope. Am J Gastroenterol 2000;95(11):3283–5.
[116] Wu L, Zaborina O, Zaborin A, et al. High-molecular-weight polyethylene glycol prevents lethal sepsis due to intestinal Pseudomonas aeruginosa. Gastroenterology 2004;126(2):488–98.
[117] Valuckaite V, Zaborina O, Long J, et al. Oral PEG 15-20 protects the intestine against radiation: role of lipid rafts. Am J Physiol Gastrointest Liver Physiol 2009;297(6):G1041–52.
[118] Shetler K, Nieuwenhuis R, Wren SM, et al. Decompressive colonoscopy with intracolonic vancomycin administration for the treatment of severe pseudomembranous colitis. Surg Endosc 2001;15(7):653–9.
[119] Turnbull RB Jr, Fazio V. Advances in the surgical technique of ulcerative colitis surgery: endoanal proctectomy and two-directional myotomy ileostomy. Surg Annu 1975;7:315–29.

The Genetic Counselor
An Important Surgical Ally in the Optimal Care of the Cancer Patient

Erin E. Salo-Mullen, MS, CGC[a], Jose G. Guillem, MD, MPH[b],*

[a]Department of Medicine, Memorial Sloan-Kettering Cancer Center, 1275 York Avenue, Box 295, New York, NY 10065, USA; [b]Department of Surgery, Memorial Sloan-Kettering Cancer Center, 1275 York Avenue, New York, NY 10065, USA

Keywords
• Genetic counselor • Hereditary cancer • Surgical oncology

Key Points
• Genetic counselors are healthcare providers specialized in the risk assessment and genetic evaluation of the cancer patient.
• Genetic counseling and genetic testing may lead to surgical-based implications for the cancer patient.
• The genetic counselor and surgeon may work together in multiple settings to enhance patient care.

With increased knowledge and greater availability of genetic testing for hereditary cancer predisposition syndromes, the role of the surgeon has further expanded. Often, surgeons are the initial treatment providers to patients recently diagnosed with cancer. This position provides the opportunity and responsibility to look beyond a patient's current disease treatment plan and consider possible future risks to patients and possible risks to their family members. Genetic counselors, equipped with specialized knowledge and skills in risk assessment and management of patients with hereditary cancer predisposition syndromes and their at-risk family members, are important allies to surgeons managing individuals and families afflicted with a hereditary cancer syndrome. Genetic counseling has been incorporated into published practice guidelines [1–4] and is now a standard recommendation for patients at increased risk for a hereditary cancer predisposition syndrome. A partnership between surgeons and genetic counselors provides a unique opportunity to identify, assess, and manage at-risk patients and their

*Corresponding author. E-mail address: guillemj@MSKCC.ORG

0065-3411/12/$ – see front matter
doi:10.1016/j.yasu.2012.03.010

family members in an optimal manner. This article discusses in detail the role of a genetic counselor, multiple settings for genetic counseling, and opportunities for coordination of care between a surgeon and genetic counselor. Although focused on patients with various forms of hereditary colorectal cancer (CRC), other hereditary cancer syndromes are discussed briefly and readers are referred to primary source documents for greater detail. Table 1 provides basic details about a few hereditary cancer predisposition syndromes. Surgeons are urged to recognize the importance of identifying and collaborating with a local genetic counselor because this relationship sets the stage for optimal care of cancer patients.

DEFINITION OF GENETIC COUNSELING AND GENETIC COUNSELORS

In 2005, the National Society of Genetic Counselors defined genetic counseling as the "process of helping people understand and adapt to the medical, psychological, and familial implications of genetic contributions to disease. This process integrates: (1) the interpretation of family and medical histories to

Table 1
Hereditary cancer predisposition syndromes—basic details

Syndrome name	Associated genes	Mode of inheritance	Associated tumors	References
Lynch syndrome/ HNPCC (hereditary non-polyposis colorectal cancer)	MLH1 MSH2 MSH6 PMS2 EPCAM	Autosomal dominant	Colorectal, endometrial, gastric, ovarian, urothelial, small bowel, biliary tract, pancreas, brain, sebaceous gland neoplasm	[32,36,43,44]
Familial adenomatous polyposis (FAP) & attenuated FAP	APC	Autosomal dominant	Colorectal, gastric, small bowel, thyroid, pancreas, hepatoblastoma	[43,45,46]
MYH-associated polyposis (MAP)	MYH	Autosomal recessive	Colorectal, gastric, small bowel	[45,47,48]
Hereditary breast and ovarian cancer syndrome	BRCA1 BRCA2	Autosomal dominant	Breast, ovarian, prostate, pancreas	[7,43,49,50]
Hereditary diffuse gastric cancer (HDGC) syndrome	CDH1	Autosomal dominant	Diffuse gastric, lobular breast, signet ring cell colorectal	[13]
Multiple endocrine neoplasia (MEN)-2A, MEN-2B, and familial medullary thyroid carcinoma (FMTC)	RET	Autosomal dominant	Medullary thyroid, pheochromocytoma (only in MEN-2A and MEN-2B)	[43,51,52]

assess the chance of disease occurrence or recurrence; (2) education about the inheritance, testing, management, prevention, resources, and research; and (3) counseling to promote informed choices and adaptation to the risk or condition" [5]. With an emphasis on education and patient empowerment, every genetic counseling encounter and diagnosis of a hereditary syndrome raises a distinct set of patient and family issues. The master's-level education and training of genetic counselors are multidisciplinary in origin, combining medical and behavioral sciences, and provides these professionals with the necessary skills to interact and connect with both the lay public/patients and other health care providers in a unique way.

ELEMENTS OF GENETIC COUNSELING
Traditionally, genetic counseling has occurred in the pre- and post-genetic testing periods (referred to as pretest and post-test, respectively, from this point on).

Pretest genetic counseling
Elements of pretest genetic counseling include collection of medical and family histories; risk assessment; education about the differential diagnoses (including genetics and inheritance, natural history of condition, penetrance, and medical management options); evaluation of the indications for, benefits of, limitations to, implications of, sensitivity of, specificity of, clinical utility of, and ability to adequately interpret the results of genetic testing; and investigation of the psychosocial consequences of the disease and possible genetic test results. The process of pretest genetic counseling is often thought of as being analogous to the informed consent process [6].

Post-test genetic counseling
Post-test genetic counseling often includes disclosure and interpretation of genetic test results; review of the test result's medical implications for the patient and family members; discussion about sharing genetic test result information with at-risk relatives; and investigation of the psychosocial and familial relationship consequences of the test result.

PRESURGICAL GENETIC COUNSELING
With increased knowledge about hereditary cancer predisposition syndromes and the awareness of medical management options, such as prophylactic surgeries that alter cancer risk, many newly diagnosed cancer patients are undergoing genetic counseling and testing before their initial surgical intervention. For example, many young women with new diagnoses of breast cancer are undergoing *BRCA1* and *BRCA2* germline genetic testing in hopes that their results are informative for surgical management and other treatment-related decisions [7,8]. With regards to CRC patients, this situation is not currently as commonplace. The potential for this practice is increasing, however, especially in situations where surgeons and genetic counselors have become partners in patient care. The multiple steps in the process of presurgical genetic testing along with a few case scenarios that describe situations in which

surgeons and specialized genetic counselors have collaborated to make presurgical genetic testing for CRC patients a reality are discussed.

Step 1: Identify who warrants genetic counseling
The first step in the process of genetic counseling is the identification of patients who warrant evaluation. The identification process may be performed by evaluating patients' personal cancer history, evaluating their family history, and/or review of pathology reports. Box 1 describes key features that should be looked for in patients and that raise red flags for a possible hereditary link to disease. The Amsterdam I and II criteria, initially developed to recruit kindreds in a standardized way for international studies designed to identify the genes associated with Lynch syndrome/hereditary nonpolyposis CRC (HNPCC), are also helpful in identifying patients and families who are at risk for Lynch syndrome (Box 2) [9,10]. Not all families with Lynch syndrome meet the Amsterdam criteria; and alternatively, not all families who meet the Amsterdam criteria have Lynch syndrome (this situation is termed, *familial CRC type X* [11]). The more recently developed revised Bethesda Guidelines, which incorporate family history, age at cancer diagnosis, and pathologic features of the tumor, were designed to be more inclusive in identifying potential individuals who may be at risk for Lynch syndrome and would benefit from further assessment [12].

With regards to review of pathology reports, certain tumor histologies have been identified as being associated with particular hereditary cancer syndromes. As discussed previously, the revised Bethesda Guidelines (see Box 2) include histologic features often seen in Lynch syndrome–associated colorectal tumors [12]. Hereditary diffuse gastric cancer syndrome is an example of a hereditary cancer predisposition syndrome that is associated with specific histopathologic forms of disease. Testing criteria for this condition require the documentation of diffuse gastric cancer, lobular breast cancer, and/or signet ring cell CRC in various familial combinations [13]. Review of endoscopic procedure and associated pathology reports are also important in the gastrointestinal polyposis conditions because there are some conditions that present with mainly adenomatous polyps, whereas others present with hamartomatous or juvenile-type polyps. The distinction between polyp types greatly influences genetic risk assessment, analysis, and medical management recommendations.

Box 1: Red flags that help identify possible hereditary cases

- Atypical age at/early-onset disease diagnosis
- Synchronous or metachronous (ie, multiple primary) diagnoses
- Bilateral tumors
- Same tumor type in multiple family members
- Multiple generations affected with cancer
- Certain histopathologic features

Box 2: Amsterdam I and II criteria and revised Bethesda Guidelines

Amsterdam I criteria [9]—for Lynch syndrome/HNPCC

There should be at least 3 relatives with CRC; all the following criteria should be present:

One should be a first-degree relative of the other 2.

At least 2 successive generations should be affected.

At least 1 CRC should be diagnosed before age 50.

Familial adenomatous polyposis should be excluded.

Tumors should be verified by pathologic examination.

Amsterdam II criteria [10]—for Lynch syndrome/HNPCC

There should be at least 3 relatives with an HNPCC-associated cancer (CRC, cancer of the endometrium, small bowel, ureter, or renal pelvis):

One should be a first-degree relative of the other 2.

At least 2 successive generations should be affected.

At least 1 should be diagnosed before age 50.

Familial adenomatous polyposis should be excluded in CRC case(s), if any.

Tumors should be verified by pathologic examination.

Revised Bethesda Guidelines for testing colorectal tumors for MSI [12]

Tumors from individuals should be tested for MSI in the following situations:

1. CRC diagnosed in a patient who is less than 50 years of age
2. Presence of synchronous, metachronous colorectal, or other HNPCC-associated tumors,[a] regardless of age
3. CRC with the MSI-H[b] histology[c] diagnosed in a patient who is less than 60 years of age[d]
4. CRC diagnosed in 1 or more first-degree relatives with an HNPCC-related tumor, with 1 of the cancers diagnosed under age 50
5. CRC diagnosed in 2 or more first-degree or second-degree relatives with HNPCC-related tumors, regardless of age

Abbreviations: MSI, microsatellite instability; MSI-H, microsatellite instability–high.

[a] HNPCC-related tumors include colorectal, endometrial, stomach, ovarian, pancreas, ureter and renal pelvis, biliary tract, and brain tumors (usually glioblastoma, as seen in Turcot syndrome), sebaceous gland adenomas and keratoacanthomas in Muir-Torre syndrome, and carcinoma of the small bowel.

[b] MSI-H in tumors refers to changes in 2 or more of the 5 National Cancer Institute–recommended panels of microsatellite markers.

[c] Presence of tumor infiltrating lymphocytes, Crohn-like lymphocytic reaction, mucinous/signet ring differentiation, or medullary growth pattern.

[d] There was no consensus among the HNPCC Workshop (held at the National Cancer Institute in Bethesda, MD, in 2002) participants on whether to include the age criteria in guideline 3; participants voted to keep less than 60 years of age in the guidelines.

Step 2: Making the referral

The next step in the process is making the referral for genetic counseling. There have been several studies looking at the effectiveness of certain referral methods. One retrospective examination of the referral process in patients recently diagnosed with early-onset (ie, <50 years old) CRC searched for determinants of variation that were associated with successful uptake of the referral [14]. Only 30% of patients followed the referral and went to a genetic counselor. In cases when a patient was referred by a surgeon and the referral was discussed between the surgeon and patient, 70% completed the genetic counseling consultation. Based on this and other studies [15,16], what seems key to making a successful referral is that the surgeon (or other referring medical provider) discusses the referral directly with the patient to explain why the referral is considered worthwhile and that the referral is unique to the patient's personal and/or familial circumstances.

The peridiagnostic/presurgical period is stressful, emotional, and overwhelming for most patients. The process of genetic counseling and testing, as illustrated in the case examples, is often intense on multiple levels. Although some patients may be motivated to pursue presurgical genetic counseling and testing for the benefit of informing surgical management decisions and risks to family members, other patients prefer to focus on one step of their treatment plan at a time and deal with potential risks for metachronous disease at a later date. The key to identifying which group a particular patient falls into lies within the discussion of the referral between the surgeon (or other referring health care provider) and the patient. If the surgeon can convey to the patient the reason for the referral (ie, which personal or familial features make this patient worthy of referral) and the ways in which genetic test results might be helpful to the patient and surgeon at the current stage of the treatment process, then a meaningful interaction has occurred and the patient's decision can be documented.

In the authors' center, a presurgical patient who warrants genetic evaluation is identified by a surgeon and the referral is discussed directly with the patient. If the patient is interested in proceeding, a genetic counselor is made aware of the referral by the surgeon or staff. The genetic counselor then reaches out to the patient directly to rediscuss the referral, answer preliminary questions about the genetic counseling process, and schedule an initial consultation. Through this collaboration between surgeon and genetic counselor, the authors find that the referral process is streamlined and that genetic counseling and genetic testing are performed in a timely manner.

Step 3: The genetic counseling consultation, testing process, and result implications

During the initial genetic counseling consultation, all elements of pretest genetic counseling (discussed previously) are executed by the genetic counselor.

Although testing for most hereditary cancer predisposition syndromes involves only germline genetic analysis, the evaluation for Lynch syndrome is more complicated. Various algorithms for the genetic evaluation of Lynch syndrome have been proposed [17–20], but the most comprehensive evaluation begins with tumor tissue screening via immunohistochemical (IHC) staining analysis and MSI analysis. The IHC staining analysis of the 4 DNA mismatch repair (MMR) proteins (MLH1, MSH2, MSH6, and PMS2) is performed by antibody staining against the mismatch repair proteins on tumor material. MSI analysis detects somatic expansion or contraction of microsatellite repetitive DNA elements and is performed using both tumor tissue and normal DNA (normal block or slides of tissue or blood DNA specimen) [21]. Because the IHC analysis can help pinpoint which of the 5 associated Lynch syndrome genes (*MLH1*, *MSH2*, *MSH6*, *PMS2*, and *EPCAM* [see Table 1]) has the highest likelihood of containing a germline mutation and it has a sensitivity and predictive value virtually equal to MSI analysis [22], this analysis is often the preferred tumor tissue screen. These analyses (IHC and MSI), however, are complementary, and some cases of Lynch syndrome are picked up only by IHC analysis whereas other cases are identified only through MSI analysis.

There are several opportunities for surgeon–genetic counselor collaboration during the evaluation process for Lynch syndrome that can help streamline and optimize the presurgical genetic counseling and testing process. For example,

- If tumor tissue is readily available in-house, a surgeon could order the IHC analysis in hopes that results will be available for the patient's initial genetic counseling consultation and direct immediate germline genetic testing. There is existing controversy over whether IHC and MSI results may be construed as genetic information. Thus, it is prudent that local regulations are applied and appropriate procedures be put into place to ensure patient understanding and consent before test orders are placed [22].
- Another possible opportunity for collaboration is when the diagnostic biopsy is performed at an outside institution. In this situation, the surgeon can request unstained tumor tissue (slides or blocks) from the outside institution during the time period between the patient's initial surgical consultation and initial genetic counseling consultation. The goal of this request is to have the unstained tumor tissue available for immediate IHC and/or MSI analysis once the initial genetic counseling consultation is complete and patient consent is obtained.
- A third opportunity for collaboration is when unstained tumor tissue is not available. In this situation, the surgeon could biopsy the tumor before the delivery of any neoadjuvant therapy that may eradicate the tumor and eliminate the possibility for tumor tissue screening via IHC and/or MSI (see case example 1 [Box 3]).

Cancerous colorectal and endometrial tissue is preferred for IHC and MSI analyses compared with colorectal adenomatous polyp material because the sensitivity of these analyses in polyp tissue may be reduced [23–27]. In addition, cancerous tissue from extracolonic primary origins (gastric, ovarian, sebaceous gland, and urothelial) can be used for the IHC and MSI analyses, but because the sensitivity and specificity of these analyses on extracolonic tissues have not been thoroughly validated, a normal result does not rule out Lynch syndrome [18]. Lastly, results from analyses in which neoadjuvantly treated tissue was used should be interpreted with caution due to concern for altered/compromised results caused by the therapy [28].

As discussed previously, germline genetic testing is the only diagnostic tool for most hereditary cancer predisposition syndromes. Several technologies for gene sequencing and large rearrangement analyses exist to detect alterations in germline DNA from peripheral blood or buccal swab samples. The turnaround time for most germline genetic analyses ranges from approximately 2 to 8 weeks.

With regards to the presurgical setting, it may be possible to have some germline genetic test results back before surgery, although the timing is often tight (down to the wire). In some ethnic populations, common founder mutations may exist. When a presurgical, newly diagnosed cancer patient presents for genetic testing, analysis of common founder mutations seen in that patient's ethnic population may provide for an expedited "biggest bang for your buck"– type of analysis. For example, testing for the *MSH2**A636P founder mutation

---

Box 3: Case example 1: presurgical evaluation for Lynch syndrome

A 40-year-old woman presents to her local surgeon with a recently diagnosed ascending colon cancer. The patient reports that her mother and maternal grandfather died from CRC in their 60s and 70s, respectively. Neither the patient nor her affected family members are known to have colorectal polyposis. Given that the patient's family history meets the Amsterdam I criteria, her surgeon mentions that there may be an inherited link between the patient's diagnosis and her family members' diagnoses. The surgeon also discusses with the patient that if Lynch syndrome is confirmed, the patient may want to consider a more extensive colon resection (subtotal colectomy instead of segmental resection) and prophylactic total abdominal hysterectomy with bilateral salpingo-oophorectomy. The patient expresses interest in pursuing genetic testing to clarify the situation and her surgical options. The patient is referred for presurgical genetic counseling.

In preparation for the patient's genetic evaluation and upcoming surgery, the surgeon performs a repeat colonoscopy to tattoo the malignant polyp and obtain additional tumor tissue for IHC analysis to help facilitate genetic evaluation.

During the patient's pretest genetic counseling consultation, Lynch syndrome and possible surgical implications are reviewed. Because the patient's surgeon had collected additional tumor tissue, evaluation for Lynch syndrome via IHC staining analysis of 4 DNA mismatch repair proteins (MLH1, MSH2, MSH6, and PMS2) and MSI analysis are ordered. Two-and-a-half weeks later, during the posttest genetic counseling session, the genetic counselor reveals that both the IHC and MSI analyses revealed normal results (all proteins expressed and no MSI detected, respectively). These results essentially rule out Lynch syndrome. The patient's personal and family histories of CRC are consistent with familial CRC type X (see reference [11]). Given these results, the patient and her surgeon decide that the most appropriate course of action is to pursue a right hemicolectomy while leaving the uterus, ovaries, and remaining colon intact.

in Ashkenazi Jewish individuals who have personal and family histories suspicious for Lynch syndrome may be useful in a presurgical setting (especially in patients who had loss of MSH2 and MSH6 protein staining on IHC analysis) [29].

Because most hereditary cancer syndromes are caused by mutations in only 1 or 2 genes, immediate germline genetic testing for those conditions is usually reasonable. With Lynch syndrome (which is thus far known to be caused by mutations in 5 genes [see Table 1]), however, up-front germline genetic testing is not as commonplace because tumor tissue screening (via IHC analysis) is used to help identify which of the 5 genes are appropriate to be analyzed on germline testing. In some presurgical cases, up-front germline genetic testing for the most common causes of Lynch syndrome (ie, germline mutations in the *MLH1* and *MSH2* genes) may be appropriate as long as patient and surgeon (or health care provider) understand that a negative/normal result does not rule out Lynch syndrome. In these situations, one may then work backwards and complete tumor tissue screening on the surgical specimen and perform germline genetic testing for the less frequent causes of Lynch syndrome (if indicated) in the postsurgical setting.

When genetic test results are available, all elements of post-test genetic counseling (described previously) are fulfilled by the genetic counselor. Germline genetic test results often return with 1 of 3 types of results: mutation identified, no mutation identified, and alteration of undetermined significance identified. Even when a mutation is identified, the implications of its finding can vary. For example, the I1307K mutation in the *APC* gene does not lead to a diagnosis of familial adenomatous polyposis (FAP) or attenuated FAP, even though other mutations in the *APC* gene do [30]. Proper test result interpretation is one of the key roles of the genetic counselor. In the presurgical setting, germline genetic test result interpretation is pivotal because patients and surgeons may use this information to make surgical management decisions.

The process of presurgical genetic counseling includes multiple steps: identification of at-risk patients; referral of at-risk patients to a genetic counselor; pretest genetic counseling consultation and genetic evaluation via tumor tissue screening and/or germline genetic testing; post-test genetic counseling with test result interpretation; and, last but not least, medical and surgical management decision-making by the patient along with the surgeon/health care provider. Surgical considerations for patients with hereditary cancer predisposition syndromes are described below. For information about recommended cancer surveillance regimes, see the articles referred to in Table 1.

CRC patients who have Lynch syndrome have increased risks for metachronous colorectal primaries [31]. Due to this increased risk, Lynch syndrome CRC patients often face the decision of pursuing segmental colectomy versus (sub)total colectomy. The need to continue regular endoscopic screening of the remaining colon may be one factor that patients take into consideration along with age at initial surgery, risk for additional/multiple surgeries, risks for urinary and sexual dysfunction, altered bowel habits, effects on fecundity, psychosocial implications, and other quality-of-life concerns. Female Lynch syndrome patients also have increased risks for endometrial and ovarian cancer [32–35]. This risk and the ability to alter it (through prophylactic surgery) is an important reason why female CRC patients who are at increased risk for Lynch syndrome should be offered presurgical genetic counseling and testing. If a diagnosis of Lynch syndrome is confirmed through genetic testing and the woman is finished with childbearing, prophylactic total abdominal hysterectomy and bilateral salpingo-oophorectomy may be considered at the same time as the CRC surgery [36].

In patients with attenuated colorectal polyposis (ie, fewer than 100 polyps), presurgical genetic counseling and testing may help clarify predisposition to polyposis, future expected burden of polyps, and most appropriate surgical management options (see case example 2 [Box 4]). In isolated, early-onset (before 40 years of age) diffuse gastric cancer patients, presurgical genetic counseling and testing can help clarify the extent of gastrectomy needed. In high-risk breast cancer patients, presurgical genetic counseling and testing may provide the opportunity to consider mastectomy versus lumpectomy, avoidance of radiation therapy, and contralateral prophylactic mastectomy. In summary, presurgical genetic counseling and testing are feasible, especially when a relationship between the genetic counselor and surgeon exists, and provide an opportunity for cancer patients who are at risk for a hereditary cancer syndrome to make optimally informed medical management and surgical management decisions.

Box 4: Case example 2: presurgical evaluation of attenuated polyposis

A 66-year-old female patient presented to her local surgeon for management of 3 large ascending colorectal adenomas. The patient reported that she had undergone colonoscopies "every couple of years" for the past 15 years and that each colonoscopy had identified "a couple of polyps." On questioning about her family history, the patient mentioned that her younger brother had "a few polyps" removed during his baseline colonoscopy 3 years ago. Due to the patient's personal and family histories of colorectal polyps, her surgeon referred her for presurgical genetic counseling.

During pretest genetic counseling, the patient's personal and family histories were found to be most consistent with MYH-associated polyposis (MAP), which is transmitted in an autosomal recessive manner. Due to the patient's Irish ancestry, the genetic counselor suggested that genetic testing for MAP begin with targeted mutation analysis for the 2 common western European founder mutations in the MYH gene. Results confirmed the presence of 2 copies (biallelic) of the MYH*G382D founder mutation and this was consistent with a diagnosis of MAP.

After test result disclosure during post-test genetic counseling, the patient returned to her surgeon to discuss surgical management of her current ascending colorectal adenomas. In light of her genetic test results confirming a diagnosis of MAP, the patient and her surgeon decided that the most appropriate procedure was a subtotal colectomy with an ileorectal anastomosis. After surgery, the patient continued to undergo close rectal surveillance.

POSTSURGICAL GENETIC COUNSELING

For some patients, presurgical genetic counseling and testing are not options or not desired. In such situations, postsurgical genetic counseling is an available alternative. The elements of postsurgical genetic counseling are similar to those in the presurgical setting.

As in the presurgical setting, the first step in the process of postsurgical genetic counseling is patient identification. Several opportunities in the postsurgical setting exist to identify individuals whose personal and/or family histories warrant genetic evaluation:

- Review of the pathology report by a surgeon is imperative not only for TNM staging and consideration of adjuvant treatment referral but also because the histologic description of the tumor may point to a possible association with a known hereditary cancer syndrome and may warrant a referral to a genetic counselor. Additionally, some institutions are automatically performing tumor tissue screening (IHC and/or MSI analysis) for Lynch syndrome on certain types of in-house surgical specimens (for example, all CRCs in patients ≤60 years of age), and results of these analyses may be imbedded in the surgical pathology report in order for the surgeon to review and take the appropriate next steps (see case example 3 [Box 5]).
- Some patients who have profuse colorectal polyposis may elect not to pursue presurgical genetic testing because the results would not have an impact on their or the surgeon's decision to perform total colectomy. Postsurgical genetic counseling and testing are appropriate in this setting because the identification of the polyposis-

---

Box 5: Case example 3: postsurgical evaluation for Lynch syndrome

A 59-year-old woman was found to have a descending CRC on colonoscopy performed for a work-up of bright red blood per rectum. A segmental colectomy was performed and surgical pathology revealed a T2N1 poorly differentiated adenocarcinoma. IHC staining analysis of the 4 DNA mismatch repair proteins (MLH1, MSH2, MSH6, and PMS2) was performed on the patient's adenocarcinoma as standard procedure at that particular institution. The IHC analysis revealed an absent staining pattern of the MLH1 and PMS2 proteins, and a normal (intact) staining pattern for the MSH2 and MSH6 proteins. After reviewing the surgical pathology report and the abnormal IHC analysis results, the patient's surgeon referred her to a genetic counselor.

Review of family history data with the genetic counselor revealed that the patient's mother died of leukemia at age 62 years and that a paternal first cousin was recently diagnosed with bladder cancer at age 65 years. Given that the family history was not concerning for Lynch syndrome, the genetic counselor decided that the first appropriate analyses to perform were for detection of MLH1 promoter hypermethylation and detection of the somatic BRAF*V600E mutation in the patient's surgical specimen. Test results confirmed that both MLH1 promoter hypermethylation and the BRAF*V600E mutation were identified in the patient's tumor and provided an explanation for the abnormal IHC analysis. Furthermore, these results, combined with the nonsignificant family history, confirmed that the patient did not have Lynch syndrome and that her tumor was of sporadic origin.

causing germline mutation in the patient would allow for presymptomatic genetic testing of at-risk relatives and informative family planning (see case example 4 [Box 6]).

• Some patients decline presurgical genetic counseling because of emotional factors or simply wanting to focus on one part of their cancer treatment at a time. After these individuals have recovered from surgery and other treatment, it is important to rediscuss the referral for genetic counseling.

• Lastly, patients who warrant a referral for genetic counseling may be identified during routine follow-up appointments several years postsurgery. Genetic counseling and testing were not widely available for individuals diagnosed with early-onset cancers 10 or more years ago. It is important to keep a patient's past cancer history and the possibility for an association with a hereditary condition in mind even if the patient is not currently dealing with disease.

After patient identification, the other steps in the process of postsurgical genetic counseling are similar to those in the presurgical setting. The referral process is exactly the same. The importance of the referring physician discussing the referral directly with the patient is as significant in the postsurgical setting as it is in the presurgical situation. Pretest and post-test genetic counseling in the postsurgical setting is also performed in a similar manner to that in the presurgical setting. The major difference between the 2 settings is that due to the absence of a major deadline (ie, the date of surgery), the actual genetic testing process can be performed in an ideal stepwise fashion (eg, when evaluating for Lynch

---

Box 6: Case example 4: postsurgical evaluation of colorectal polyposis

At age 19 years, the patient underwent baseline colonoscopy due to a change in bowel habits and frequent abdominal pain; profuse colorectal polyposis was identified. The patient then underwent total colectomy with ileal pouch-anal anastomosis; surgical pathology identified more than 100 adenomatous polyps without malignancy. The patient's family history was largely nonsignificant: both of his parents had undergone colonoscopy with normal findings; the patient was an only child; and there was no extended family history of colorectal polyposis or cancer.

At 28 years of age, this otherwise healthy man explained to his genetic counselor that he and his wife wanted to have children. He presented for genetic counseling to learn about the risks of his future offspring also having polyposis.

During the pretest genetic counseling consultation, the genetic counselor discussed the differential diagnoses and the possibility for the patient and his wife to use preimplantation genetic diagnosis (PGD) technology to select for unaffected embryos. The patient and his wife expressed interest in this technology. After thorough pretest genetic counseling, the patient pursued germline genetic testing of the *APC* and *MYH* genes. A pathogenic *APC* germline mutation was identified in the patient's DNA sample. The patient's parents were later tested for the same *APC* mutation and neither was found to carry the mutation. These results indicated that the patient's *APC* mutation was of de novo origin. Because each of the patient's offspring would have a 50% risk of also carrying the pathogenic allele, he and his wife pursued PGD for family planning purposes.

syndrome, tumor tissue screening can be performed before any germline genetic testing is undertaken). With regards to medical management decision-making, the postsurgical setting allows for patients and health care providers to focus on implementing specific organ-focused surveillance regimes in the immediate near future with time for consideration of prophylactic surgeries.

As highlighted in these case examples, through surgeon and genetic counselor collaborations, the identification, referral, and genetic evaluation of appropriate patients can be optimized in both presurgical and postsurgical settings.

OTHER CONSIDERATIONS

Some of the most common concerns patients express during the genetic counseling process relate to insurance coverage of testing / possible financial responsibility and concern for genetic discrimination. In general, many group health insurance carriers include cancer genetic testing as a covered benefit. The authors find it worthy to note that even if genetic testing is not pursued by the patient (perhaps due to lack of insurance coverage), the actual genetic counseling and education is still important for the patient and family. With regards to genetic discrimination, many patients are surprised to learn that federal (Genetic Information Nondiscrimination Act [37]) and often state legislation exists to protect individuals against the use of genetic test result information for discriminatory purposes by employers and by health insurance providers.

The issue of duty to warn is also worth discussion. *Pate v Threlkel* [38] and *Safer v Estate of Pack* [39] are 2 malpractice suits that highlight the issue of a physician's duty to warn family members about risks for inherited disease. The main conflict within the duty to warn issue lies between a "physician's ethical obligations to respect the privacy of genetic information versus the potential legal liabilities resulting from the physician's failure to notify at-risk relatives" due to the possible availability of medical interventions that may reduce risk of disease [40]. It has been suggested that "healthcare professionals have a responsibility to encourage but not to coerce the sharing of genetic information in families, while respecting the boundaries imposed by the law and by the ethical practice of medicine" [40].

Lastly, opportunities for collaboration between genetic counselors and surgeons exist in other capacities. Some institutions run multidisciplinary clinics focusing on patients with particular hereditary conditions. These multidisciplinary teams may include surgeons, genetic counselors, medical geneticists, gastroenterologists, medical oncologists, pathologists, nurses, nutritionists, social workers, psychologists, radiologists, and ethicists. Multidisciplinary clinics create a system for comprehensive care because timely communication between a patient's health care providers may be central in ensuring continuity of care and a reduction in appointment attendances for the patient [41]. The multidisciplinary approach to risk assessment and disease management (discussed previously) will become increasingly important as genomic technology continues to expand and "personalized genomic information" becomes integrated "into the practice of cancer medicine" [42]. In addition to the multidisciplinary clinic, some institutions may have registries for patients with certain conditions. Along

Box 7: Resources to find a genetic counselor

National Society of Genetic Counselors
  http://www.nsgc.org
  "Find a Genetic Counselor" tab
American Board of Genetic Counseling, Inc.
  http://www.abgc.net
  "Find a Certified Genetic Counselor" tab
GeneTests
  http://www.ncbi.nlm.nih.gov/sites/GeneTests/
  "Clinic Directory" tab
The Collaborative Group of the Americas on Inherited Colorectal Cancer
  http://www.cgaicc.com/
  "Find a Registry" tab
National Cancer Institute/NCI Cancer Genetics Services Directory
  http://www.cancer.gov/cancertopics/genetics/directory

with other health care providers, genetic counselors may be key players in the development of, organization of, and maintenance of these registries, which help optimize the care of the individual and family as well as facilitate translational, multi-institutional research.

SUMMARY

Genetic counselors and surgeons both have important roles in the care of patients with hereditary cancer predisposition syndromes. Surgeons have the initial responsibility to identify and refer high-risk patients. Genetic counselors' specialized skill sets are then used in the risk assessment and genetic evaluation of such patients and their at-risk family members, and this may be performed in multiple settings. As discussed in this article, these roles and the processes of genetic counseling and genetic testing may be enhanced through multiple surgeon and genetic counselor collaborations. Continued medical management of patients and families with hereditary cancer predisposition syndromes becomes the responsibility of patients and their multiple health care providers. Box 7 provides a list of resources to assist in finding a local genetic counselor. Because there are various opportunities for surgeons and genetic counselors to collaborate, the authors urge surgeons to recognize the importance of, identify, and work in partnership with a local genetic counselor because that relationship sets the stage for optimal care of the cancer patient.

Acknowledgments

We would like to thank Kenneth Offit, MD, MPH, Zsofia Stadler, MD, and Megan Harlan Fleischut, MS, CGC for their critical reading of this article.

References

[1] Robson ME, Storm CD, Weitzel J, et al. American Society of Clinical Oncology policy statement update: genetic and genomic testing for cancer susceptibility. J Clin Oncol 2010;28(5):893–901.

[2] American Gastroenterological Association. American Gastroenterological Association medical position statement: hereditary colorectal cancer and genetic testing. Gastroenterology 2001;121(1):195–7.

[3] Trepanier A, Ahrens M, McKinnon W, et al. Genetic cancer risk assessment and counseling: recommendations of the national society of genetic counselors. J Genet Couns 2004;13(2):83–114.

[4] National Comprehensive Cancer Network. NCCN Practice Guidelines V.1. 2011. Genetic/ Familial High-risk Assessment: Breast and Ovarian. 2011. Available at: http://www.nccn.org/ professionals/physician_gls/pdf/genetics_screening.pdf. Accessed April 7, 2011.

[5] National Society of Genetic Counselors. Genetic Counseling as a Profession. 2005. Available at: http://www.nsgc.org/About/FAQsDefinitions/tabid/97/Default.aspx. Accessed August 20, 2011.

[6] Offit K, Thom P. Ethicolegal aspects of cancer genetics. Cancer Treat Res 2010;155:1–14.

[7] Robson M, Offit K. Clinical practice. Management of an inherited predisposition to breast cancer. N Engl J Med 2007;357(2):154–62.

[8] Stolier AJ, Fuhrman GM, Mauterer L, et al. Initial experience with surgical treatment planning in the newly diagnosed breast cancer patient at high risk for BRCA-1 or BRCA-2 mutation. Breast J 2004;10(6):475–80.

[9] Vasen HF, Mecklin JP, Khan PM, et al. The International Collaborative Group on Hereditary Non-Polyposis Colorectal Cancer (ICG-HNPCC). Dis Colon Rectum 1991;34(5):424–5.

[10] Vasen HF, Watson P, Mecklin JP, et al. New clinical criteria for hereditary nonpolyposis colorectal cancer (HNPCC, Lynch syndrome) proposed by the International Collaborative group on HNPCC. Gastroenterology 1999;116(6):1453–6.

[11] Lindor NM, Rabe K, Petersen GM, et al. Lower cancer incidence in Amsterdam-I criteria families without mismatch repair deficiency: familial colorectal cancer type X. JAMA 2005;293(16):1979–85.

[12] Umar A, Boland CR, Terdiman JP, et al. Revised Bethesda Guidelines for hereditary nonpolyposis colorectal cancer (Lynch syndrome) and microsatellite instability. J Natl Cancer Inst 2004;96(4):261–8.

[13] Fitzgerald RC, Hardwick R, Huntsman D, et al. Hereditary diffuse gastric cancer: updated consensus guidelines for clinical management and directions for future research. J Med Genet 2010;47(7):436–44.

[14] Overbeek LI, Hoogerbrugge N, van Krieken JH, et al. Most patients with colorectal tumors at young age do not visit a cancer genetics clinic. Dis Colon Rectum 2008;51(8):1249–54.

[15] Keller M, Jost R, Kadmon M, et al. Acceptance of and attitude toward genetic testing for hereditary nonpolyposis colorectal cancer: a comparison of participants and nonparticipants in genetic counseling. Dis Colon Rectum 2004;47(2):153–62.

[16] Vadaparampil ST, Quinn GP, Miree CA, et al. Recall of and reactions to a surgeon referral letter for BRCA genetic counseling among high-risk breast cancer patients. Ann Surg Oncol 2009;16(7):1973–81.

[17] Weissman SM, Burt R, Church J, et al. Identification of Individuals at Risk for Lynch Syndrome Using Targeted Evaluations and Genetic Testing: National Society of Genetic Counselors and the Collaborative Group of the Americas on Inherited Colorectal Cancer Joint Practice Guideline. J Genet Couns 2011. [Epub ahead of print].

[18] Weissman SM, Bellcross C, Bittner CC, et al. Genetic counseling considerations in the evaluation of families for Lynch syndrome—a review. J Genet Couns 2011;20(1):5–19.

[19] Ladabaum U, Wang G, Terdiman J, et al. Strategies to identify the Lynch syndrome among patients with colorectal cancer: a cost-effectiveness analysis. Ann Intern Med 2011;155(2):69–79.

[20] Burt RW. Who should have genetic testing for the Lynch syndrome? Ann Intern Med 2011;155(2):127–8.

[21] Zhang L. Immunohistochemistry versus microsatellite instability testing for screening colorectal cancer patients at risk for hereditary nonpolyposis colorectal cancer syndrome. Part II. The utility of microsatellite instability testing. J Mol Diagn 2008;10(4):301–7.

[22] Shia J. Immunohistochemistry versus microsatellite instability testing for screening colorectal cancer patients at risk for hereditary nonpolyposis colorectal cancer syndrome. Part I. The utility of immunohistochemistry. J Mol Diagn 2008;10(4):293–300.

[23] Velayos FS, Allen BA, Conrad PG, et al. Low rate of microsatellite instability in young patients with adenomas: reassessing the Bethesda guidelines. Am J Gastroenterol 2005;100(5):1143–9.

[24] Stoffel EM, Syngal S. Adenomas in young patients: what is the optimal evaluation? Am J Gastroenterol 2005;100(5):1150–3.

[25] Shia J, Klimstra DS, Nafa K, et al. Value of immunohistochemical detection of DNA mismatch repair proteins in predicting germline mutation in hereditary colorectal neoplasms. Am J Surg Pathol 2005;29(1):96–104.

[26] Pino MS, Mino-Kenudson M, Wildemore BM, et al. Deficient DNA mismatch repair is common in Lynch syndrome-associated colorectal adenomas. J Mol Diagn 2009;11(3):238–47.

[27] Recommendations from the EGAPP Working Group: genetic testing strategies in newly diagnosed individuals with colorectal cancer aimed at reducing morbidity and mortality from Lynch syndrome in relatives. Genet Med 2009;11(1):35–41.

[28] Choi MY, Lauwers GY, Hur C, et al. Microsatellite instability is frequently observed in rectal cancer and influenced by neoadjuvant chemoradiation. Int J Radiat Oncol Biol Phys 2007;68(5):1584.

[29] Guillem JG, Glogowski E, Moore HG, et al. Single-amplicon MSH2 A636P mutation testing in Ashkenazi Jewish patients with colorectal cancer: role in presurgical management. Ann Surg 2007;245(4):560–5.

[30] Laken SJ, Petersen GM, Gruber SB, et al. Familial colorectal cancer in Ashkenazim due to a hypermutable tract in APC. Nat Genet 1997;17(1):79–83.

[31] Aarnio M, Mecklin JP, Aaltonen LA, et al. Life-time risk of different cancers in hereditary nonpolyposis colorectal cancer (HNPCC) syndrome. Int J Cancer 1995;64(6):430–3.

[32] Aarnio M, Sankila R, Pukkala E, et al. Cancer risk in mutation carriers of DNA-mismatch-repair genes. Int J Cancer 1999;81(2):214–8.

[33] Vasen HF, Wijnen JT, Menko FH, et al. Cancer risk in families with hereditary nonpolyposis colorectal cancer diagnosed by mutation analysis. Gastroenterology 1996;110(4):1020–7.

[34] Hendriks YM, Wagner A, Morreau H, et al. Cancer risk in hereditary nonpolyposis colorectal cancer due to MSH6 mutations: impact on counseling and surveillance. Gastroenterology 2004;127(1):17–25.

[35] Stoffel E, Mukherjee B, Raymond VM, et al. Calculation of risk of colorectal and endometrial cancer among patients with Lynch syndrome. Gastroenterology 2009;137(5):1621–7.

[36] Schmeler KM, Lynch HT, Chen LM, et al. Prophylactic surgery to reduce the risk of gynecologic cancers in the Lynch syndrome. N Engl J Med 2006;354(3):261–9.

[37] Genetic Information Nondiscrimination Act H.R. 493 (2008).

[38] Pate v Threlkel, 661 So 2d 278 (Fla 1995).

[39] Safer v Estate of Pack, 677 A2d 1188 (NJ App 1996).

[40] Offit K, Groeger E, Turner S, et al. The "duty to warn" a patient's family members about hereditary disease risks. JAMA 2004;292(12):1469–73.

[41] White HD, Blair J, Pinkney J, et al. Improvement in the care of multiple endocrine neoplasia type 1 through a regional multidisciplinary clinic. QJM 2010;103(5):337–45.

[42] Weitzel JN, Blazer KR, Macdonald DJ, et al. Genetics, genomics, and cancer risk assessment: state of the art and future directions in the era of personalized medicine. CA Cancer J Clin 2011;61:327–59.

[43] Guillem JG, Wood WC, Moley JF, et al. ASCO/SSO review of current role of risk-reducing surgery in common hereditary cancer syndromes. J Clin Oncol 2006;24(28):4642–60.

[44] Vasen HF, Moslein G, Alonso A, et al. Guidelines for the clinical management of Lynch syndrome (hereditary non-polyposis cancer). J Med Genet 2007;44(6):353–62.

[45] Steinhagen E, Markowitz AJ, Guillem JG. How to manage a patient with multiple adenomatous polyps. Surg Oncol Clin N Am 2010;19(4):711–23.

[46] Church J. Familial adenomatous polyposis. Surg Oncol Clin N Am 2009;18(4):585–98.

[47] Sieber OM, Lipton L, Crabtree M, et al. Multiple colorectal adenomas, classic adenomatous polyposis, and germ-line mutations in MYH. N Engl J Med 2003;348(9):791–9.

[48] Peterlongo P, Mitra N, Chuai S, et al. Colorectal cancer risk in individuals with biallelic or monoallelic mutations of MYH. Int J Cancer 2005;114(3):505–7.

[49] Rebbeck TR, Kauff ND, Domchek SM. Meta-analysis of risk reduction estimates associated with risk-reducing salpingo-oophorectomy in BRCA1 or BRCA2 mutation carriers. J Natl Cancer Inst 2009;101(2):80–7.

[50] Chen S, Parmigiani G. Meta-analysis of BRCA1 and BRCA2 penetrance. J Clin Oncol 2007;25(11):1329–33.

[51] Traugott AL, Moley JF. Multiple endocrine neoplasia type 2: clinical manifestations and management. Cancer Treat Res 2010;153:321–37.

[52] Guillem JG, Berchuck A, Moley JF, et al. Role of surgery in cancer prevention. In: DeVita VT Jr, Lawrence TS, Rosenberg SA, et al, editors. DeVita, Hellman, and Rosenberg's cancer: principles & practice of oncology. 9th edition. Lippincott Williams and Wilkins; 2011. p. 543–57.

Readmission Rates after Abdominal Surgery: Can They Be Decreased to a Minimum?

Thomas J. Lee, MD, Robert C.G. Martin II, MD, PhD*

Division of Surgical Oncology, University of Louisville School of Medicine, Louisville, KY, USA

Keywords
• Readmission • Surgery • Complications • Quality

Key Points
• The reader should begin to understand the key factors to readmission rates in the current literature for patients undergoing abdominal surgery.
• The reader will understand the differences of readmission for different types of abdominal procedures.
• Understand the lack of consistency for reporting of readmissions in abdominal procedures.

INTRODUCTION

A recent demand by the Medicare Payment Advisory Commission (MedPAC) that hospital readmission rates be captured has caught the attention of policymakers and is a component of currently proposed healthcare reforms. Recent recommendations from MedPAC that the Centers for Medicare and Medicaid Services report on and determine payments based in part on readmission rates have led to an attendant interest by payers, hospital administrators, and far-sighted physicians. The proposed use of readmission rates as a measure of quality has implications that extend beyond proximal financial concerns and could potentially affect credentialing, referral patterns, medical education, and the continued fragmentation of the specialty of general surgery.

Readmission after any hospitalization has been advocated to reflect the physician quality of clinical care. In the British National Health Service, acute readmission has been termed a "failed discharge" and an increased effort to prevent failed discharges has recently spawned interest in implementation of novel guidelines, which may provide an unidentified benefit. Significant cost is associated with any readmission or failed discharge: a cost to the patient (physiologic,

*Corresponding author. Division of Surgical Oncology, Department of Surgery, University of Louisville School of Medicine, 315 East Broadway, Suite 313, Louisville, KY 40202. E-mail address: robert.martin@louisville.edu

0065-3411/12/$ – see front matter
doi:10.1016/j.yasu.2012.04.003

psychological, and monetary); a financial cost to the institution; and a potential cost to the practicing surgeon (when higher readmission rates are used as surrogates for substandard care in quality improvement circles). The medical community has come under increased pressure to reduce costs as healthcare expenditures have risen during the last decade.

Readmissions after hospitalization have been shown to increase the financial burden to patients and providers, and they have been seen more and more as a measurement to judge quality of care. MedPAC estimated that in 2005, readmissions cost Medicare an additional $15 billion in expenditures. They found that more than 75% of 30- and 15-day readmissions and 84% of 7-day readmissions were potentially preventable. The medical community has come under increased pressure to reduce costs as healthcare expenditures have steadily risen during the last several decades. Developing proposals to reduce payments for an excess of potentially preventable readmissions [1] have led to a component of the Affordable Care Act and the implementation of the Hospital Value-Based Purchasing Program, which are scheduled to start in October 2012. An analysis of the Medicare claims database by Jencks and colleagues [2] is frequently cited as presenting the severity of this problem. Surgical readmissions account for 22.4% of the total readmissions; however, the only abdominal operation mentioned within this study was for "major bowel surgery," which accounted for only 1% of the total and a 30-day readmission rate of 16.6%. This category hardly addresses the breadth of procedures performed in the abdomen, because general surgeons and several subspecialties, urologists, and gynecologists operate in this region. Some of the potential reasons for rehospitalization have most commonly included postoperative infection, nutrition, and gastrointestinal obstruction.

Differences in operative complexity, involved anatomy, patient demographics, and pathology likely affect readmission rates in a similar fashion to other frequently measured outcomes, such as morbidity and mortality. Within each abdominal operation one must address individually that there are variations in relevant anatomy, preoperative pathology, and population demographics. Given this wide variety in pathophysiology of the abdominal cavity, one cannot expect that all risk factors for readmissions are generalizable to all abdominal procedures. To minimize future readmissions, there is a need to first identify an estimate of what rates exist for the most common abdominal operations. From those established estimates, cause of readmission needs to be evaluated and then what risk factors contributed to readmission analyzed. This article evaluates the seven most common abdominal operations, summarizes the rates and risks for readmission, and provides potential guidelines as to where the operating surgeon can have an impact on readmission.

METHODS
The English literature searches were conducted through Medline, Embase, Science Citation Index, Current Contents, and PubMed databases from January 1, 2001 to January 1, 2011. The outline of articles reviewed is

presented in a Quality of Reporting of Meta-Analysis flow chart showing the number of studies screened and included in the meta-analysis (Fig. 1). Search items were "readmission," "unplanned hospitalization," "hernia," "colectomy," "esophagectomy," "gastrectomy," "bariatrics," "hepatobiliary," "abdominal aortic aneurysm," and "pancreatectomy." Restrictions were placed on language of publication, and only English was included. Studies lacking readmission rates and presentation of established data sets were excluded. Case reports were excluded. These restrictions were placed to have consistency among the reports reviewed.

HERNIA

Abdominal wall hernia repairs are among the most common general surgery procedures currently performed in the United States. Despite that, there have been few studies specifically looking at readmission outcomes on US populations (Table 1) [3–6]. Bisgaard and colleagues [6] reviewed the Denmark national patient registry for 3431 ventral hernia repair with an overall 5.3%

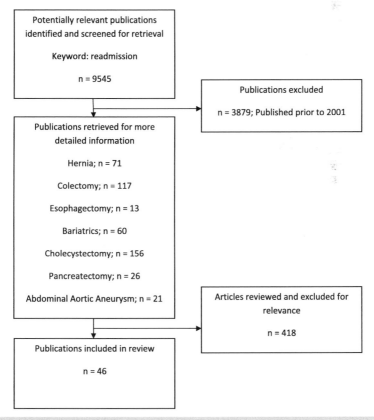

Fig. 1. Quality of Reporting of Meta-Analysis distribution of articles reviewed and then selected for presentation.

Table 1
Thirty day readmission rates for ventral hernia repair

Operation	Type	30-day readmission rate	Patient number	Authors
VHR (laparoscopic)	UHC database	5.15%	45,007	Tiwari et al [3,4]
VHR (laparoscopic)	Institution	5.00%	221	Blatnik et al [5]
VHR (laparoscopic)	National	10.50%	266	Bisgaard et al [6]
VHR (open)	UHC database	8.21%	685	Tiwari et al [3,4]
VHR (open)	Institution	20.00%	198	Blatnik et al [5]
VHR (open)	National	4.90%	3165	Bisgaard et al [6]

Abbreviations: UHC, University HealthSystem Consortium; VHR, ventral hernia repair.

readmission rate. Open repairs had a rate of 4.9% for 3165 patients, and laparoscopic repairs had a rate of 10% for 266 patients. These data only examined elective primary repair of umbilical and epigastric hernias; it excludes acute repairs and secondary hernias. Wound problems, seroma, and pain were the major causes for readmission. Blatnik and colleagues [5] performed a retrospective review of 420 laparoscopic and open ventral hernia repairs performed by a single surgeon in Ohio over a period of 4 years. Differences in preoperative diagnoses were significant predictors for readmission, such as previous abdominal surgeries (odds ratio [OR], 1.23); defect size greater than 300 cm^2 (OR, 5.35); existing fistula (OR, 8.55); and active abdominal infection (OR, 4.37). Operative risk factors include open repairs (OR, 4.27); operative times longer than 250 minutes (OR, 3.52); and concurrent panniculectomy (OR, 2.59). Helgstrand and colleagues [7] also looked at elective ventral hernia repairs using the nationwide database in Denmark. In their sample, wound issues were the dominant factor for readmission, and no analysis was performed in regards to demographic and preoperative risk factors for readmission.

ESOPHAGUS AND STOMACH
Currently, the reported readmission rates after esophagectomy and gastrectomy range from 5% to 25% (Table 2) [3,4,8–11]. Goodney and colleagues

Table 2
Thirty day readmission rates for esophagectomy and gastric surgery

Operation	Type	30-day readmission rate	Patient number	Authors
Esophagectomy	Washington	12.2%–16.6%	2605	Massarweh et al [8]
Esophagectomy	Washington	16.5%–24.9%	1352	Varghese et al [9]
Esophagectomy	Medicare	17.9%–19.1%		Goodney et al [10]
Esophagectomy	UHC database	5%–7.2%	5236	Reavis et al [11]
Gastrectomy	Medicare	16.3%–16.8%		Goodney et al [10]
Reflux surgery (open)	UHC database	4.05%	1942	Tiwari et al [3,4]
Reflux surgery (laparoscopic)	UHC database	1.94%	6966	Tiwari et al [3,4]

Abbreviation: UHC, University HealthSystem Consortium.

[10] performed a large Medicare claims database review of high-risk procedures on patients from 1994 to 1999. Readmission rates for esophagectomy ranged from 18.2% to 20.1%, and high-volume centers (>19 cases per year) had the lowest readmission rate. A review by Reavis and colleagues [11] performed on the University HealthSystem Consortium Clinical Database on patients undergoing esophagectomy from 2003 to 2008 showed readmission rates from 5% to 7.2% between high- (>12 cases per year) and low-volume centers. Both reviews showed that higher-volume centers have decreased readmission rates. However, the mechanism for this is likely multifactorial, and one of the largest confounding variables is that high-volume centers are usually tertiary referral centers that do not capture all of their readmissions that may occur in smaller rural hospitals based on the patient's location. Auerbach and colleagues [12] performed an observational cohort study of 14,170 patients who underwent various procedures, including esophagectomy. They analyzed several factors including hospital and physician volume (OR, 1.01); β-blocker use (OR, 1.04); antibiotic use (OR, 1.08); and venous thromboembolism prophylaxis (OR, 0.88). However, they were not able to show that differences in any of these measures had a significant effect on readmission rates.

In 2000, the Leapfrog group started an initiative based on volume-based referral. Initially, their recommendations were to have hospitals perform at least seven esophagectomies yearly; that figure was adjusted to 13 in 2003 because of the evidence of volume on mortality. Massarweh and colleagues [8] performed a cohort study using the Washington State Comprehensive Hospital Abstract Reporting System to assess the effect of the Leapfrog initiative. Before the Leapfrog initiative was implemented, the hospitals that met evidence-based hospital referral (EBHR) criteria had a readmission rate of 16.6%, which was found to be statistically different than the 12.2% at non-EBHR hospitals. Interestingly, after the Leapfrog initiative started, the readmission rates changed to 14.2% and 13.1% in the EBHR and non-EBHR hospitals, respectively. Theoretically, the higher-risk patients should have shifted with the initiative; however, there is no obvious explanation for this shift in the statistics. Varghese and colleagues [9] performed another analysis on specific hospitals compliant with the Leapfrog system, which showed significant decreases in mortality, reintervention rates, and length of stay. However, 30-day readmission rates actually increased compared with the non-Leapfrog compliant hospitals in four out of five Leapfrog hospitals. They hypothesize that this may be caused by the regionalization of the Leapfrog system, again demonstrating that readmission rates in larger tertiary referral centers may be higher than reported simply because there is a larger distance back to that tertiary referral center and readmission can occur at the local smaller rural or suburban hospital. Given the large heterogeneity in patients with esophageal cancer, and the significant heterogeneity in esophageal cancer histologies, established predictors of readmission are not available at this time and continue to be a need of ongoing research as the incidence of this disease continues to rise.

BARIATRIC

The reported readmission rates after the various types of bariatric operations range from 0% to 13% (Table 3) [3,4,13–24]. Tiwari and colleagues [3] studied 37,765 laparoscopic gastric bypass patients in the University HealthSystem Consortium database and found several differences based on demographics; although there were no differences in gender, overall African Americans showed an increase at 3% over their white counterparts at 2.3% ($P<.01$). They also found that increasing age ($P<.001$) and University HealthSystem Consortium severity score ($P<.05$) showed increasing rates of readmission. Weller and colleagues [14] used New York State's discharge database to find factors affecting 30-day readmission rates for all bariatric procedures.

Table 3
Thirty day readmission rates for bariatric and gastric bypass surgeries

Operation	Type	30-day readmission rate	Patient number	Authors
Bariatric procedures	Institution	6.70%	1939	Saunders et al [13]
Bariatric procedures	New York	7.60%	7868	Weller et al [14]
Bariatric procedures	MarketScan	11.30%	2522	Encinosa et al [15]
Bariatric procedures (COE)	Multipractice	3.4%–7.6%		Bradley et al
Bariatric procedures (non-COE)	Multipractice	8.3%–16.5%		Bradley et al
Gastric band	Institution	0%	86	Nguyen et al [16]
Gastric band	UHC database	0.70%	20,543	Hinojosa et al [17]
Gastric band	Institution	3.10%	862	Saunders et al [13]
Gastric bypass	Institution	5.40%	111	Nguyen et al [16]
Gastric bypass	Institution	6.10%	1886	Dumon et al [18]
Gastric bypass	Institution	6.70%	1222	Kellogg et al [19]
Gastric bypass	Institution	1.7/8.5%	2416	Blackstone et al [20,21]
Gastric bypass	Institution	6–7.4%	1474	Willkomm et al [22]
Gastric bypass (open)	UHC database	6.00%	4400	Tiwari et al [3,4]
Gastric bypass (laparoscopic)	UHC database	2.43%	26,585	Tiwari et al [3,4]
Gastric bypass (laparoscopic)	UHC database	2.50%	4226	Hinojosa et al
Gastric bypass (laparoscopic)	Institution	7.30%	1185	Saunders et al [13]
Gastric bypass (laparoscopic)	Institution	1.4–1.7%	2000	McCarty et al
Gastric bypass (laparoscopic)	Institution	2.4/13.1%	250	Baker et al [23]
Gastric bypass (with VBG)	Institution	6.80%	776	Saunders et al [13]
Sleeve gastrectomy (laparoscopic)	Institution	1.70%	529	Bellanger and Greenway [24]

Abbreviations: COE, Center of Excellence; UHC, University HealthSystem Consortium; VBG, vertical band gastroplasty.

Demographic differences in the readmissions group were increasing age ($P<.05$); male gender ($P<.01$); increasing number of comorbidities ($P<.03$); history of cardiac arrhythmia ($P<.01$); uncomplicated diabetes ($P<.04$); and peptic ulcer disease ($P<.01$). From the provider perspective, longer hospital stays ($P<.01$), surgeon volume ($P<.01$), and hospital volume ($P<.01$) significantly affected readmission rates. Another insurance claims–based study on all bariatric procedures performed by Encinosa and colleagues [15] showed that the actual percentage of readmission rates had increased from 2001 to 2002, to 2005 to 2006; however, when the populations were risk adjusted, the overall readmission rates had dropped from 9.78% to 6.79%. The authors attribute this primarily to an increase of the use of laparoscopy and gastric banding. They also attribute this improvement to the effects of increased volume. Saunders and colleagues [13] examined their high volume center for all bariatric operations, revealing an overall readmission rate over 1 year of 16.7%; 36% of these readmissions were within the first 30 days. The leading cause of readmission at 30 days was technical complication (42%), followed by gastrointestinal complaints (23.4%). The use of routine cholecystectomy for gallstones at the time of index operation decreased the rate of readmission from 2.9% to 1.2%. On multivariate analysis, initial admission length more than 5 days (OR, 2.12; $P<.005$), laparoscopic gastric bypass (OR, 1.50; <0.002), and asthma (OR, 1.55; $P<.005$) proved to be significant risk factors.

Willkomm and colleagues [22] showed evidence that at their institution age was not predictive. They specifically examined a group of patients older than age 65 that had a higher prevalence of comorbid conditions and found comparable readmission rates between high and low age groups. In 2010, Blackstone and Cortes [20] developed the metabolic acuity score that stratifies bariatric patients using age, body mass index, history of deep venous thrombosis or pulmonary embolism, severity of sleep apnea, diabetes, hypertension, mobility, cardiac status, and psychological classification. Their results showed that this management tool decreased the rates for readmission to 1.7% from 8.5%. Another study by Blackstone and colleagues [21] showed that readmission rates were comparable between patients with favorable psychological expectations and those that had AXIS I disorders that had appropriate psychological support. Dumon and colleagues [18] showed at their institution how a dedicated bariatric surgery program with a dedicated staff and defined preoperative, perioperative, and postoperative pathways led to a reduction of readmission rates from 13.7% to 9.27%.

Hinojosa and colleagues [17] performed a large review on the University HealthSystem clinical database specifically looking at outcomes between laparoscopic gastric banding and gastric bypass. The complication rates were 2.8% and 7.5%, but there are no specifics on which complications led to readmission. Nguyen and colleagues [16] performed a randomized prospective trial on 250 bariatric patients assigned between gastric bypass and gastric banding. The bypass group has a 5.4% readmission rate, whereas the band group has 0%. Wound infection (29.1%), dehydration (16.7%), and obstruction

(16.7) were the most common early complications requiring readmission. Kellogg and colleagues [19] did a retrospective review of 1222 patients who underwent gastric bypass performed at their hospital. This study was also one of the few that evaluated regional hospitals and the index facility. There were no demographic differences between the readmitted and non-readmitted patients, but those who were readmitted more likely had an open gastric bypass. There was no differentiation between causes for emergency room visits and visits that ended in readmission. Nausea, vomiting, and dehydration (26%), abdominal pain (20%), and wound issues (8%) were the most common reasons for patients seeking emergency care. Baker and colleagues [23] studied a group of patients undergoing laparoscopic gastric bypass. They found that patients who had an inpatient stay longer than the expected 2 days after their operation had a higher readmission rate, 13.1% compared with 2.4%. Bellanger and Greenway [24] performed an institutional review that showed a 1.7% 30-day readmission rate in 529 laparoscopic sleeve gastrectomies. Their most frequent complications were vomiting, dehydration, mesenteric venous thrombosis, deep venous thrombosis, and severe reflux esophagitis. There was no differentiation on which complications led to readmissions. The factors that lead to readmission rates remain multifactorial, with the most common being gastrointestinal complaints.

CHOLECYSTECTOMY

The readmission rates for patients undergoing cholecystectomy have ranged between 2% and and 8% (Table 4) [3,4,25,26]. Tiwari and colleagues [4] showed that overall, patients who undergo laparoscopic cholecystectomy (2.3%) have lower readmission rates than those who undergo open cholecystectomy (6.1%). Sanjay and colleagues [25] performed a review of 1523 elective laparoscopic cholecystectomies, and they found an unexpected side effect of segregation of the patient populations receiving an open versus the

Table 4
Thirty day readmission rates for cholecystectomy

Operation	Type	30-day readmission rate	Patient number	Authors
Cholecystectomy (laparoscopic)	UHC database	2.31%	35,872	Tiwari et al [3,4]
Cholecystectomy (laparoscopic)	Institution	2.82%	1523	Sanjay et al [25]
Cholecystectomy (laparoscopic)	Institution	3.00%	1210	Wolf et al [26]
Cholecystectomy (converted)	Institution	8.80%	68	Wolf et al [26]
Cholecystectomy (open)	UHC database	6.06%	13,268	Tiwari et al [3,4]
Cholecystectomy (open)	Institution	8.10%	136	Wolf et al [26]

Abbreviation: UHC, University HealthSystem Consortium.

laparoscopic procedure. They showed a 2.8% readmission rate at 6 weeks, and almost half of these readmissions were caused by nonbiliary-related abdominal pain. The rest were directly caused by the procedure itself, namely obstructive jaundice, pancreatitis, bile leaks, and wound issues. Wolf and colleagues [26] reviewed 1629 cholecystectomies performed by a single surgeon during a 10-year period. They found that patients who had an open or laparoscopic converted to open cholecystectomy had substantially higher readmission rates than the laparoscopic group. These patients were older, had a higher American Society of Anesthesiologists (ASA) class, and had a higher frequency of having a history of abdominal surgery. The readmission rates from cholecystectomy are predominantly driven by the incision type, with laparoscopic cholecystectomy having substantially lower rates, with the age of the patient and underlying comorbidities playing the largest role in readmission after laparoscopic cholecystectomy.

PANCREAS

Early in the decade, articles examining readmission rates were more long term, because readmission for tumor recurrence is a substantial concern for pancreatectomy for cancer. However, increasing interest in the Medicare proposals has led to more focused investigations of 30-day readmission rates, which can be seen in Table 5 [8,10,27–30]. Yermilov and colleagues [30] showed what seems to be an unusually high readmission rate at 59%; however, this study included readmissions to hospitals outside the facility where the primary operation was performed. They note that almost half of these readmissions occurred outside the primary hospital.

On multivariate analysis, Kent and colleagues [27] found that of the preoperative demographics, physiologic variance, or intraoperative factors only pancreatic duct size less than 3 mm ($P<.03$) was significantly different between the readmitted and non-readmitted groups. However, Yermilov and colleagues [30] showed that age greater than 73 (OR, 1.37), T4 stage (OR, 1.69), and a Charlson score greater than 3 (OR, 1.62) were found in greater proportions

Table 5
Thirty day readmission rates for pancreatectomy

Operation	Type	30-day readmission rate	Patient number	Authors
Pancreatectomy (distal)	Institution	22.80%	187	Kent et al [27]
Pancreatectomy	SEER-Medicare	16.00%	1730	Reddy et al
Pancreatectomy	Washington	13.2%–17.6%	2829	Massarweh et al [8]
Pancreatectomy	Medicare	16.6%–20.3%		Goodney et al [10]
Pancreatoduodenectomy	Institution	13.28%	436	Zhu et al [28]
Pancreatoduodenectomy	Institution	22.10%	371	Kent et al [27]
Pancreatoduodenectomy	Institution	26.00%	1643	Emick et al [29]
Pancreatoduodenectomy	Institution	38.00%	280	Geenen et al
Pancreatoduodenectomy	CCR database	59.00%	2023	Yermilov et al [30]

in readmitted patients. Reddy and colleagues [31] found that a length of stay greater than 10 days (hazard ratio 1.46) were predictive of readmission. Emick and colleagues [29] showed that their readmissions were younger (OR, 1.6) and likely to be African American (OR, 1.6). Additionally, this study found that the readmissions group was associated with estimated blood loss more than a liter (OR, 1.4) and use of percutaneous bile stent (OR, 1.4). Index admission disposition was associated with readmission rates, with 30% of those discharged with home health services, 12% to home only, and 16% to a rehabilitation facility. Goodney and colleagues [10] showed in their Medicare study that readmission rates increased at an inverse proportion to hospital volume.

Surgery-specific complications were found consistently in higher proportion. Kent and colleagues [27] showed 65% of readmissions were caused by surgery-related problems, with 47% specific to pancreatic resection and 18% caused by general postoperative complications. These include primarily pancreatic fistulae, delayed gastric emptying, bile leaks, and wound infection. The remainder was divided among failure to thrive, medical problems, and complaints with a negative diagnostic workup. Emick and colleagues [29] also showed that intra-abdominal infections (19%), delayed gastric emptying (15%), and cholangitis (13%) were most of the readmitting diagnoses. Reddy and colleagues [31] also found that 80% of 30-day readmissions were caused by surgical complications. After the first 30 days, recurrence of disease was found at higher proportions compared with surgical complications. At 1 year, Yermilov and colleagues [30] showed that 24.3% were caused by progression of disease, 14% by surgery-related complications, and 12% by infection. Zhu and colleagues [28] found that surgical complications and infection accounted for 14% of readmissions at 1 year, compared with progression of disease, radiation, and chemotherapy at 60%.

COLON

The breadth of colorectal surgery creates a wide potential of readmission rates, which are summarized in Table 6 [3,4,32–35], because of the differences in pathology, types and methods for resection, and techniques for reconstruction. Kiran and colleagues [36] reviewed 628 patients who underwent colorectal procedures in a 6-month period at a single institution. They tried to minimize confounding by searching other hospitals for readmissions and contacting patients lost to follow-up by telephone. Demographically, there were no differences between the two groups in terms of age, gender, diagnosis, or operation type. For the immediate postoperative course, the readmitted group had a higher percentage of perioperative steroid use ($P<.03$) and a median length of stay 1 day longer ($P<.049$). In the readmitted group, the most frequent complications included bowel obstruction or ileus (33%); infection (35%); and anastomotic leak (5.4%). The total length of hospital stay for patients who were readmitted, which included the days for index admission and days for readmission from the complication, was similar to the time taken for patients who developed these complications during their inpatient stay.

Table 6
Thirty day readmission rates for colectomy and low rectal surgeries

Operation	Type	30 day readmission rate	Patient number	Authors
Colectomy (elective)	MEDPAR	11.90%	29,552	Lidor et al [32]
Colectomy (emergent)	MEDPAR	21.40%	23,764	Lidor et al [32]
Colectomy (laparoscopic)	Institution	2.90%	235	Larson et al
Colectomy (laparoscopic)	UHC database	4.38%	32,555	Tiwari et al [3,4]
Colectomy (laparoscopic)	Institution	7.60%	99	Larson et al
Colectomy (laparoscopic)	Institution	10.00%	820	O'Brien et al [38]
Colectomy (left)	Institution	12.00%	108	Abarca et al [33]
Colectomy (open)	UHC database	6.50%	972	Tiwari et al [3,4]
Colectomy (right)	Institution	14.00%	155	Abarca et al [33]
Colonic surgery	Institution	11.30%	541	Andersen et al
Ileal pouch anal anastamosis	Institution	30.00%	195	Datta et al [34]
Ileostomy closure	Institution	9.50%	42	Joh et al [35]
Intestinal surgery	Institution	12.70%	1180	Kariv et al
LAR/APR	Institution	26.00%	27	Abarca et al [33]
Appendectomy (open)	UHC database	2.97%/5.93%	14,356	Tiwari et al [3,4]
Appendectomy (open)	UHC database	4.10%	14,222	Tiwari et al [3,4]
Appendectomy (laparoscopic)	UHC database	1.86%/5.04%	25,981	Tiwari et al [3,4]
Appendectomy (laparoscopic)	UHC database	2.51%	25,840	Tiwari et al [3,4]

Abbreviations: APR, abdominal perineal resection; LAR, low anterior resection; UHC, University Health System Consortium.

Datta and colleagues [34] examined specifically ileal pouch–anal anastomosis and found that 30% of 195 patients required readmission. The most frequent admitting diagnoses were small bowel obstruction (33%) and anastomotic leak (33%). On univariate analysis they found that younger age, two stage, and urgent procedures were predictive of readmission, but only perioperative steroid use ($P<.001$) was found to be predictive on multivariate analysis. The authors speculate that the univariate findings may present themselves in a larger sample size. Guinier and colleagues [37] performed a prospective study on 1421 patients undergoing colorectal procedures and found that 7.5% had an unplanned readmission, 50% of whom were secondary to surgical complications. Of these, anastomotic leak (17%), wound infection (17%), and intracavitary abscess (17%) were the most prevalent. On multivariate analysis, they showed that operative field contamination (OR, 2.56), long operation time (OR, 1.34), performance of an associated procedure (OR, 1.65), initial hemoglobin less than 12 g/dL (OR, 1.59), and air-testing not performed (OR, 1.72) were risk factors for readmission.

O'Brien and colleagues [38] performed a retrospective study on 820 patients specifically looking at readmission rates and causes for laparoscopic colon surgery. These operations included partial and total colectomies, small bowel resections, ileocecal resections, stoma procedures, and prolapse repairs. Most of the indications for these procedures were diverticulitis; however, some were indicated for inflammatory bowel diseases and colon or rectal cancer. The primary readmitting diagnoses were bowel obstruction and ileus (36.7%); abscess (11.4%); and anastomotic leak (8.8%). There were no differences found in demographics, but pulmonary comorbidities ($P<.028$) and inflammatory bowel disease ($P<.001$) were found more frequently in the readmission group. Use of perioperative steroids ($P<.012$) and conversion from laparoscopic to open ($P<.017$) were also found more frequently in the readmitted patients. Abarca and colleagues [33] reviewed 358 patients at their institution who underwent laparoscopic colectomy by two surgeons. Of these readmissions, nausea and vomiting (23%) were most prevalent, followed by wound infection (20%), pain (16%), and dehydration (12.5%). Of note, they had 19 hernias necessitating reoperation, with seven causing obstructions requiring reoperation within the first 30 days. Joh and colleagues [35] studied 42 patients who underwent ileostomy closure by a single surgeon. Four of these patients were readmitted, with one each for small bowel obstruction, postoperative ileus, wound infection, and dehydration. Lidor and colleagues [32] reviewed the Medicare database from 2004 to 2007 in a study regarding diverticulitis. Their primary endpoint was mortality between emergent or urgent and elective colectomies, but they also found that readmission rates for emergent colectomy were much higher than elective colectomy at all age groups.

ABDOMINAL AORTIC ANEURYSM

Most of the longitudinal reviews on postoperative outcomes for abdominal aortic aneurysm (AAA) were measured in person years; the statistics relevant for readmission data in the first 30 days postdischarge are listed in Table 7 [8,10,39]. Holt and colleagues [39] used the English National Health Service administrative dataset, the hospital episode statistics data, to specifically study readmissions and reinterventions in patients who underwent AAA repair. Readmission rates at 1 year were 12% for open repair and 13% for endovascular aneurysm repair (EVAR). They found that octogenarians had a higher risk for readmission at 30 days and at 1 year. Jetty and colleagues [40] performed a comparative review of patients undergoing operative repair for nonruptured

Table 7
Thirty day readmission rates for abdominal aortic aneurysm rates

Operation	Type	30-day readmission rate	Patient number	Authors
AAA	Washington	8.3–10.5%	7723	Massarweh et al [8]
AAA	Medicare	10.1–11.4%		Goodney et al [10]
AAA - open	Hospital episode statistics	12.00%	18,060	Holt et al [39]
AAA - EVAR	Hospital episode statistics	13.00%	18,060	Holt et al [39]

Abbreviation: EVAR, endovascular aneurysm repair.

AAA. Mortality was the primary focus for this study, but reinterventions and readmissions were secondary outcomes evaluated. They found that patients undergoing EVAR had more urgent and vascular readmissions, and more interventions overall. Giles and colleagues [41] studied the Medicare database to compare outcomes between open and endovascular abdominal aneurysm repair. Unlike the other studies discussed here, outcomes were measured in events per person-years with the primary focus on postoperative reinterventions, not readmissions. They found that endovascular repair had a higher overall reintervention rate at 7.56 events per person-year, compared with the open rate of 6.96. The endovascular group had more overall reinterventions including rupture; however, most of the AAA-related reinterventions were minor. Open repairs required more laparotomy-related intervention, and they also had more hospitalizations for nonoperative gastrointestinal symptoms.

Gioia and colleagues [42] performed a thorough analysis on 206 patients who underwent elective and nonelective open AAA repair at two hospitals. They found that 50% were readmitted within the first 2 weeks after discharge and more than 75% occurred by the first 2 months. Of the elective patients, the only difference between readmitted and nonreadmitted patients was that more nonreadmitted patients were discharged to self care (64.8%–40%). For the nonelective patients, the readmitted group had a higher proportion of females and African Americans.

DISCUSSION

MedPAC [43,44] characterizes a readmission as potentially preventable if expert panels determined that the readmission could be avoided by the following:

1. Provision of quality of care in the hospital
2. Adequate discharge planning
3. Adequate postdischarge follow-up
4. Improved coordination between hospitals and providers outside of the hospital setting.

From a previous discussion [45], an analysis of risk factors based on the patient' demographics, medical history, hospital course, and disposition could give providers insight on how to anticipate who may require readmission. Not surprisingly, surgeons can improve readmission rates by reducing technical complications, and the risk factors described previously may be used for adjustments to discharge criteria and could potentially be used as justification for a prolonged index hospital stay. Earlier follow-up with the surgeon and primary care provider could address potential problems before they require a hospital admission. One study showed that only 25% of readmitted patients were seen by the treating physician before the readmission [46].

The two main types of study that have been used in the United States to evaluate readmission are institutional and insurance database based. Both have specific strengths and weaknesses that need to be considered if their data are to be applicable from individual cases to a nation-wide level. Institutional studies have the advantage of eliminating confounders by focusing on a single surgeon at a single facility and having the capability of reviewing individual medical records for specific characteristics in demographics and postoperative care that can be investigated. The biggest problem is that these studies may not have the power to show that risk factors on univariate analysis are significant on multivariate analysis. In the case of colon operations, steroid use was cited by multiple authors as a risk factor for readmission. For pancreatectomy, however, demographic risk factors were inconsistently significant.

The large database studies have the advantage in volume; however, they are primarily created for billing purposes and data are dependent on *International Classification of Diseases, Ninth Revision* codes. Errors are difficult to evaluate because reference to patient charts are unavailable.

The study by Yermilov and colleagues [30] using the California Cancer Registry Database tried to capture readmissions to hospitals other than the index admission and found that 47% occurred at outside facilities. This study was among the few that tried to capture readmission rates outside of the index facility, and their rates were considerably higher than similar institutional reviews for pancreatectomy. This finding is likely as pronounced with other operations that are performed primarily at tertiary referral centers that draw from a large geographic region.

Posthospital disposition has also been associated with readmission rates. At one institution, patients sent home with home health represented 62% [46] of the readmitted group. Providers may be underestimating patients' needs or overestimating their ability for self-care. Standardization of discharge disposition may be a useful tool to direct patients to the appropriate level of posthospital care and reduce this group of readmissions. Hospital specialization for specific procedures, such as esophagectomy and bariatrics, has been shown to improve inpatient outcomes, so it is reasonable that specialization by home health agencies and posthospital rehabilitation centers could have a similarly positive effect on readmission rates.

The increasing awareness of the cost of readmissions has complicated the evaluation for good clinical practice and overall cost management. The current data estimate what current readmission rates are for many operations, but the number of these that are preventable is debatable. The challenge to minimize readmission rates requires further investigation and a coordinated approach among providers, patients, and posthospital organizations. Currently, surgeons can play a role in only one of the four factors, which is providing quality care in the hospital. However, the three other factors are currently not under surgeon control or even the understanding of how quality is measured. Given the increased pressure for early hospital discharge, great emphasis on posthospital disposition will become increasing important to achieve minimal readmission rates.

References

[1] Averill RF, McCullough EC, Hughes JS, et al. Redesigning the Medicare inpatient PPS to reduce payments to hospitals with high readmission rates. Health Care Financ Rev 2009;30(4):1–15.

[2] Jencks SF, Williams MV, Coleman EA. Rehospitalizations among patients in the Medicare fee-for-service program. N Engl J Med 2009;360(14):1418–28.

[3] Tiwari MM, Goede MR, Reynoso JF, et al. Differences in outcomes of laparoscopic gastric bypass. Surg Obes Relat Dis 2011;7(3):277–82.

[4] Tiwari MM, Reynoso JF, High R, et al. Safety, efficacy, and cost-effectiveness of common laparoscopic procedures. Surg Endosc 2011;25(4):1127–35.

[5] Blatnik JA, Harth KC, Aeder MI, et al. Thirty-day readmission after ventral hernia repair: predictable or preventable? Surg Endosc 2011;25(5):1446–51.

[6] Bisgaard T, Kehlet H, Bay-Nielsen M, et al. A nationwide study on readmission, morbidity, and mortality after umbilical and epigastric hernia repair. Hernia 2011;15(5):541–6.

[7] Helgstrand F, Rosenberg J, Kehlet H, et al. Nationwide analysis of prolonged hospital stay and readmission after elective ventral hernia repair. Dan Med Bull 2011;58(10):A4322.

[8] Massarweh NN, Flum DR, Symons RG, et al. A critical evaluation of the impact of Leapfrog's evidence-based hospital referral. J Am Coll Surg 2011;212(2):150–159 e151.

[9] Varghese TK Jr, Wood DE, Farjah F, et al. Variation in esophagectomy outcomes in hospitals meeting Leapfrog volume outcome standards. Ann Thorac Surg 2011;91(4):1003–9 [discussion: 1009–10].

[10] Goodney PP, Stukel TA, Lucas FL, et al. Hospital volume, length of stay, and readmission rates in high-risk surgery. Ann Surg 2003;238(2):161–7.

[11] Reavis KM, Smith BR, Hinojosa MW, et al. Outcomes of esophagectomy at academic centers: an association between volume and outcome. Am Surg 2008;74(10):939–43.

[12] Auerbach AD, Maselli J, Carter J, et al. The relationship between case volume, care quality, and outcomes of complex cancer surgery. J Am Coll Surg 2010;211(5):601–8.

[13] Saunders JK, Ballantyne GH, Belsley S, et al. 30-day readmission rates at a high volume bariatric surgery center: laparoscopic adjustable gastric banding, laparoscopic gastric bypass, and vertical banded gastroplasty-Roux-en-Y gastric bypass. Obes Surg 2007;17(9): 1171–7.

[14] Weller WE, Rosati C, Hannan EL. Relationship between surgeon and hospital volume and readmission after bariatric operation. J Am Coll Surg 2007;204(3):383–91.

[15] Encinosa WE, Bernard DM, Chen CC, et al. Healthcare utilization and outcomes after bariatric surgery. Med Care 2006;44(8):706–12.

[16] Nguyen NT, Hohmann S, Slone J, et al. Improved bariatric surgery outcomes for Medicare beneficiaries after implementation of the Medicare national coverage determination. Arch Surg 2010;145(1):72–8.

[17] Hinojosa MW, Varela JE, Parikh D, et al. National trends in use and outcome of laparoscopic adjustable gastric banding. Surg Obes Relat Dis 2009;5(2):150–5.

[18] Dumon KR, Edelson PK, Raper SE, et al. Implementation of designated bariatric surgery program leads to improved clinical outcomes. Surg Obes Relat Dis 2011;7(3):271–6.

[19] Kellogg TA, Swan T, Leslie DA, et al. Patterns of readmission and reoperation within 90 days after Roux-en-Y gastric bypass. Surg Obes Relat Dis 2009;5(4):416–23.

[20] Blackstone RP, Cortes MC. Metabolic acuity score: effect on major complications after bariatric surgery. Surg Obes Relat Dis 2010;6(3):267–73.

[21] Blackstone RP, Cortes MC, Messer LB, et al. Psychological classification as a communication and management tool in obese patients undergoing bariatric surgery. Surg Obes Relat Dis 2010;6(3):274–81.

[22] Willkomm CM, Fisher TL, Barnes GS, et al. Surgical weight loss >65 years old: is it worth the risk? Surg Obes Relat Dis 2010;6(5):491–6.

[23] Baker MT, Lara MD, Larson CJ, et al. Length of stay and impact on readmission rates after laparoscopic gastric bypass. Surg Obes Relat Dis 2006;2(4):435–9.

[24] Bellanger DE, Greenway FL. Laparoscopic sleeve gastrectomy, 529 cases without a leak: short-term results and technical considerations. Obes Surg 2011;21(2):146–50.

[25] Sanjay P, Weerakoon R, Shaikh IA, et al. 5-year analysis of readmissions following elective laparoscopic cholecystectomy: cohort study. Int J Surg 2011;9(1):52–4.

[26] Wolf AS, Nijsse BA, Sokal SM, et al. Surgical outcomes of open cholecystectomy in the laparoscopic era. Am J Surg 2009;197(6):781–4.

[27] Kent TS, Sachs TE, Callery MP, et al. Readmission after major pancreatic resection: a necessary evil? J Am Coll Surg 2011;213(4):515–23.

[28] Zhu ZY, He JK, Wang YF, et al. Multivariable analysis of factors associated with hospital readmission following pancreaticoduodenectomy for malignant diseases. Chin Med J (Engl) 2011;124(7):1022–5.

[29] Emick DM, Riall TS, Cameron JL, et al. Hospital readmission after pancreaticoduodenectomy. J Gastrointest Surg 2006;10(9):1243–52 [discussion: 1252–3].

[30] Yermilov I, Bentrem D, Sekeris E, et al. Readmissions following pancreaticoduodenectomy for pancreas cancer: a population-based appraisal. Ann Surg Oncol 2009;16(3):554–61.

[31] Reddy DM, Townsend CM Jr, Kuo YF, et al. Readmission after pancreatectomy for pancreatic cancer in Medicare patients. J Gastrointest Surg 2009;13(11):1963–74 [discussion: 1974–5].

[32] Lidor AO, Schneider E, Segal J, et al. Elective surgery for diverticulitis is associated with high risk of intestinal diversion and hospital readmission in older adults. J Gastrointest Surg 2010;14(12):1867–73 [discussion: 1873–4].

[33] Abarca F, Saclarides TJ, Brand MI. Laparoscopic colectomy: complications causing reoperation or emergency room/hospital readmissions. Am Surg 2011;77(1):65–9.

[34] Datta I, Buie WD, Maclean AR, et al. Hospital readmission rates after ileal pouch-anal anastomosis. Dis Colon Rectum 2009;52(1):55–8.

[35] Joh YG, Lindsetmo RO, Stulberg J, et al. Standardized postoperative pathway: accelerating recovery after ileostomy closure. Dis Colon Rectum 2008;51(12):1786–9.

[36] Kiran RP, Delaney CP, Senagore AJ, et al. Outcomes and prediction of hospital readmission after intestinal surgery. J Am Coll Surg 2004;198(6):877–83.

[37] Guinier D, Mantion GA, Alves A, et al. Risk factors of unplanned readmission after colorectal surgery: a prospective, multicenter study. Dis Colon Rectum 2007;50(9):1316–23.

[38] O'Brien DP, Senagore A, Merlino J, et al. Predictors and outcome of readmission after laparoscopic intestinal surgery. World J Surg 2007;31(12):2430–5.

[39] Holt PJ, Poloniecki JD, Hofman D, et al. Re-interventions, readmissions and discharge destination: modern metrics for the assessment of the quality of care. Eur J Vasc Endovasc Surg 2010;39(1):49–54.

[40] Jetty P, Hebert P, van Walraven C. Long-term outcomes and resource utilization of endovascular versus open repair of abdominal aortic aneurysms in Ontario. J Vasc Surg 2010;51(3):577–83, 583. e571–3.

[41] Giles KA, Landon BE, Cotterill P, et al. Thirty-day mortality and late survival with reinterventions and readmissions after open and endovascular aortic aneurysm repair in Medicare beneficiaries. J Vasc Surg 2011;53(1):6–12, 13. e11.

[42] Gioia LC, Filion KB, Haider S, et al. Hospital readmissions following abdominal aortic aneurysm repair. Ann Vasc Surg 2005;19(1):35–41.

[43] Payment policy for inpatient readmissions. In: Medicare Payment Advisory Commission. Report to the Congress: Promoting greater efficiency in Medicare. Washington, DC: MedPAC; 2007. p. 103–20. Available at: http://www.medpac.gov/documents/jun07_entirereport.pdf.

[44] Stone J, Hoffman GJ. Medicare hospital readmissions: issues, policy options and PPACA. Washington, DC: U.S. Congressional Research Service; 2010. R40972; Sept 21, 2010.

[45] Brown RE, Qadan M, Martin RC II, et al. The evolving importance of readmission data to the practicing surgeon. J Am Coll Surg 2010;211(4):558–60.

[46] Martin RC, Brown R, Puffer L, et al. Readmission rates after abdominal surgery: the role of surgeon, primary caregiver, home health, and subacute rehab. Ann Surg 2011;254(4):591–7.

Superiority of Minimally Invasive Parathyroidectomy

John W. Kunstman, MD[a], Robert Udelsman, MD, MBA[a,b,*]

[a]Yale University School of Medicine, New Haven, CT, USA; [b]Yale-New Haven Hospital, New Haven, CT, USA

Keywords
- Parathyroidectomy • Primary hyperparathyroidism
- Minimally invasive parathyroidectomy

Key Points
- Conventional bilateral cervical exploration has been the gold standard for the surgical treatment of primary hyperparathyroidism (PHPT).
- Minimally invasive parathyroidectomy (MIP) has become the preferred approach in select patients.
- Cure and complication rates are more favorable following MIP.
- In addition, length of stay, total costs and cosmetic outcomes all favor MIP.

INTRODUCTION

Primary hyperparathyroidism (PHPT) is a common endocrine disorder with an incidence of 21.6 per 100,000 person-years in the United States [1,2]. Its effects are manifested by autonomous hypersecretion of parathyroid hormone (PTH) from 1 or more parathyroid glands, resulting in hypercalcemia. It is more common in women and those of advanced age. As serum calcium measurement became routine in the 1970s after development of the multichannel serum autoanalyzer, prevalence of the disease increased from 0.1% to 0.4% in the United States [2]. As a result, classic symptoms reflecting long-term PTH overexpression (osteitis fibrosa cystica, nephrocalcinosis, peptic ulcer disease, and pancreatitis) are now rarely encountered in clinical practice outside the developing world. Instead, after ruling out alternate causes of hypercalcemia, the diagnosis is made via biochemical confirmation of an inappropriately normal or increased serum PTH concentration in the setting of normal renal function. Milder signs and symptoms, such as neurocognitive deficits, osteopenia, nephrolithiasis, and dyspepsia, are still common. Although only 20% of patients have clear signs or symptoms of

*Corresponding author. Department of Surgery, Yale University School of Medicine, New Haven, CT 06520. E-mail address: robert.udelsman@yale.edu

0065-3411/12/$ – see front matter
doi:10.1016/j.yasu.2012.04.004

PHPT at diagnosis [3], more rigorous investigations, such as dexa bone scans to evaluate osteopenia and a careful assessment of neurocognitive symptoms, greatly increases the fraction of symptomatic patients [4].

Surgery remains the only curative modality for PHPT. Although medical therapy with calcimimetics for secondary hyperparathyroidism is well established, its role in PHPT is limited to refractory disease and those who are not surgical candidates [5]. As described later, the dominant surgical approach since the first successful parathyroidectomy in 1925 has been bilateral cervical exploration (BCE) because of its exemplary cure rate and morbidity profile. However, because the causative lesion in greater than 80% of PHPT is a single adenoma, a unilateral approach is feasible for many patients. New developments in imaging, surgical techniques, and operative adjuncts have made focused parathyroidectomy a reality. Minimally invasive open parathyroidectomy [6,7] and endoscopic/video-assisted [8–10] techniques have been described and validated. Numerous investigators have shown equivalence in outcomes between minimally invasive parathyroidectomy (MIP) and BCE [7,11,12]. Although equivalence alone is notable given the durability and efficacy of conventional BCE, enough experience with MIP has now been accrued to show that its advantages translate into superior clinical results [4]. The improved rate of cure and decreased frequency of complications argue for adoption of minimally invasive techniques in appropriately selected patients with sporadic PHPT.

HISTORICAL PERSPECTIVE AND RATIONALE FOR FOCUSED PARATHYROIDECTOMY

After the initial description of glandulae parathyreoideae in humans by the Swedish medical student Ivar Sandstrom [13] in 1880, understanding of the parathyroid's role in calcium metabolism was slow in coming. An important clue was the frequent occurrence of tetany following thyroid surgery, causing Halsted and Evans [14] to remark in 1907, "With our present knowledge, scant as it is, of the function of the parathyroid bodies comes the recognition of the necessity for [the] preservation...of these little life sustaining organs." In that same article, Halsted and Evans [14] (unknowingly describing iatrogenic hypoparathyroidism) noted the preference of many surgeons to perform thyroid resections 1 lobe at a time to prevent tetany; he also asserted that this is unnecessary if the parathyroids are identified and preserved. Understanding of parathyroid physiology gradually improved and the first successful parathyroidectomy was performed in Vienna by Felix Mandl [15] in 1925. The patient presented with osteitis fibrosa cystica and a single enlarged parathyroid gland was removed resulting in a cure; the case was notable because it was performed under local anesthesia. As hyperparathyroidism was better defined by Fuller Albright and colleagues [16] in the 1930s, parathyroid surgery gradually gained acceptance as the preferred treatment of PHPT. During this time, subtotal or total parathyroidectomy with autotransplantation was advocated, because many had noted persistent disease despite resection of a dominant adenoma. This finding was clarified in 1958 by Cope and colleagues [17] who recognized 4-gland hyperplasia and double adenomas as distinct clinical entities and attributed ~80% of PHPT cases to single adenomas. BCE therefore became the operative approach of choice, because it allowed identification of the cause of PHPT followed by appropriate resection of the causative lesion or lesions. As Cope [18] stated in 1966, "The only way a surgeon can be sure [of the diagnosis] is to see at least 2 glands...It is obviously more helpful if all 4 glands are exposed."

The durability of BCE under general anesthesia in the next half-century as the gold standard for treating sporadic PHPT is the result of its unqualified success. Large, modern cases series show cure rates in excess of 95%, morbidity of less than 4%, and essentially no mortality when performed by a high-volume endocrine surgeon [19]. However, despite the success of BCE, it has been challenged of late because approximately 85% of patients harbor only a single adenoma, resection of which achieves a durable cure. Unilateral exploration was first advocated in the 1970s using a variety of preoperative localization studies such as video esophagography, vascular PTH sampling, neck palpation, or a simple guess [20]. In 1982, Tibblin and colleagues [21] advocated unilateral exploration with intraoperative oil-red-O staining of the resected gland to determine whether multigland hyperplasia was present. If not, the operation was terminated without further exploration. Both approaches were vulnerable to missing contralateral double adenomas. Moreover, because the described modalities for localization were all poor, the choice of which side to initially explore was often left to chance. As interventional radiologist John L. Doppman [22] noted in 1986, "In my opinion, the only localizing study indicated in a patient with untreated PHPT is to localize an experienced parathyroid surgeon." Even so, the potential advantages of unilateral surgery, including a lower incidence of postoperative hypocalcemia with 2 unmolested parathyroids left in situ and decreased risk for nerve damage, were enticing. Also, by leaving 1 hemisphere of the neck unexplored, a more favorable operative field would be preserved in the event of reexploration. These hypothesized benefits encouraged further effort.

Preoperative localization of the causative lesion in PHPT is a requirement for focused parathyroidectomy. Ultrasound for parathyroid tumors was initially reported in the late 1970s [23,24] and successful radioisotope scintigraphy was first described in 1983 [25]. The development of sestamibi-technetium 99m (Tc^{99m}) scintigraphy in 1989 [26] increased both the use and sensitivity of nuclear imaging. Thus, although not yet widely used, most patients with PHPT were at least candidates for effective preoperative localization by the early 1990s. However, even modern ultrasonography and scintigraphy are subject to missing double adenomas, parathyroid hyperplasia, and ectopically located glands. In these cases, focused parathyroidectomy guided by preoperative localization alone would fail in a significant subset of patients. To overcome this deficit, postresection measurement of PTH was first suggested as an adjunct to show cure by Nussbaum and colleagues [27] in 1988. Because of its brief circulating half-life (3.3 ± 0.9 minutes [28]), postresection measurement of PTH could potentially indicate whether PHPT cure was achieved or further exploration for another adenoma or hyperplastic glands would be required. In 1991, Irvin and colleagues [29] began using the PTH assay as an intraoperative adjunct to assess adequacy of resection. This crucial improvement meant that the surgeon, after noting a rapid decline in serum PTH following resection of a single adenoma, could forgo visual inspection of the remaining glands and expect a durable cure before leaving the operating room. In contrast, persistence of an increased serum PTH concentration would prompt further exploration. The combination of preoperative localization and confirmation of cure via intraoperative PTH (IOPTH) assay suggested a viable approach to unilateral, focused parathyroidectomy and was validated by Irvin and colleagues [30] in 1994. Since then, many investigators have modified the basic approach and rendered focused parathyroidectomy a reliable treatment modality for PHPT.

DEFINING MIP

Minimally invasive surgery can be defined as the performance of a traditional surgical procedure in a novel way to minimize the trauma of surgical exposure [31]. Using this broad definition, multiple surgical approaches to parathyroid-ectomy in current clinical practice are variants of minimally invasive tech-niques, especially when juxtaposed to BCE. This definition includes open, radio-guided, and endoscopic or video-assisted techniques; all are focused, in that they do not attempt to visualize all 4 parathyroid glands via BCE. Thus, regardless of modality, MIP universally requires:

1. An unequivocal diagnosis of PHPT meeting proper indications for surgery
2. With positive or suggestive noninvasive, preoperative localization
3. Resulting in focused, unilateral exploration
4. Via a limited incision.

Furthermore, for open MIP, we routinely use:

5. Surgeon-administered locoregional anesthesia with conscious sedation via monitored anesthesia care (MAC)
6. IOPTH measurement to assess adequacy of resection
7. An ambulatory day surgery venue.

We first reported our assimilation of preoperative localization, IOPTH assay, and use of regional (cervical block) anesthesia in 1999 [6]. This approach allowed flexible, focused exploration with same-day discharge, and maintained the capacity for bilateral exploration through the same incision when necessary. Our initial experience offered validation of both the safety and efficacy of MIP, as well as showing several advantages compared with BCE [32]. Ambulatory parathyroidectomy has been shown to decrease operative times and length of stay (LOS) [33] by using the IOPTH assay, which can provide direct biochemical evidence of cure before leaving the operating room. Precision of point of care PTH testing during parathyroid surgery has been validated, allowing the surgeon to use it with confidence [34]. In addition, a locoregional block avoids general anesthesia with instant confirmation of recurrent laryngeal nerve integrity by prompting the patient to phonate. Unlike MIP, other techniques of focused parathyroidectomy, such as endoscopic or video-assisted approaches, usually require general anesthesia. MIP permits bilateral exploration if required and, when necessary, conversion to conventional BCE. BCE can be accomplished with bilateral locoregional cervical blocks, and conversion to general anesthesia is also possible.

INDICATIONS FOR MIP

Patient selection for surgical intervention in PHPT is similar whether a minimally invasive approach or a bilateral exploration is planned. All symptomatic patients should be considered for operative exploration. Consensus guidelines most recently published in 2009 identify asymptomatic patients with PHPT who are operative candidates [35]. Careful evaluation of more subtle or subjective symptoms of PHPT may increase the fraction of patients falling into the symptomatic category. For instance, a large number of patients exhibit PHPT-associated neurocognitive symptoms, and a recent large, prospective study showed improvement in mood, anxiety, and neurocognitive function following parathyroidectomy [36]. These data have not yet been incorporated into consensus guidelines; nevertheless, it is an important consideration for surgical intervention. Recent novel findings regarding cardiovascular implications of PHPT are intriguing, but have not been systematically incorporated into clinical practice [37,38].

Contraindications for MIP are few. In rare cases of suspected or confirmed parathyroid carcinoma, patients should undergo traditional exploration and en bloc resection [39]. However, we have performed extensive parathyroid and thyroid resections using cervical block anesthesia. The role of MIP in familial or syndromic hyperparathyroidism is limited; most patients should undergo bilateral exploration because of the high frequency of multiglandular disease. However, MIP does have a limited role in carefully selected patients when uniglandular disease is clearly identified on preoperative localization studies [40]. Reoperative exploration in cases of persistent or recurrent PHPT can also use a minimally invasive approach in properly selected patients because up to 40% of missed parathyroid adenomas are ultimately found in eutopic positions [41]. MIP can be used as the initial approach and converted to conventional exploration should the need arise.

PREOPERATIVE IMAGING

Numerous noninvasive modalities for identifying the causative lesion of PHPT exist, each with distinct advantages and disadvantages. With regard to MIP, accuracy in predicting both lesion location and the presence of multigland disease (MGD) is of foremost concern because focused exploration is predicated on correctly lateralizing a single, causative adenoma. Secondary considerations include exposure to ionizing radiation, operator dependence, and cost.

Scintigraphy

Nuclear scintigraphy is one of the most widely used methods for identifying parathyroid adenomas. Earlier techniques, such as thallium-201/technetium-99m

(Tc^{99m}) pertechnetate subtraction scintigraphy, are still occasionally used, but these have largely been supplanted by Tc^{99m}-sestamibi imaging. Sestamibi is a monovalent lipophilic cation that localizes to the mitochondria because of negative membrane potential. Differential accumulation occurs in parathyroid because of their high mitochondrial density and rich blood supply; typically, normal parathyroid glands do not meet the threshold for detection because of their small size. However, this can sometimes result in a falsely negative scan in smaller parathyroid adenomas (<600 mg) [42]. Overall sensitivity of sestamibi scanning ranges from 80% to 95% [43], with one meta-analysis of 6331 cases reporting a sensitivity and specificity of 90.7% and 98.8%, respectively [44]. These impressive results are rarely obtained in clinical practice where quality control and operator expertise may not be robust. The concurrent presence of other abnormal metabolically active tissues in the neck is the most frequent cause of false-positive scans. A nodular thyroid can reduce sestamibi sensitivity by 15% to 39% [45,46], whereas lymph node metastases, malignant disease, and other lesions can have equally deleterious effects. Multigland hyperplasia also reduces sestamibi sensitivity, with only 62% to 84% of hyperplastic glands correctly identified by sestamibi imaging [47,48]. Despite this, sestamibi scintigraphy is often used as a first-line imaging study for parathyroid localization because of its lessened operator dependence, comparatively modest cost, minimal amount of ionizing radiation exposure (~15–25 mCi), and wide field of view (including the mediastinum) that facilitates identification of ectopically located glands. In addition, sestamibi can be used with single-photon emission computed tomography (SPECT), allowing generation of multiplanar, three-dimensional imaging. This method can increase sestamibi sensitivity and provide additional anatomic detail that is critical for MIP planning [49,50].

Ultrasound

Sonography is another commonly used parathyroid imaging technique that can be used in a primary or complementary role. It provides excellent anatomic detail, is inexpensive and widely available, and is able to assess concurrent thyroid disease seen in up to 40% of patients with PHPT [51]. However, ultrasound has limited capability to assess small or hyperplastic glands because smaller adenomas (or normal glands) are rarely visualized. An adenoma appears as a homogenous, hypoechoic ovoid mass with a characteristic fat plane separating it from the thyroid and a peripheral rim of vascularity. Despite this distinctive appearance, parathyroid ultrasound is notoriously operator dependent and is also affected by patient characteristics such as body habitus [52]. In addition, ectopic glands are difficult to visualize with sonography; for instance, low mediastinal glands cannot be assessed because of the inability of ultrasound to penetrate osseous structures such as the sternum. In several large case series performed by experienced parathyroid sonographers, sensitivity for detection of solitary adenomas range from 72% to –89% [53–56]. However, this decreases to only 35% for patients with diffuse hyperplasia and 16% for those with double adenomas [57]. When used singly by an experienced practitioner, ultrasound has a true-positive rate of 74% to 77% for solitary adenomas and increases to 90% to 95% when coupled with sestamibi scintigraphy [56,58]. As a result, many centers use the 2 techniques in a complementary role. Others reserve nuclear imaging for patients with a negative sonogram or vice versa. In addition, it has been reported that preoperative sestamibi scintigraphy coupled with surgeon-performed ultrasound has also yielded superior results [59].

Axial imaging

Tomographic imaging in the form of computed tomography (CT) and magnetic resonance imaging (MRI) are particularly useful in cases requiring reoperation or localizing of ectopic glands. CT imaging has reported sensitivities for parathyroid localization of 46% to 87% but has the disadvantage of increased ionizing radiation exposure; accordingly, it has been largely limited to a secondary role until recently [60]. Four-dimensional CT imaging (4DCT, with the additional dimension being time) is a promising new modality that highlights the perfusion gradient present in parathyroid adenomas (ie, rapid uptake and washout of contrast). Matched studies have shown an improvement in true-positive adenoma localization versus Tc^{99m}-sestamibi and ultrasound [61]. 4DCT has also shown an improved sensitivity in detecting multigland hyperplasia (85.7%) and some investigators have suggested using 4DCT as the initial localization study before MIP in patients with newly diagnosed PHPT [62]. However, 4DCT generates even greater ionizing radiation than ordinary CT, which is especially crucial because the innately radiation-sensitive thyroid is within the field of exposure. CT should therefore be used with caution for parathyroid localization, especially in younger patients. MRI provides axial imaging without ionizing radiation exposure, with adenomatous glands appearing hyperintense on T2-weighted images. However, MRI is costly and most centers that use MRI do so in a complementary or secondary fashion only, because the anatomic detail is inferior compared with high-quality CT scans [63,64].

Invasive localization

Invasive modalities of parathyroid localization, such as angiographic PTH sampling, should be reserved for selected patients with remedial disease.

SURGICAL PROCEDURE

After a verified diagnosis of PHPT and positive or suggestive preoperative localization, the patient is offered MIP. Preoperative laryngoscopy is performed on all patients. Although most parathyroid explorations in the United States are still performed under general anesthesia with a secured airway via either endotracheal or laryngeal mask intubation, many centers have long used MAC for standard BCE for PHPT with success [65]. We routinely use surgeon-administered locoregional anesthesia with MAC for MIP. The awake patient is brought to the operating room and placed in a semi-Fowler position. The upper drape is elevated over the patient's face and air is circulated beneath it to minimize claustrophobia (Fig. 1). Intravenous access in an antecubital fossa is obtained and a baseline plasma PTH level drawn. Vascular access is

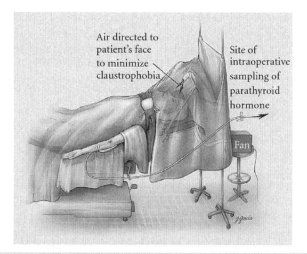

Fig. 1. The patient has a large-bore peripheral intravenous line inserted, which is used for medication and fluid administration, as well as sampling for PTH levels. The patient is awake, and a fan is used to blow room air gently toward the face to minimize the sensation of claustrophobia. (*From* Udelsman R. Unilateral neck exploration under local or regional anesthesia. In: Gagner M, Inabnet WB, editors. Minimally invasive endocrine surgery. Philadelphia: Lippincott, Williams & Wilkins; 2002. p. 93–102; with permission.)

maintained by anesthesia personnel to facilitate intraoperative PTH measurement. After mild intravenous sedation, the surgeon performs a locoregional block. We use 1% lidocaine with 1:100,000 epinephrine and routinely infuse a total volume of 15 to 25 mL. Unilateral infiltration at a depth of 1 to 2 cm along the posterior border of the sternocleidomastoid muscles midway (Erb point) between the mastoid process and its sternoclavicular insertion as well as serial infiltrations along the anterior border of the sternocleidomastoid muscle (SCM) provides excellent regional anesthesia to the neck (Fig. 2). Care must be taken to avoid intravascular administration. We then locally anesthetize the anterior neck. An abbreviated Kocher incision (2–3 cm) is made and the anterior compartment of the neck is entered. The strap muscles are dissected along the median raphe. Unilateral, focused dissection visualizes the parathyroid adenoma. After ensuring the integrity of the recurrent laryngeal nerve, the adenoma is excised (Fig. 3). Serial PTH measurements commence at the time of resection and are performed every 5 minutes. Initial postresection measurement may exceed the patient's baseline PTH because of mobilization of the adenoma. Cure is confirmed when PTH is both within normal limits and less than 50% of the baseline PTH level [7,30,33,66,67].

In some cases, the PTH does not decrease to a level consistent with a durable cure, which indicates residual abnormal parathyroid tissue and mandates additional exploration. The most suitable time to address inadequate resection is during the initial surgery when anatomic planes are pristine. We evaluate

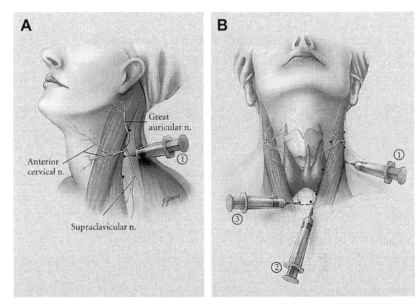

Fig. 2. Cervical block anesthesia. (A) A superficial cervical block is administered posterior and deep to the SCM (1). (B) Local infiltration is also performed along the anterior border of the SCM (2), followed by a local field block (3). (*From* Udelsman R. Unilateral neck exploration under local or regional anesthesia. In: Gagner M, Inabnet WB, editors. Minimally invasive endocrine surgery. Philadelphia: Lippincott, Williams & Wilkins; 2002. p. 93–102; with permission.)

the ipsilateral parathyroid gland first and convert to a bilateral exploration to fully explore both eutopic and ectopic sites when appropriate. The need for bilateral exploration is not itself an indication for conversion to general anesthesia, because BCE can safely be performed under MAC with bilateral locoregional anesthesia [68]. During MIP, we have observed a conversion rate to general anesthesia of 10.2%, most often because of ectopic gland location [4]. Patient discomfort required conversion in only 0.6% of cases. Most patients are discharged home the same day.

OUTCOMES FOLLOWING MIP
Cure rate
Because the rate of cure for patients with sporadic PHPT undergoing conventional BCE exceeds 95% when performed in a high-volume setting [19], it is crucial that MIP meet that threshold. Numerous groups have established that biochemical cure following MIP matches that of BCE. Equivalent outcomes have been shown in large, retrospective reviews and validated in numerous prospective trials directly comparing MIP with BCE [4,7,12,32,69–71]. Because outcomes are similar and additional features of MIP compare favorably with BCE (see later discussion), MIP has seen growing adoption among endocrine

KUNSTMAN & UDELSMAN

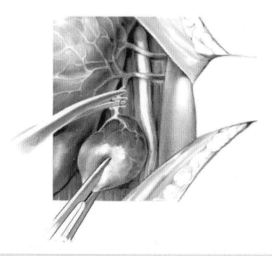

Fig. 3. The parathyroid adenoma is identified, its blood supply ligated, the recurrent laryngeal nerve is protected, and the adenoma is removed. (*From* Udelsman R. Unilateral neck exploration under local or regional anesthesia. In: Gagner M, Inabnet WB, editors. Minimally invasive endocrine surgery. Philadelphia: Lippincott, Williams & Wilkins; 2002. p. 93–102; with permission.)

surgeons [72]. Moreover, in the nearly 2 decades since its first report, enough experience has been accrued at high-volume centers to suggest that MIP conveys a superior, rather than equivalent, cure rate compared with BCE. In the largest study addressing this topic, we recently reported a consecutive case series of 1650 patients with sporadic PHPT who underwent either BCE or MIP during a 19-year time period [4]. Cure, defined by postoperative normalization of both serum PTH and calcium, was achieved in 97.1% of 613 patients who underwent BCE and 99.4% of the 1037 patients who underwent MIP (Fig. 4). Because of the power of this study, this small incremental improvement was statistically significant ($P<.001$). Aside from the inherent nonrandomized nature of the study, it was also subject to both referral and selection bias; the setting of the study was at a tertiary referral center and a large number of patients had negative or questionable preoperative localization studies. In addition, patients with syndromic disease and those requiring reexploration were preferentially offered a bilateral approach (21% of BCEs were reoperative cases vs 5% of MIPs). However, reoperative cases made up only 11.3% of the total.

Complications

Postoperative complications of MIP mirror those of conventional BCE and include injury to the recurrent laryngeal nerve (RLN), hematoma formation, and postoperative hypocalcemia. A key reason why focused parathyroidectomy, such as MIP, was initially advocated was to decrease the incidence of RLN injuries and postoperative hypocalcemia by leaving 1 side of the neck unexplored. Experienced endocrine surgeons report a frequency of RLN injury of less than

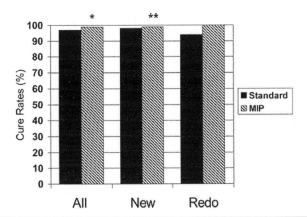

Fig. 4. Cure rates in patients undergoing standard BCEs or MIP procedures. *$P<.001$; **$P<.05$. (*From* Udelsman R, Lin Z, Donovan P. The superiority of minimally invasive parathyroidectomy based on 1650 consecutive patients with primary hyperparathyroidism. Ann Surg 2011;253(3):585–91; with permission.)

2%. In a comparison of BCE and MIP, Beyer and colleagues [73] noted 2 cases of permanent RLN injury in 109 patients undergoing BCE, whereas none of the 111 patients having MIP had an injury to the RLN, although this difference was not statistically significant. Recently, 1 study evaluating both laryngeal physiology and vocal capacity found no significant difference between preoperative and postoperative function in 104 patients undergoing MIP [74].

Postoperative hypocalcemia caused by hungry bone syndrome following parathyroidectomy for PHPT can occur regardless of surgical approach. However, a bilateral exploration resulting in mobilization of all 4 parathyroid glands can worsen this phenomenon because of iatrogenic hypoparathyroidism from surgical trauma. This effect is mitigated by the unilateral exploration performed during MIP. Bergenfelz and colleagues [75] showed in a prospective, randomized controlled trial of BCE versus MIP in 91 patients with sporadic PHPT that patients undergoing BCE had more frequent symptomatic hypocalcemia, decreased serum calcium concentration, and increased need for oral calcium consumption in the postoperative setting. All of these findings reached statistical significance. Our own study of 1650 patients with sporadic PHPT found RLN injury in 0.99% versus 0.77% of patients and hypocalcemia in 0.49% versus 0.10% of patients undergoing BCE versus MIP, respectively. Although neither of these findings reached statistical significance, when all-cause surgical morbidity was evaluated, patients undergoing BCE had an overall complication rate of 3.10% compared with 1.45% of patients undergoing MIP; this was found to be statistically significant ($P<.05$) [4].

Durability of cure

A concern regarding a focused, unilateral approach to parathyroidectomy is the possibility of missed MGD, because all 4 glands are not visualized. During MIP, this is functionally addressed by using IOPTH measurements to ensure biochemical cure before termination of the case [6,30]. When comparing frequency of MGD in patients undergoing BCE and MIP, several studies have noted a higher incidence of MGD in those treated with BCE, contributing to concerns that focused parathyroidectomy may underdiagnose MGD. One large meta-analysis of 4261 patients undergoing parathyroidectomy for nonsyndromic PHPT noted MGD in 19.3% of patients undergoing BCE compared with only 5.3% of those undergoing focused parathyroidectomy [76]. Because patients with preoperative localizing studies suggesting MGD invariably undergo BCE, a large portion of this disparity can be attributed to case selection bias. Studies evaluating the durability of cure following MIP do not support a statistically significant increase in recurrent PHPT following MIP. In a 5-year follow-up of 71 patients randomized to BCE or MIP, Westerdahl and Bergenfelz [77] noted no significant difference in biochemical recurrence between the 2 groups when analyzed by intent to treat. Of the 4 patients who recurred in the MIP group (n = 45), 3 were explored bilaterally during the initial case and 2 were later found to have MEN2 in the absence of prior family history. Aspinall and colleagues [78] evaluated long-term symptom relief using a validated survey tool assessing symptoms of hyperparathyroidism in patients undergoing MIP or BCE; again, no significant difference between the 2 was shown, although follow-up time was longer for the BCE group (41 vs 61 months). Multiple additional studies support IOPTH monitoring as the single most important adjunct for achieving successful cure during MIP [73,79,80], and, given the demonstrated durability of that cure, most endocrine surgeons routinely use IOPTH monitoring [72]. A small number of recent studies have asserted that IOPTH monitoring may not be necessary in carefully selected patients who have concordant Tc^{99m}-sestamibi scintigraphy and cervical ultrasound studies before surgery that clearly identify a single adenoma [81,82]. However, long-term outcomes following this approach have not been reported.

Economic considerations

Several investigators have evaluated the cost-effectiveness of the focused approach to parathyroidectomy. For MIP, the cost of preoperative localization and IOPTH testing is offset by potentially decreased operative times and lengths of stay. Several investigators using MIP have shown superior operative times compared with BCE [11,12]. On average, exploration takes 15 to 25 minutes less when MIP is used. Similarly, both LOS and total cost seem to favor MIP (Fig. 5). In our own experience with 1650 patients, patients who underwent BCE had a mean LOS of 1.3 days versus 0.2 days for MIP. The median LOS for patients undergoing MIP was zero, because 85% of MIP cases were performed on an ambulatory basis. Reflecting this, total hospital charges per patient (including IOPTH monitoring and preoperative localizing studies) were $1471 less for patients undergoing MIP. Currently, there is a paucity of rigorous cost-effectiveness analyses comparing MIP with BCE for PHPT; however, a recent meta-review of existing articles strongly advocated the overall

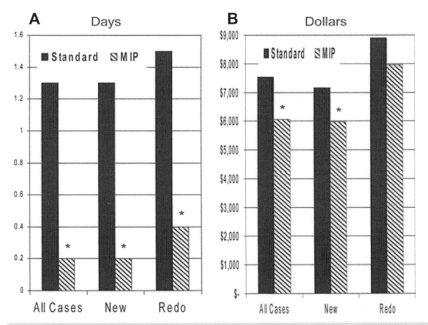

Fig. 5. (A) Mean length of hospital stay and (B) total hospital charges for patients having standard bilateral exploration. *P<.0001. New, previously unexplored patients; Redo, patients who underwent remedial surgical exploration. (*From* Udelsman R, Lin Z, Donovan P. The superiority of minimally invasive parathyroidectomy based on 1650 consecutive patients with primary hyperparathyroidism. Ann Surg 2011;253(3):585–91; with permission.)

cost-effectiveness of surgery in general for treating PHPT and favored focused parathyroidectomy as the treatment of choice [83].

Patient satisfaction

Despite the near equivalence of biochemical cure rate conveyed by both BCE and MIP approaches to parathyroidectomy for PHPT, secondary factors of patient satisfaction seem to favor MIP. Because MIP is limited to unilateral exploration, an abbreviated incision can be used compared with BCE. Brunaud and colleagues [84] noted a decrease in mean incision length from 4.1 cm to 2.8 cm when comparing BCE with focused parathyroidectomy in a case series of 67 patients (*P*<0.001). A randomized controlled trial of 48 patients comparing BCE with MIP also noted a statistically significant decrease in incision length (8.0 vs 1.9 cm) and also an increase in patient cosmetic satisfaction at 6 months after surgery, although satisfaction later equalized at 1 year [12]. The same study also documented significant decreases in pain scores, analgesia requests, and analgesia consumption in patients undergoing MIP. The intangible improvements in patient satisfaction and quality of life in patients undergoing MIP is best shown in a 2008 study by Adler and colleagues [85] comparing 98 patients undergoing MIP versus 48 that underwent BCE. The rate of complications was not significantly different between the 2 study arms. Each patient was administered a validated survey tool (SF-36, Medical Outcome Trusts) 1 week before, 1 week after, and 1 year after surgery. All patients experienced improved quality of life, but, at 1 week, patients undergoing MIP improved in 4 of 8 survey scales, whereas BCE improved in only 2. At 1 year, the MIP arm improved in all 8 categories, whereas the BCE group did so only in 4 ($P<.05$ for all).

Additional considerations

Much like other minimally invasive surgical techniques, a significant advantage of MIP is its flexibility. Conversion to BCE is easily performed when needed, such as persistently increased IOPTH measurements, because the abbreviated Kocher incision used in MIP is able to access the contralateral neck without making a second incision. Similarly, although most patients successfully tolerate MIP when performed under MAC with locoregional anesthesia, conversion to general anesthesia can be performed in a controlled fashion when necessary with protection of the surgical field [86]. Avoidance of general anesthesia also allows real-time intraoperative assessment of RLN integrity by asking the patient to phonate, and abrogates the independent 5% risk of vocal cord damage or injury conferred by endotracheal intubation or instrumentation [87].

MIP has not been formally compared with alternate focused techniques such as totally endoscopic and video-assisted parathyroidectomy, or open parathyroidectomy via a lateral neck approach. MIP has the advantage of presenting the operating surgeon with the familiar anatomy of the midline neck and a reduced learning curve. Most endocrine procedures in the United States, including parathyroidectomy, remain more frequently performed by general surgeons rather than endocrine-specific surgeons at academic centers [88], which makes this benefit more significant. MIP has been successfully used in the community hospital setting [89]. Furthermore, although exposure to parathyroidectomy during residency training varies between institutions, exposure of graduating surgical residents to endocrine cases may be severely limited in volume [90,91]. The familiar anatomy and faster learning curve of MIP for focused parathyroidectomy may mitigate some of these concerns.

SUMMARY

Because greater than 80% of spontaneous cases of primary hyperparathyroidism are caused by a single adenoma, BCE of the neck, which has long been the approach of choice, is being replaced. Focused parathyroidectomy has been made possible by advances in preoperative parathyroid localization and IOPTH monitoring, which allows confirmation of cure and confirmation of the absence of MGD without visualizing all 4 parathyroids. Several techniques for focused parathyroidectomy exist, but open MIP through an incision of 2 to 3 cm with surgeon-administered locoregional anesthesia seems to improve on the already high success rate and low morbidity associated with bilateral exploration. In addition, MIP is associated with numerous secondary benefits such as decreased hospital cost, improved patient satisfaction, decreased operative time, and same-day discharge. Bilateral exploration will remain the standard of care for most patients with multigland or syndromic disease. Most patients with sporadic PHPT are candidates for MIP.

References

[1] Melton LJ 3rd. The epidemiology of primary hyperparathyroidism in North America. J Bone Miner Res 2002;17(Suppl 2):N12–7.

[2] Wermers RA, Khosla S, Atkinson EJ, et al. Incidence of primary hyperparathyroidism in Rochester, Minnesota, 1993-2001: an update on the changing epidemiology of the disease. J Bone Miner Res 2006;21(1):171–7.

[3] Bilezikian JP, Silverberg SJ. Clinical practice. Asymptomatic primary hyperparathyroidism. N Engl J Med 2004;350(17):1746–51.

[4] Udelsman R, Lin Z, Donovan P. The superiority of minimally invasive parathyroidectomy based on 1650 consecutive patients with primary hyperparathyroidism. Ann Surg 2011;253(3):585–91.

[5] Rothe HM, Liangos O, Biggar P, et al. Cinacalcet treatment of primary hyperparathyroidism. Int J Endocrinol 2011;2011:415719.

[6] Chen H, Sokoll LJ, Udelsman R. Outpatient minimally invasive parathyroidectomy: a combination of sestamibi-SPECT localization, cervical block anesthesia, and intraoperative parathyroid hormone assay. Surgery 1999;126(6):1016–21 [discussion: 1021–2].

[7] Udelsman R. Six hundred fifty-six consecutive explorations for primary hyperparathyroidism. Ann Surg 2002;235(5):665–70 [discussion: 670–2].

[8] Gagner M. Endoscopic subtotal parathyroidectomy in patients with primary hyperparathyroidism. Br J Surg 1996;83(6):875.

[9] Miccoli P, Bendinelli C, Vignali E, et al. Endoscopic parathyroidectomy: report of an initial experience. Surgery 1998;124(6):1077–9 [discussion: 1079–80].

[10] Miccoli P, Berti P, Materazzi G, et al. Results of video-assisted parathyroidectomy: single institution's six-year experience. World J Surg 2004;28(12):1216–8.

[11] Bergenfelz A, Kanngiesser V, Zielke A, et al. Conventional bilateral cervical exploration versus open minimally invasive parathyroidectomy under local anaesthesia for primary hyperparathyroidism. Br J Surg 2005;92(2):190–7.

[12] Slepavicius A, Beisa V, Janusonis V, et al. Focused versus conventional parathyroidectomy for primary hyperparathyroidism: a prospective, randomized, blinded trial. Langenbecks Arch Surg 2008;393(5):659–66.

[13] Sandström I. Om en ny körtel hos menniskan och åtskilliga däggdjur. Ups Läk Forh 1880;15:441–71.

[14] Halsted WS, Evans HM. I. The parathyroid glandules. Their blood supply and their preservation in operation upon the thyroid gland. Ann Surg 1907;46(4):489–506.

[15] Mandl F. Versuch bei Ostitis fibrosa generalisata mittels Exstirpation eines Epithelkörperchentumors. Wien Klin Wehnschr 1925;50:1343.

[16] Albright F, Aub JC, Bauer W. Hyperparathyroidism: a common and polymorphic condition as illustrated by seventeen proved cases from one clinic. JAMA 1934;102(16):1276–87.

[17] Cope O, Keynes WM, Roth SI, et al. Primary chief-cell hyperplasia of the parathyroid glands: a new entity in the surgery of hyperparathyroidism. Ann Surg 1958;148(3):375–88.

[18] Cope O. The study of hyperparathyroidism at the Massachusetts General Hospital. N Engl J Med 1966;274(21):1174–82.

[19] Allendorf J, DiGorgi M, Spanknebel K, et al. 1112 consecutive bilateral neck explorations for primary hyperparathyroidism. World J Surg 2007;31(11):2075–80.

[20] Roth SI, Wang CA, Potts JT Jr. The team approach to primary hyperparathyroidism. Hum Pathol 1975;6(6):645–8.

[21] Tibblin S, Bondeson AG, Ljungberg O. Unilateral parathyroidectomy in hyperparathyroidism due to single adenoma. Ann Surg 1982;195(3):245–52.

[22] Doppman JL. Reoperative parathyroid surgery; localization procedures. Prog Surg 1986;18:117–32.

[23] Arima M, Yokoi H, Sonoda T. Preoperative identification of tumor of the parathyroid by ultra-sonotomography. Surg Gynecol Obstet 1975;141(2):242–4.

[24] Sample WF, Mitchell SP, Bledsoe RC. Parathyroid ultrasonography. Radiology 1978;127(2):485–90.

[25] Young AE, Gaunt JI, Croft DN, et al. Location of parathyroid adenomas by thallium-201 and technetium-99m subtraction scanning. Br Med J (Clin Res Ed) 1983;286(6375):1384–6.

[26] Coakley AJ, Kettle AG, Wells CP, et al. 99Tcm sestamibi–a new agent for parathyroid imaging. Nucl Med Commun 1989;10(11):791–4.

[27] Nussbaum SR, Thompson AR, Hutcheson KA, et al. Intraoperative measurement of parathyroid hormone in the surgical management of hyperparathyroidism. Surgery 1988;104(6): 1121–7.

[28] Davies C, Demeure MJ, St John A, et al. Study of intact (1-84) parathyroid hormone secretion in patients undergoing parathyroidectomy. World J Surg 1990;14(3):355–9 [discussion: 360].

[29] Irvin GL 3rd, Dembrow VD, Prudhomme DL. Operative monitoring of parathyroid gland hyperfunction. Am J Surg 1991;162(4):299–302.

[30] Irvin GL 3rd, Prudhomme DL, Deriso GT, et al. A new approach to parathyroidectomy. Ann Surg 1994;219(5):574–9 [discussion: 579–81].

[31] Hunter JG. Minimally invasive surgery: the next frontier. World J Surg 1999;23(4):422–4.

[32] Udelsman R, Donovan PI, Sokoll LJ. One hundred consecutive minimally invasive parathyroid explorations. Ann Surg 2000;232(3):331–9.

[33] Irvin GL 3rd, Sfakianakis G, Yeung L, et al. Ambulatory parathyroidectomy for primary hyperparathyroidism. Arch Surg 1996;131(10):1074–8.

[34] Sokoll LJ, Drew H, Udelsman R. Intraoperative parathyroid hormone analysis: a study of 200 consecutive cases. Clin Chem 2000;46(10):1662–8.

[35] Bilezikian JP, Khan AA, Potts JT Jr. Guidelines for the management of asymptomatic primary hyperparathyroidism: summary statement from the third international workshop. J Clin Endocrinol Metab 2009;94(2):335–9.

[36] Roman SA, Sosa JA, Pietrzak RH, et al. The effects of serum calcium and parathyroid hormone changes on psychological and cognitive function in patients undergoing parathyroidectomy for primary hyperparathyroidism. Ann Surg 2011;253(1):131–7.

[37] Bollerslev J, Rosen T, Mollerup CL, et al. Effect of surgery on cardiovascular risk factors in mild primary hyperparathyroidism. J Clin Endocrinol Metab 2009;94(7):2255–61.

[38] Broulik PD, Broulikova A, Adamek S, et al. Improvement of hypertension after parathyroidectomy of patients suffering from primary hyperparathyroidism. Int J Endocrinol 2011;2011:309068.

[39] Carling T, Udelsman R. Parathyroid tumors. Curr Treat Options Oncol 2003;4(4):319–28.

[40] Carling T, Udelsman R. Parathyroid surgery in familial hyperparathyroid disorders. J Intern Med 2005;257(1):27–37.

[41] Brennan MF, Doppman JL, Marx SJ, et al. Reoperative parathyroid surgery for persistent hyperparathyroidism. Surgery 1978;83(6):669–76.

[42] Erbil Y, Barbaros U, Tukenmez M, et al. Impact of adenoma weight and ectopic location of parathyroid adenoma on localization study results. World J Surg 2008;32(4):566–71.

[43] Sandrock D, Merino MJ, Norton JA, et al. Parathyroid imaging by Tc/Tl scintigraphy. Eur J Nucl Med 1990;16(8–10):607–13.

[44] Denham DW, Norman J. Cost-effectiveness of preoperative sestamibi scan for primary hyperparathyroidism is dependent solely upon the surgeon's choice of operative procedure. J Am Coll Surg 1998;186(3):293–305.

[45] Erbil Y, Barbaros U, Yanik BT, et al. Impact of gland morphology and concomitant thyroid nodules on preoperative localization of parathyroid adenomas. Laryngoscope 2006;116(4):580–5.

[46] Sukan A, Reyhan M, Aydin M, et al. Preoperative evaluation of hyperparathyroidism: the role of dual-phase parathyroid scintigraphy and ultrasound imaging. Ann Nucl Med 2008;22(2):123–31.

[47] Blanco I, Carril JM, Banzo I, et al. Double-phase Tc-99m sestamibi scintigraphy in the preoperative location of lesions causing hyperparathyroidism. Clin Nucl Med 1998;23(5):291–7.

[48] Kasai ET, da Silva JW, Mandarim de Lacerda CA, et al. Parathyroid glands: combination of sestamibi-(99m)Tc scintigraphy and ultrasonography for demonstration of hyperplasic parathyroid glands. Rev Esp Med Nucl 2008;27(1):8–12.

[49] Pappu S, Donovan P, Cheng D, et al. Sestamibi scans are not all created equally. Arch Surg 2005;140(4):383–6.

[50] Thomas DL, Bartel T, Menda Y, et al. Single photon emission computed tomography (SPECT) should be routinely performed for the detection of parathyroid abnormalities utilizing technetium-99m sestamibi parathyroid scintigraphy. Clin Nucl Med 2009;34(10):651–5.

[51] Milas M, Mensah A, Alghoul M, et al. The impact of office neck ultrasonography on reducing unnecessary thyroid surgery in patients undergoing parathyroidectomy. Thyroid 2005;15(9):1055–9.

[52] Berber E, Parikh RT, Ballem N, et al. Factors contributing to negative parathyroid localization: an analysis of 1000 patients. Surgery 2008;144(1):74–9.

[53] Haber RS, Kim CK, Inabnet WB. Ultrasonography for preoperative localization of enlarged parathyroid glands in primary hyperparathyroidism: comparison with (99m)technetium sestamibi scintigraphy. Clin Endocrinol 2002;57(2):241–9.

[54] Rickes S, Sitzy J, Neye H, et al. High-resolution ultrasound in combination with colour-Doppler sonography for preoperative localization of parathyroid adenomas in patients with primary hyperparathyroidism. Ultraschall Med 2003;24(2):85–9.

[55] Siperstein A, Berber E, Mackey R, et al. Prospective evaluation of sestamibi scan, ultrasonography, and rapid PTH to predict the success of limited exploration for sporadic primary hyperparathyroidism. Surgery 2004;136(4):872–80.

[56] Solorzano CC, Carneiro-Pla DM, Irvin GL 3rd. Surgeon-performed ultrasonography as the initial and only localizing study in sporadic primary hyperparathyroidism. J Am Coll Surg 2006;202(1):18–24.

[57] Ruda JM, Hollenbeak CS, Stack BC Jr. A systematic review of the diagnosis and treatment of primary hyperparathyroidism from 1995 to 2003. Otolaryngol Head Neck Surg 2005;132(3):359–72.

[58] Lumachi F, Ferretti G, Povolato M, et al. Usefulness of 99m-Tc-sestamibi scintimammography in suspected breast cancer and in axillary lymph node metastases detection. Eur J Surg Oncol 2001;27(3):256–9.

[59] Melton GB, Somervell H, Friedman KP, et al. Interpretation of 99mTc sestamibi parathyroid SPECT scan is improved when read by the surgeon and nuclear medicine physician together. Nucl Med Commun 2005;26(7):633–8.

[60] Johnson NA, Tublin ME, Ogilvie JB. Parathyroid imaging: technique and role in the preoperative evaluation of primary hyperparathyroidism. AJR Am J Roentgenol 2007;188(6):1706–15.

[61] Rodgers SE, Hunter GJ, Hamberg LM, et al. Improved preoperative planning for directed parathyroidectomy with 4-dimensional computed tomography. Surgery 2006;140(6):932–40 [discussion: 940–1].

[62] Starker LF, Mahajan A, Bjorklund P, et al. 4D parathyroid CT as the initial localization study for patients with de novo primary hyperparathyroidism. Ann Surg Oncol 2011;18(6):1723–8.

[63] Gotway MB, Reddy GP, Webb WR, et al. Comparison between MR imaging and 99mTc MIBI scintigraphy in the evaluation of recurrent of persistent hyperparathyroidism. Radiology 2001;218(3):783–90.

[64] Ruf J, Lopez Hanninen E, Steinmuller T, et al. Preoperative localization of parathyroid glands. Use of MRI, scintigraphy, and image fusion. Nuklearmedizin 2004;43(3):85–90.

[65] Ditkoff BA, Chabot J, Feind C, et al. Parathyroid surgery using monitored anesthesia care as an alternative to general anesthesia. Am J Surg 1996;172(6):698–700.

[66] Chen H, Pruhs Z, Starling JR, et al. Intraoperative parathyroid hormone testing improves cure rates in patients undergoing minimally invasive parathyroidectomy. Surgery 2005;138(4):583–7 [discussion: 587–90].

[67] Fraker DL, Harsono H, Lewis R. Minimally invasive parathyroidectomy: benefits and requirements of localization, diagnosis, and intraoperative PTH monitoring. long-term results. World J Surg 2009;33(11):2256–65.

[68] Lo Gerfo P. Bilateral neck exploration for parathyroidectomy under local anesthesia: a viable technique for patients with coexisting thyroid disease with or without sestamibi scanning. Surgery 1999;126(6):1011–4 [discussion: 1014–5].

[69] Aarum S, Nordenstrom J, Reihner E, et al. Operation for primary hyperparathyroidism: the new versus the old order. A randomised controlled trial of preoperative localisation. Scand J Surg 2007;96(1):26–30.

[70] Grant CS, Thompson G, Farley D, et al. Primary hyperparathyroidism surgical management since the introduction of minimally invasive parathyroidectomy: Mayo Clinic experience. Arch Surg 2005;140(5):472–8 [discussion: 478–9].

[71] Seving AI, Derici ZS, Bekis R, et al. Success of minimally invasive single-gland exploration using the quick intraoperative parathyroid assay. Acta Chir Belg 2010;110(4): 463–6.

[72] Sackett WR, Barraclough B, Reeve TS, et al. Worldwide trends in the surgical treatment of primary hyperparathyroidism in the era of minimally invasive parathyroidectomy. Arch Surg 2002;137(9):1055–9.

[73] Beyer TD, Solorzano CC, Starr F, et al. Parathyroidectomy outcomes according to operative approach. Am J Surg 2007;193(3):368–72 [discussion: 372–3].

[74] Leder SB, DP, Acton LM, et al. Laryngeal physiology and voice acoustics are maintained after minimally invasive parathyroidectomy. Ann Surg 2012, in press.

[75] Bergenfelz A, Lindblom P, Tibblin S, et al. Unilateral versus bilateral neck exploration for primary hyperparathyroidism: a prospective randomized controlled trial. Ann Surg 2002;236(5):543–51.

[76] Lee NC, Norton JA. Multiple-gland disease in primary hyperparathyroidism: a function of operative approach? Arch Surg 2002;137(8):896–9 [discussion: 899–900].

[77] Westerdahl J, Bergenfelz A. Unilateral versus bilateral neck exploration for primary hyperparathyroidism: five-year follow-up of a randomized controlled trial. Ann Surg 2007;246(6):976–80 [discussion: 980–1].

[78] Aspinall SR, Boase S, Malycha P. Long-term symptom relief from primary hyperparathyroidism following minimally invasive parathyroidectomy. World J Surg 2010;34(9): 2223–7.

[79] Chen H, Mack E, Starling JR. A comprehensive evaluation of perioperative adjuncts during minimally invasive parathyroidectomy: which is most reliable? Ann Surg 2005;242(3): 375–80 [discussion: 380–3].

[80] Nagar S, Reid D, Czako P, et al. Outcomes analysis of intraoperative adjuncts during minimally invasive parathyroidectomy for primary hyperparathyroidism. Am J Surg 2012;203(2):177–81.

[81] Gawande AA, Monchik JM, Abbruzzese TA, et al. Reassessment of parathyroid hormone monitoring during parathyroidectomy for primary hyperparathyroidism after 2 preoperative localization studies. Arch Surg 2006;141(4):381–4 [discussion: 384].

[82] Smith N, Magnuson JS, Vidrine DM, et al. Minimally invasive parathyroidectomy: use of intraoperative parathyroid hormone assays after 2 preoperative localization studies. Arch Otolaryngol Head Neck Surg 2009;135(11):1108–11.

[83] Zanocco K, Heller M, Sturgeon C. Cost-effectiveness of parathyroidectomy for primary hyperparathyroidism. Endocr Pract 2011;17(Suppl 1):69–74.

[84] Brunaud L, Zarnegar R, Wada N, et al. Incision length for standard thyroidectomy and para-thyroidectomy: when is it minimally invasive? Arch Surg 2003;138(10):1140–3.

[85] Adler JT, Sippel RS, Chen H. The influence of surgical approach on quality of life after para-thyroid surgery. Ann Surg Oncol 2008;15(6):1559–65.

[86] Carling T, Donovan P, Rinder C, et al. Minimally invasive parathyroidectomy using cervical block: reasons for conversion to general anesthesia. Arch Surg 2006;141(4):401–4 [discussion: 404].

[87] Stojadinovic A, Shaha AR, Orlikoff RF, et al. Prospective functional voice assessment in patients undergoing thyroid surgery. Ann Surg 2002;236(6):823–32.

[88] Saunders BD, Wainess RM, Dimick JB, et al. Who performs endocrine operations in the United States? Surgery 2003;134(6):924–31 [discussion: 931].

[89] Vaid S, Pandelidis S. Minimally invasive parathyroidectomy: a community hospital experience. Arch Surg 2011;146(7):876–8.

[90] Chen H, Hardacre JM, Martin C, et al. Do future general surgery residents have adequate exposure to endocrine surgery during medical school? World J Surg 2002;26(1):17–21.

[91] Udelsman R. Unilateral neck exploration under local or regional anesthesia. In: Gagner M, Inabnet WB, editors. Minimally invasive endocrine surgery. Philadelphia: Lippincott, Williams & Wilkins; 2002. p. 93–102.

Current Treatment of Papillary Thyroid Microcarcinoma

Xiao-Min Yu, MD, PhD[a], Ricardo Lloyd, MD, PhD[b],
Herbert Chen, MD[c],*

[a]Department of Surgery, University of Wisconsin, 600 Highland Avenue, K3-705 Clinical Science Center, Madison, WI 53792, USA; [b]Department of Pathology, University of Wisconsin, 600 Highland Avenue, K3-705 Clinical Science Center, Madison, WI 53792, USA; [c]Division of General Surgery, Department of Surgery, University of Wisconsin, 600 Highland Avenue, K3-705 Clinical Science Center, Madison, WI 53792, USA

Keywords
• Papillary thyroid microcarcinoma • Thyroid cancer • Prognostic factors
• Treatment • ATA guidelines

Key Points
• Papillary thyroid microcarcinoma (PTMC) is being diagnosed with increasing frequency.
• Better prognostic stratification, especially for high-risk patients, helps to optimize surgical care.
• Total or near-total thyroidectomy is advocated as the initial therapy for most primary PTMCs.
• Neck dissection is only recommended by ATA with the presence of cervical lymphadenopathy or T4 tumors.
• Post-operative RAI ablations are suggested be administrated to patients with gross extrathyroidal invasion or distant metastases.

According to World Health Organization, Papillary thyroid microcarcinomas (PTMCs) are papillary thyroid cancers (PTCs) measuring 1 cm or less. The increase in incidence of PTMC to more than 400% during the last 3 decades [1] makes it to be the most commonly occurring PTC in the United States [2]. Despite the notable increasing incidence of PTMC, the optimal treatment of these patients remains controversial, ranging from observation to total thyroidectomy [3]. Recently, several evidence-based guidelines for the management of thyroid cancer have been published, including the consensus statements from the American Thyroid Association (ATA) and European Thyroid Association (ETA) [4,5]. These guidelines

*Corresponding author. K3/705 Clinical Science Center, 600 Highland Avenue, Madison, WI 53792. E-mail address: chen@surgery.wisc.edu

0065-3411/12/$ – see front matter
doi:10.1016/j.yasu.2012.03.002

recommend that the initial surgery type and postoperative care need to be determined depending on the different features of PTMC. The current treatment modality for PTMC has emphasized more on the individualized therapy based on a better prognosis stratification, especially for high-risk patients.

DIAGNOSIS

PTMC, as a subtype of PTC, originates from thyroid follicular cells and has been estimated to account for 30% to 40% of all PTC cases [6]. Depending on the circumstances of detection, PTMC has been broadly classified into 3 categories (Box 1) [7].

Among these 3 categories of PTMC, the first 2 are common clinical scenarios that surgeons encounter. The diagnosis of PTMC, unlike that of other malignancies, is mostly based on imaging and cytologic examinations because PTMCs are usually asymptomatic and rarely detected by physical examinations. Physical examinations including palpation of the thyroid gland are dependent on the patient's characteristics and the experience of the examiner. Thyroid nodule with a diameter of 0.5 cm may be palpable in a patient with a long thin neck, whereas nodules greater than 2.0 cm could be missed in a short fat neck. By palpation even individuals with experienced hands miss 76% of the nodules that were detected by pathologic examinations. In these impalpable nodules, 85% were large nodules with diameters greater than 1.0 cm [8]. Therefore, imaging studies and cytologic examinations are the most common and reliable way to diagnose PTMC preoperatively.

Neck ultrasonography, because of its noninvasive nature and improved technology, is now used as the first option in all the imaging studies for the screening of thyroid diseases. Ultrasonography facilitates the detection of small thyroid nodules measuring 3.0 mm or larger. On ultrasonography, the composition of PTMC typically appears to be completely or predominantly solid (Fig. 1). Some PTMCs present as irregular-shaped small nodules with ill-defined nodule margins

---

Box 1: Classification of PTMC based on the methods of detection

- Incidental PTMC
  - PTMC incidentally detected by pathologic examination of the surgical specimens from the thyroid resected for other diseases; or
  - PTMC incidentally detected by imaging studies for other purposes such as screening studies for thyroid diseases
- Occult PTMC
  - PTMC discovered as the origin of lymph node and/or distant metastases
- Latent PTMC
  - PTMC incidentally detected in autopsy specimens

Data from Ito Y, Miyauchi A. A therapeutic strategy for incidentally detected papillary microcarcinoma of the thyroid. Nat Clin Pract Endocrinol Metab 2007;3(3):240–8.

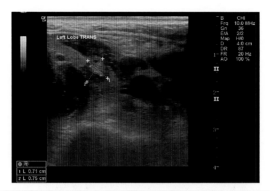

Fig. 1. Neck ultrasonography revealing a microcarcinoma measuring around 0.7 cm in the left lobe of thyroid (*indicated by the dotted lines*). (*Courtesy of* Dr Rebecca S. Sippel, Madison, WI.)

or punctate calcifications, which are helpful to differentiate malignant nodules from benign ones. However, the diagnostic sensitivity and specificity of ultrasonography alone are not satisfactory.

Ultrasonography-guided fine-needle aspiration biopsy (FNAB) has been widely accepted as the most crucial step in the preoperative assessment of a thyroid nodule because it provides the most specific information about the cellular composition of a nodule. Between 250,000 and 300,000 of FNABs were estimated to be performed annually in the United States alone [9]. Although practice guidelines set forth by the ATA state that FNAB should be used as one of the initial diagnostic tests for thyroid nodules because of its high diagnostic reliability and cost-effectiveness, FNAB is not indicated routinely for thyroid nodules less than 1 cm by the guidelines [10]. The decision regarding the biopsy of suspicious small lesions is dependent on the performer. Surgeon-performed ultrasonography (SPUS) or ultrasonography-guided FNAB has become a new trend during recent years. Mazzaglia [11] has reported that SPUS in patients referred for thyroid disease improves patient care by minimizing the use of unnecessary procedures. Among 364 consecutive patients referred for endocrine surgical evaluation of thyroid disease, 64 (19.2%) had findings on the SPUS that significantly differed from those on the pre-referral study. Those differences led to a change in the management of 58 patients (17.4%) [11]. In another study, features defined by SPUS can predict benignity in thyroid nodules with a specificity as high as 98.5% [12]. Because SPUS substantially benefits patient care and affects surgical decision making, it is highly recommended as a valuable adjunct to endocrine surgical practice [13].

Onsite cytopathologic review is usually performed to ensure the adequacy of the samples from FNAB. The characteristic cytologic features of papillary lesions include irregular nuclei, nuclear clearing, and prominent nuclear grooves (Fig. 2). The other important diagnostic standard for PTMC is the histopathological evaluation of a surgical specimen. Incidental or occult PTMCs can sometimes be as

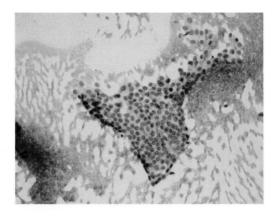

Fig. 2. Fine-needle aspiration biopsy of a papillary thyroid microcarcinoma showing sheets of tumor cells with irregular nuclei, nuclear clearing, and prominent nuclear grooves. Many red blood cells are present in the background (Papanicolaou stain, original magnification ×60).

small as a single follicle but has the architectural and cytologic features of papillary carcinoma. Fig. 3 shows a typical microscopic view of an encapsulated PTMC, showing papillae with fibrovascular cores, prominent nuclear clearing, and enlarged overlapping nuclei in a background containing nonneoplastic thyroid follicles. Histopathological evaluations also provide specific information on whether PTMC shows extrathyroidal invasion, multifocality, or lymph node metastases. These data are essential to predict the prognosis and helpful to direct the treatment plan as well.

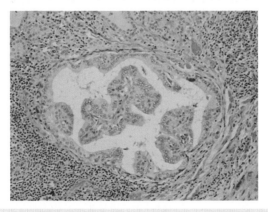

Fig. 3. Histopathologic view of a papillary thyroid microcarcinoma. Hematoxylin-Eosin–stained section of an encapsulated papillary thyroid microcarcinoma showing papillae with fibrovascular cores, prominent nuclear clearing and enlarged overlapping nuclei. The background contains nonneoplastic thyroid follicles and many lymphocytes (original magnification ×100).

PROGNOSIS AND PROGNOSTIC FACTORS

The overall survival for well-differentiated thyroid carcinoma including papillary carcinoma is greater than 90% [14] and is even better for PTMC. In a recent study of more than 18,000 PTMC cases using a large national cancer database, the 10-year and 15-year overall survivals for PTMC was reported to be 95% and 91%, respectively. In addition, the 10-year disease-specific survival is approximately 99.5%, which suggests that 0.5% patients may die of PTMC [15]. There is no doubt that PTMC is not homogeneous, and better prognosis stratification, especially for high-risk patients, optimizes surgical care. During the past 3 decades, a group of valuable prognostic factors have been identified and validated based on multifactorial analysis of many retrospective studies. These factors, with different combinations, were developed into several well-known prognostic scoring systems including AMES, MACIS, which are commonly used perioperatively to guide surgical therapy (Box 2).

Age and gender

Unique to differentiated thyroid cancer is the fact that age is a key prognostic indicator for these patients. A recent report from the Surveillance, Epidemiology, and End Results program showed that the death rate from thyroid cancer is 2.7/100,000 in patients older than 65 whereas it is only 0.1/100,000 in patients younger than 65, a difference of greater than 25 fold. This phenomenon is reflected in almost all of the current staging systems including AMES, MACIS, and pTNM systems [16–19]. Patient age has been confirmed to significantly affect survival in a population-based study recently. In the multivariate analysis, patients older than 45 years exhibited a much worse survival with overwhelmingly high hazard

---

Box 2: Prognostic scoring systems for PTMC. Prognostic factors such as age and distant metastases are commonly shared among these systems developed by different institutions

Center (where the system was developed)	Scoring system	Year of publication
MSKCC	GAMES: grade, age, distant metastasis, extrathyroidal extension, size	1992
Mayo Clinic	AGES: age, grade, extrathyroidal extension, size	1987 1993
	MACIS: distant metastasis, age, completeness of resection, invasion, size	
Lahey Clinic	AMES: age, distant metastasis, extrathyroidal extension, size	1988
Karolinska Hospital and Institute	DAMES: DNA ploidy, age, distant metastasis, extrathyroidal extension, size	1992

Abbreviation: MSKCC, Memorial Sloan-Kettering Cancer Center.
Data from Mazeh H, Chen H. Advances in surgical therapy for thyroid cancer. Nat Rev Endocrinol 2011;7(10):581–8.

ratio of 6.18, which made age stand out as the most powerful prognostic factor among all the factors analyzed [15]. Gender is regarded as a risk factor only in AMES system. AMES defines its high-risk patients as men older than 40 years or women older than 50 years, which obviously suggests a less favorable prognosis in the male gender [18]. In our study, male patients revealed less than twice of the hazard ratio compared with female patients which may explain why gender is not usually considered as a prognostic factor in other staging systems, because it is a relatively weak factor.

Size

The average size of PTMC is 5 to 6 mm according to the literature [20]. Size does matter for a lot of malignancies including classical PTC. Most of the current staging systems use 2 cm and 4 cm as the cut-off value to differentiate between low- and high-risk tumors. However, it remains controversial whether size serves as a prognostic factor for PTMC. As early as in 1987, the terms tiny referring to 5 to 10 mm diameter foci and minute to foci of 5 mm diameter or less were proposed because of the difference in the incidences of lymph node metastasis in these 2 groups (59% vs 13%) and the incidence for extrathyroidal invasion (10% vs 3%) [21]. Although tumor size larger than 5 mm was found to be associated with recurrent PTMC in a univariate model, it was not significantly related either with disease-free survival or with overall survival in the multivariate analysis [15,22,23].

Extrathyroidal invasion

This is another important risk factor that all of the staging algorithms take into account. The occurrence rate of extrathyroidal invasion for PTMC varies a lot from different studies, which range from 2% to 21% [20,24]. This large variation may be accounted for by different locations of the PTMC. Microcarcinomas close to the thyroid capsule may be more likely to show extrathyroidal invasion. TNM system defines T4 disease as tumor of any size extending beyond thyroid capsule. Depending on the location of tumor extension, T4 disease can be further categorized into T4a or T4b.

Multifocality

When PTMC is detected, it is often multifocal in nature (20%–46% of cases) with no clear tendency to be localized to the same lobe [20,25], especially in patients with 2 or more foci in the resected lobe who will have an increased risk of additional foci in the contralateral lobe. Although multifocality is not considered as a prognostic factor in any of the current staging systems, the literature to date indicates that multifocality is associated with a higher rate of tumor recurrence. In one study, only 1.2% of patients with unifocal disease had recurrent cancer, whereas the recurrence rate reached 8.6% in patients with multifocal disease [26]. Similar observations were reported in another study showing a 5.6-fold increased risk for cervical lymph node recurrence when multifocal disease was present at diagnosis [27].

Lymph node metastasis

A variety of studies have been focused on the importance and prognostic value of lymph node metastases in PTMC. Approximately 25% to 43% of all patients with PTMC have been reported to have lymph node involvement without lymph node dissection routinely performed in the study cohorts [20]. This rate can be as high as 64% if all of the patients with PTMC undergo lymph node dissection at the time of thyroidectomy [28]. The correlation between lymph node metastases and tumor recurrence has been confirmed in different aspects by many studies [29–31]. In addition, lymph node involvement has prognostic value in predicting survival as well [32,33]. Recent findings showed that patients with PTMC also with lymph node metastases had a poorer overall survival than those without lymph node metastases [15].

Distant metastasis

The rate of distant metastasis seems to be very low in patients with PTMC and has been reported to be between 0.2% and 2.85% based on 3 studies in patients with PTMC [10,26,27]. Patients with distant metastasis have a significantly worse prognosis than patients without distant metastasis, which is similar to those associated with PTMC.

Molecular biomarkers

DNA ploidy has been shown to be a powerful prognostic factor, with aneuploidy conferring increased risk of distant metastasis and death. DNA ploidy was added to AMES system and renamed as DAMES in 1992 [34]. Although DNA ploidy is undoubtedly useful, it is very time-consuming and expensive, which prevents it from being widely adopted. Other molecular markers such as BRAF mutations have been extensively investigated recently with more and more evidence showing their usefulness to predict PTMC aggressiveness [35,36]. However, none of them has been incorporated with any of the staging systems as of yet. Future studies are urged to investigate the prognostic value of these markers and their use in decision-making algorithm.

Based on the above discussion, the American Joint Committee on Cancer (AJCC)/pTNM staging system has incorporated the 4 most potent prognostic factors (age, extrathyroidal invasion, lymph node, and distant metastasis) with a simple algorithm. According to its algorithm for well-differentiated thyroid cancer, PTMCs can be ranged from stage I to the highest stage of IVC (Box 3). Age is a key prognostic factor in pTNM staging system. For example, the tumor stage will be stage II if a PTMC patient with distant metastasis is younger than 45 years, whereas it will be more advanced to stage IVC if the patient is older than 45 years. AJCC/pTNM is the most widely adopted cancer staging system and is strongly recommend by ATA guidelines as a necessary evaluation for disease mortality.

TREATMENT

Because of the indolent nature of most PTMCs, there used to be a lot of debate on the appropriate treatment of PTMC, including the necessity for surgery, the

Box 3: TNM classification system for PTMC

Stage	Patient age <45 year	Patient age 45 years or older
Stage I	Any T, any N, M0	T1, N0, M0
Stage II	Any T, any N, M1	
Stage III		T1, N1a, M0
Stage IVA		T4a, N0, M0
		T4a, N1a, M0
		T4a, N1b, M0
Stage IVB		T4b, Any N, M0
Stage IVC		Any T, Any N, M1

T1, tumor diameter 2 cm or smaller; T4a: tumor of any size extending beyond the thyroid capsule to invade subcutaneous soft tissues, larynx, trachea, esophagus, or recurrent laryngeal nerve; T4b: tumor invades prevertebral fascia or encases carotid artery or mediastinal vessels.

N0, no metastatic nodes; N1a: metastases to level VI (pretracheal, paratracheal, and prelaryngeal/Delphian lymph nodes; N1b: metastases to unilateral, bilateral, contralateral cervical or superior mediastinal nodes.

M0, no distant metastases; M1: distant metastases.

Data from Greene FL, Page DL, Fleming ID, et al. AJCC Cancer Staging Manual. 6th edition. New York: Springer-Verlag; 2002.

extent of the surgery, and the proper indications for adjuvant therapies, such as radioactive iodine (RAI) ablation. The recently released ATA guidelines for patients with thyroid nodules and differentiated thyroid cancer present a range of views in relation to the management of PTMC, which try to clarify some misunderstandings and set up certain standards for the treatment of PTMC based on evidence from contemporary literature. Fig. 4 demonstrates a simplified flow chart summarizing the recommended treatment strategy for PTMC according to ATA guidelines.

Surgery

Surgery is recommended as the initial treatment of primary PTMC by guidelines of both ATA and ETA. Some studies found that close observation alone can also result in satisfactory patient outcomes [7]. In one study that followed 162 patients with PTMC who chose observation, 70% of tumors were stable over a mean follow-up time of 3.8 years [37]. Then, is surgicHematoxylinmor resection required at all? The answer is definitely yes. In the same study, the rest of the 570 patients preferred surgery to observation and another 56 patients who initially elected observation ultimately underwent surgery. Most patients would prefer therapy to observation once carcinoma is diagnosed. Some targeted drug therapies, such as histone deacetylase inhibitors, can inhibit the growth of well-differentiated thyroid cancer [38], which might be promising as the adjuvant treatment of more advanced thyroid cancer, but no evidence to date shows they can replace surgery as the initial treatment of PTMC.

The next question is regarding the type of the surgery and whether total or near-total thyroidectomy (leaving <3 gm of thyroid tissue) is preferable to

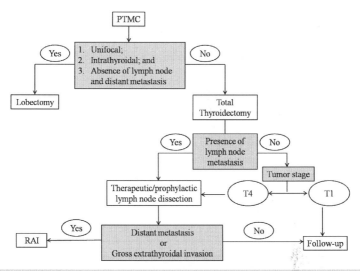

Fig. 4. Simplified flow chart of therapeutic strategy for PTMC. (*Data from* Cooper DS, Doherty GM, Haugen BR, et al. Revised American Thyroid Association management guidelines for patients with thyroid nodules and differentiated thyroid cancer. Thyroid 2009;19(11):1167–214.)

thyroid lobectomy for the treatment of PTMC. As mentioned in the previous section, PTMC is characterized by a high incidence of multifocality. In addition, some studies also revealed a 15% to 20% rate of contralateral lobe involvement with at least 1 other focus found in patients initially thought to have just 1 focus before total thyroidectomy was done [23,26]. The surprisingly high proportion of patients in these series with bilateral or multifocal disease suggests that residual tumor may frequently be left behind in the contralateral lobe if lobectomy is performed. The recurrence rate for patients with multifocality undergoing total thyroidectomy has been found to be between 2.3% and 5%, whereas patients who had lobectomy and/or isthmusectomy revealed a much higher recurrence rate between 8.2% and 25%. In contrast, only 3% to 4% of patients with unifocal PTMCs had recurrence if managed by lobectomy and isthmusectomy [10,26,27]. Similar findings were reported in another study, which recruited more than 600 patients with PTMC [39]. Based on this evidence, total or near-total thyroidectomy is preferred for most patients with PTMC as the initial surgery type especially for those present with multifocal lesions, which helps to avoid the risk of tumor recurrence. Thyroid lobectomy should only be performed in patients in whom it is certainly known that the tumor is unifocal and intrathyroidal without the presence of any lymph node or distant metastases [10].

The extent of surgery is another debated issue because of the high frequency of lymph node metastases of PTMC. Lymph node metastasis is closely associated with increased risk of tumor recurrence in PTC. The average recurrence rate in patients with metastatic lymph nodes is around 25%, whereas it is only 10% in patients without metastatic lymph nodes [33,40,41]. In addition, the risk of distant metastasis is also increased with the presence of cervical lymphade-nopathy [27]. Modified radical neck dissection in patients with PTMC also with ultrasonography-documented abnormal lymph nodes has been shown to potentially improve recurrence-free survival [42]. Thus, patients found to have abnormal cervical lymph nodes preoperatively, especially palpable nodes, should undergo total thyroidectomy together with therapeutic lymph node dissection. But, is there a role for prophylactic neck dissection in the surgical treatment for PTMC patients? Wada and colleagues [28] reported that 64% of all PTMCs had central node involvement after they followed a group of 259 patients, all of whom underwent lymph node dissection at the time of thyroid-ectomy. The investigators concluded that routine therapeutic lymph node dissec-tion at the time of thyroidectomy was necessary in patients with PTMC with palpable lymph nodes at presentation and that prophylactic lymph node dissection was not useful in patients without palpable lymphadenopathy. On the contrary, in a more recent study, prophylactic central lymph node dissection was shown to successfully manage the subclinical central lymph node metastases in PTMC with 0% recurrent rate during a 3-year follow-up [43]. Recommendation 27 from ATA guidelines suggests that prophylactic central compartment neck dissec-tion may be performed in patients with clinically uninvolved central neck lymph nodes, especially for advanced primary tumors (T3 or T4). Therefore, prophy-lactic neck dissection could be considered for the patients with PTMC with gross extrathyroidal extension, but not for the majority of patients.

RAI ablation

Ablation with RAI after surgery is used to destroy any remaining thyroid remnant after total/near-total thyroidectomy. Although RAI ablation may improve the sensitivity of thyroglobulin (Tg) levels and whole body scan (WBS) imaging in follow-up monitoring for PTMC progression, the adminis-tration of RAI ablation to patients with PTMC is generally not recommended because it has not been shown to reduce mortality or recurrence, especially for low-risk cases. Multifocality and cervical lymphadenopathy are associated with an increased recurrence rate, but it remains unproven that RAI decreases the risk. Studies have not found any benefit for the use of RAI in patients with PTMC when multiple foci are present [24]. RAI is recommended to be used in patients in whom worrisome features are present and especially in patients with gross extrathyroidal extension and distant metastasis [10].

Postoperative monitoring

Patients with PTMC older than 45 years, extrathyroidal invasion, and lymph node or distant metastasis are considered as at high risk, and thus require more intensive postoperative monitoring. The workup for postoperative monitoring is mainly dependent on neck ultrasonography because RAI ablation is not universally done in patients with PTMC. Laboratory testing for Tg as well as Tg antibody (Tg Ab) levels and WBS can be performed after RAI ablation if necessary. Tg and Tg Ab levels help to detect persistent or recurrent dis-ease when the results of ultrasonography are negative. In addition, for Tg

Ab-negative patients, thyrotropin (TSH)-stimulated serum Tg values are highly predictive of long-term outcome. A recent study has shown a 1% relapse rate and no distant metastases in the patients with initial TSH-stimulated Tg less than 1 ng/mL; a 16% relapse rate in those with Tg levels ranging within 1– to 10 ng/mL; and a 68% recurrence rate in those with serum Tg values greater than 10 ng/mL [23]. Therefore, patients with PTMC who are Tg Ab-negative and have an undetectable initial stimulated serum Tg values, can be regarded as cured and require only minimal long-term monitoring. Patients with a higher initial stimulated serum Tg values than 10 ng/mL may have persistent tumor and should be followed closely [44].

SUMMARY

PTMC is being diagnosed with increasing frequency and generally has an excellent prognosis with less than 0.5% disease-specific mortality. Better prognostic stratification, especially for high-risk patients, helps to optimize surgical care. Older age, extrathyroidal invasion, lymph node involvement, and distant metastases are usually regarded as the most potent risk factors for patients with PTMC. Total or near-total thyroidectomy is advocated as the initial therapy for most primary PTMCs, whereas neck dissection is only recommended with the presence of cervical lymphadenopathy or T4 tumors. ATA suggests that postoperative RAI ablations be administered to patients with gross extrathyroidal invasion or distant metastases. RAI ablation may also facilitate the use of serum Tg concentrations for postoperative risk assessment.

References

[1] Cramer JD, Fu P, Harth KC, et al. Analysis of the rising incidence of thyroid cancer using the Surveillance, Epidemiology and End Results national cancer data registry. Surgery 2010;148(6):1147–52 [discussion: 1152–3].

[2] Hughes DT, Haymart MR, Miller BS, et al. The most commonly occurring papillary thyroid cancer in the United States is now a microcarcinoma in a patient older than 45 years. Thyroid 2011;21(3):231–6.

[3] Haymart MR, Cayo M, Chen H. Papillary thyroid microcarcinomas: big decisions for a small tumor. Ann Surg Oncol 2009;16(11):3132–9.

[4] Cooper DS, Doherty GM, Haugen BR, et al. Management guidelines for patients with thyroid nodules and differentiated thyroid cancer. Thyroid 2006;16(2):109–42.

[5] Pacini F, Schlumberger M, Dralle H, et al. European consensus for the management of patients with differentiated thyroid carcinoma of the follicular epithelium. Eur J Endocrinol 2006;154(6):787–803.

[6] Mazeh H, Chen H. Advances in surgical therapy for thyroid cancer. Nat Rev Endocrinol 2011;7(10):581–8.

[7] Ito Y, Miyauchi A. A therapeutic strategy for incidentally detected papillary microcarcinoma of the thyroid. Nat Clin Pract Endocrinol Metab 2007;3(3):240–8.

[8] Witterick IJ, Abel SM, Noyek AM, et al. Nonpalpable occult and metastatic papillary thyroid carcinoma. Laryngoscope 1993;103(2):149–55.

[9] Gharib H. Fine-needle aspiration biopsy of thyroid nodules: advantages, limitations, and effect. Mayo Clin Proc 1994;69(1):44–9.

[10] Cooper DS, Doherty GM, Haugen BR, et al. Revised American Thyroid Association management guidelines for patients with thyroid nodules and differentiated thyroid cancer. Thyroid 2009;19(11):1167–214.

[11] Mazzaglia PJ. Surgeon-performed ultrasound in patients referred for thyroid disease improves patient care by minimizing performance of unnecessary procedures and optimizing surgical treatment. World J Surg 2010;34(6):1164–70.

[12] Goldfarb M, Gondek S, Solorzano C, et al. Surgeon-performed ultrasound can predict benignity in thyroid nodules. Surgery 2011;150(3):436–41.

[13] Milas M, Stephen A, Berber E, et al. Ultrasonography for the endocrine surgeon: a valuable clinical tool that enhances diagnostic and therapeutic outcomes. Surgery 2005;138(6): 1193–200 [discussion: 1200–1].

[14] Sherman SI. Thyroid carcinoma. Lancet 2003;361(9356):501–11.

[15] Yu XM, Wan Y, Sippel RS, et al. Should all papillary thyroid microcarcinomas be aggressively treated? An analysis of 18,445 cases. Ann Surg 2011;254(4):653–60.

[16] Hay ID, Grant CS, Taylor WF, et al. Ipsilateral lobectomy versus bilateral lobar resection in papillary thyroid carcinoma: a retrospective analysis of surgical outcome using a novel prognostic scoring system. Surgery 1987;102(6):1088–95.

[17] Hay ID, Bergstralh EJ, Goellner JR, et al. Predicting outcome in papillary thyroid carcinoma: development of a reliable prognostic scoring system in a cohort of 1779 patients surgically treated at one institution during 1940 through 1989. Surgery 1993;114(6):1050–7 [discussion: 1057–8].

[18] Cady B, Rossi R. An expanded view of risk-group definition in differentiated thyroid carcinoma. Surgery 1988;104(6):947–53.

[19] Greene FL, Page DL, Fleming ID, et al. AJCC cancer staging manual. 6th edition. New York: Springer-Verlag; 2002.

[20] Bernet V. Approach to the patient with incidental papillary microcarcinoma. J Clin Endocrinol Metab 2010;95(8):3586–92.

[21] Kasai N, Sakamoto A. New subgrouping of small thyroid carcinomas. Cancer 1987;60(8): 1767–70.

[22] Giordano D, Gradoni P, Oretti G, et al. Treatment and prognostic factors of papillary thyroid microcarcinoma. Clin Otolaryngol 2010;35(2):118–24.

[23] Pellegriti G, Scollo C, Lumera G, et al. Clinical behavior and outcome of papillary thyroid cancers smaller than 1.5 cm in diameter: study of 299 cases. J Clin Endocrinol Metab 2004;89(8):3713–20.

[24] Hay ID, Hutchinson ME, Gonzalez-Losada T, et al. Papillary thyroid microcarcinoma: a study of 900 cases observed in a 60-year period. Surgery 2008;144(6):980–7 [discussion: 987–8].

[25] Piersanti M, Ezzat S, Asa SL. Controversies in papillary microcarcinoma of the thyroid. Endocr Pathol 2003;14(3):183–91.

[26] Baudin E, Travagli JP, Ropers J, et al. Microcarcinoma of the thyroid gland: the Gustave-Roussy Institute experience. Cancer 1998;83(3):553–9.

[27] Chow SM, Law SC, Chan JK, et al. Papillary microcarcinoma of the thyroid-Prognostic significance of lymph node metastasis and multifocality. Cancer 2003;98(1):31–40.

[28] Wada N, Duh QY, Sugino K, et al. Lymph node metastasis from 259 papillary thyroid microcarcinomas: frequency, pattern of occurrence and recurrence, and optimal strategy for neck dissection. Ann Surg 2003;237(3):399–407.

[29] Mercante G, Frasoldati A, Pedroni C, et al. Prognostic factors affecting neck lymph node recurrence and distant metastasis in papillary microcarcinoma of the thyroid: results of a study in 445 patients. Thyroid 2009;19(7):707–16.

[30] Besic N, Zgajnar J, Hocevar M, et al. Extent of thyroidectomy and lymphadenectomy in 254 patients with papillary thyroid microcarcinoma: a single-institution experience. Ann Surg Oncol 2009;16(4):920–8.

[31] Lombardi CP, Bellantone R, De Crea C, et al. Papillary thyroid microcarcinoma: extrathyroidal extension, lymph node metastases, and risk factors for recurrence in a high prevalence of goiter area. World J Surg 2010;34(6):1214–21.

[32] Sellers M, Beenken S, Blankenship A, et al. Prognostic significance of cervical lymph node metastases in differentiated thyroid cancer. Am J Surg 1992;164(6):578–81.

[33] Mazzaferri EL, Young RL. Papillary thyroid carcinoma: a 10 year follow-up report of the impact of therapy in 576 patients. Am J Med 1981;70(3):511–8.
[34] Pasieka JL, Zedenius J, Auer G, et al. Addition of nuclear DNA content to the AMES risk-group classification for papillary thyroid cancer. Surgery 1992;112(6):1154–9 [discussion: 1159–60].
[35] Xing M. BRAF mutation in papillary thyroid microcarcinoma: the promise of better risk management. Ann Surg Oncol 2009;16(4):801–3.
[36] Melck AL, Yip L, Carty SE. The utility of BRAF testing in the management of papillary thyroid cancer. Oncologist 2010;15(12):1285–93.
[37] Ito Y, Uruno T, Nakano K, et al. An observation trial without surgical treatment in patients with papillary microcarcinoma of the thyroid. Thyroid 2003;13(4):381–7.
[38] Xiao X, Ning L, Chen H. Notch1 mediates growth suppression of papillary and follicular thyroid cancer cells by histone deacetylase inhibitors. Mol Cancer Ther 2009;8(2):350–6.
[39] Ross DS, Litofsky D, Ain KB, et al. Recurrence after treatment of micropapillary thyroid cancer. Thyroid 2009;19(10):1043–8.
[40] Jukkola A, Bloigu R, Ebeling T, et al. Prognostic factors in differentiated thyroid carcinomas and their implications for current staging classifications. Endocr Relat Cancer 2004;11(3): 571–9.
[41] Sugitani I, Kasai N, Fujimoto Y, et al. A novel classification system for patients with PTC: addition of the new variables of large (3 cm or greater) nodal metastases and reclassification during the follow-up period. Surgery 2004;135(2):139–48.
[42] Ito Y, Tomoda C, Uruno T, et al. Preoperative ultrasonographic examination for lymph node metastasis: usefulness when designing lymph node dissection for papillary microcarcinoma of the thyroid. World J Surg 2004;28(5):498–501.
[43] So YK, Son YI, Hong SD, et al. Subclinical lymph node metastasis in papillary thyroid microcarcinoma: a study of 551 resections. Surgery 2010;148(3):526–31.
[44] Pearce EN, Braverman LE. Papillary thyroid microcarcinoma outcomes and implications for treatment. J Clin Endocrinol Metab 2004;89(8):3710–2.

Use of Computed Tomography in the Emergency Room to Evaluate Blunt Cerebrovascular Injury

Nancy A. Parks, MD, Martin A. Croce, MD*

Department of Surgery, University of Tennessee Health Science Center, 910 Madison Avenue, #219, Memphis, TN 38163, USA

Keywords
• Blunt cerebrovascular injury • Diagnosis • Screening • Computed tomography

Key Points
• Early diagnosis and treatment of blunt cerebrovascular injury (BCVI) improves outcomes.
• Even aggressive screening protocols miss approximately 20% of patients with BCVI.
• CT Angiography (CTA) is currently not reliable enough to definitively diagnose BCVI.
• Digital subtraction angiography remains the gold standard for diagnosis of BCVI.
• Adding abnormal CTA to standard screening criteria captures nearly all patients with BCVI.

lunt cerebrovascular injury (BCVI) was historically thought to be an exceedingly rare, and unavoidably morbid, consequence of significant blunt-force trauma. Originally described in 1872, it was not until the second half of the twentieth century, with increasing numbers of high-speed motor vehicle accidents and the availability of new diagnostic technology, that these injuries were identified regularly [1]. Although during the last 30 years there have been significant advances with regard to the diagnosis and treatment of BCVI, there remain several key questions regarding the optimal screening and best method to diagnose these potentially devastating injuries.

Before the 1990s, BCVIs were only recognized clinically once the patient had developed symptoms of the ischemic neurologic insult. The underlying pathophysiology is that blunt-force trauma causes intimal disruption of the carotid or vertebral artery. Hypothesized mechanisms for this intimal tear include direct blow to the neck, hyperextension with contralateral rotation of the head, laceration of the artery by adjacent bony fractures, and intraoral trauma [2]. The

*Corresponding author. *E-mail address:* mcroce@uthsc.edu

0065-3411/12/$ – see front matter
doi:10.1016/j.yasu.2012.03.003

damaged intima may serve as a lead point of a dissection or pseudoaneurysm (Figs. 1–3), which can occlude flow in the true lumen, or may cause platelet aggregation leading to distal emboli. Regardless of the mechanism, the classic presenting symptoms of BCVI were consistent with cerebral ischemia in the distribution of the injured vessel. Blunt carotid injury (BCI) typically causes contralateral hemiparesis or hemiplegia, aphasia, dysphasia, or Horner syndrome. Blunt vertebral injury (BVI) can present as ataxia, dizziness, or visual field deficits. Carotid-cavernous sinus fistula may present with orbital pain or exophthalmos, and can lead to permanent vision loss [3].

Early studies of BCVI found a low incidence of injury, occurring in less than 1 in 1000 blunt trauma patients [4]. However, in 1996 Fabian and colleagues [1] published a series of 67 patients with BCI. This article was significant for several reasons. First, their incidence of BCI, 0.67% of all blunt trauma patients, was higher than previously reported. In addition, it introduced the idea of screening and that appropriate treatment of BCVI can improve neurologic outcomes, which is important because once patients have developed symptoms of ischemia, BCVI has significant associated morbidity and mortality. However, in their series of 67 patients with BCI, treating injuries with a low-dose heparin drip (target partial thromboplastin time 40–50 seconds) independently improved survival and neurologic outcome. Early BCI-related mortality ranged from 23% to 31% [1], and nearly half of all survivors were left with permanent neurologic sequelae [5]. Classically BVI were not thought to be significant; however, in 2000 Biffl and colleagues [6] showed that BVI is more common than previously thought, that the incidence of associated posterior stroke is 24%, and that BVI-related mortality in their series was 8%. In addition, the posterior fossa strokes associated with BVI are generally catastrophic [7].

In the mid 1990s, trauma centers began aggressive screening in an effort to identify patients with BCVI before the development of symptoms. Whereas some

A   B

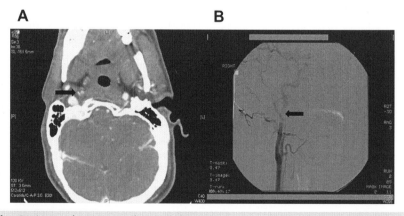

Fig. 1. Arrows denote internal carotid dissection on computed tomographic angiography (CTA) (A) and digital subtraction angiography (DSA) (B).

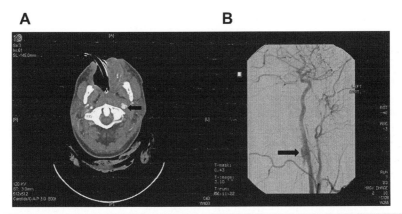

Fig. 2. Arrows denote internal carotid pseudoaneurysm on CTA (A) and DSA (B).

patients present with neurologic symptoms, most do not. There is typically a latent period, commonly between 10 and 72 hours after injury, before symptoms begin [8]. Identifying the BCVI and initiating treatment with anticoagulation or antiplatelet therapy before onset of neurologic symptoms has been shown to improve outcomes in this population. Stein and colleagues [9] studied their blunt trauma patients for 30 months and found 147 patients (1.2%) with BCVI. In their series, the stroke rate for untreated patients with BCVI was 25.8%; treated patients had a significantly lower stroke rate of 3.9%. This reduction is crucial not only because of the avoidable neurologic sequelae but also because the stroke-related mortality was 50%. Similarly, the Denver group demonstrated in 2004 that in their series of

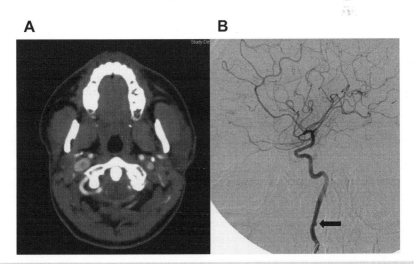

Fig. 3. (A) False-negative CTA. (B) Arrow denotes internal carotid pseudoaneurysm on DSA.

114 patients, 73 received anticoagulation and none of these patients had a stroke. Unfortunately, in the remaining 41 patients who did not receive anticoagulation, 46% developed an ischemic neurologic event [10].

To better classify and study BCVI, the Denver group has graded the various types of BCVI (Table 1). The stroke rate of BCI increases with increasing grade, and the overall stroke rate of BVI is approximately 20% regardless of injury grade [8]. Even grade I injuries do incur a finite risk of stroke and therefore should be treated accordingly. Current treatment recommendations are that all injuries should be treated with either low-dose heparin drip or antiplatelet therapy for 7 to 10 days. Repeat imaging of the injury is done after 7 to 10 days of therapy [5]. In a review of 171 patients from Denver, grade I injuries healed 57% of the time and grade II injuries healed 8% of the time. Healed injuries require no further treatment. By contrast, 8% of grade I and 43% of grade II lesions progressed to pseudoaneurysm formation [11]. The Memphis group has shown that pseudoaneurysms do not typically improve with time, and therefore recommend endovascular stent placement for grade III injuries as well as extensive grade II injuries [12]. Endovascular stents should not be placed until the patient has been treated with several days of heparin, all major surgical procedures have been completed, and the patient has received preprocedural aspirin and clopidogrel. Dual antiplatelet therapy is continued for 6 months after placement of endovascular stents [13].

Over the past decades, knowledge of BCVI has increased greatly. Current strategies for best management of these injuries include early diagnosis and institution of treatment before onset of neurologic symptoms. The goal should be to accurately diagnose patients with BCVI, before becoming symptomatic, to avoid the devastating neurologic consequences of these injuries.

SCREENING CRITERIA FOR BCVI

For screening to be optimally effective, there must be a latent stage of the disorder during which, if the condition is identified and appropriate treatment instituted, outcome can be positively influenced. With its typical initial silent period and improved neurologic outcomes with appropriate treatment, BCVI seems to be an ideal condition for attempts at screening.

Initial screening guidelines developed in Denver and Memphis remain largely unchanged today. To identify risk factors for BCVI, each group studied their injured population. In 1999, Biffl and colleagues [14] published their initial analysis

Table 1
Blunt cerebrovascular injury grading scale

Grade I	Luminal irregularity or dissection with <25% luminal narrowing
Grade II	Dissection or intramural hematoma with ≥25% luminal narrowing, intraluminal thrombus, or raised intimal flap
Grade III	Pseudoaneurysm
Grade IV	Occlusion
Grade V	Vessel transection or arteriovenous fistula

of independent risk factors for BCVI. Since 1996, they had been screening asymptomatic patients that met the following criteria with digital subtraction angiography (DSA): injury mechanism associated with severe cervical hyperextension/rotation, displaced midface fractures or complex mandibular fractures, closed head injury consistent with diffuse axonal injury, near-hanging resulting in anoxic brain injury, basilar skull fracture, cervical vertebral body fracture, seat-belt abrasion, or other soft-tissue injury of the anterior neck. In addition, DSA was performed in patients with any of the following signs or symptoms of BCVI: severe hemorrhage from mouth, nose, ears, or wounds, an expanding cervical hematoma, cervical bruit in a patient younger than 50 years, patients with evidence of cerebral infarction on CT scan, unexplained neurologic deficit, transient ischemic attack, amaurosis fugax, or Horner syndrome. After analyzing 249 patients, independent predictors of BCVI were: Glasgow Coma Scale score of 6 or less, petrous bone fracture, diffuse axonal brain injury, and LeFort fracture II or III. Of note, 39% of patients with a cervical spine fracture were found to have a vertebral artery injury.

Several subsequent studies then independently validated the need for aggressive screening of asymptomatic patients at risk for BCVI. In 2000, Berne and colleagues [15] at East Texas Medical Center examined their series of 17 patients with BCVI. Ten of these 17 patients died, and 8 of these deaths were a direct consequence of the BCVI. In analyzing their data, the investigators found that median time to diagnosis was 12.5 hours in survivors and 19.5 hours in nonsurvivors, underscoring the need for aggressive screening and institution of anticoagulation before the onset of neurologic symptoms.

Kerwin and colleagues [16] also evaluated their early experience with an aggressive screening protocol for BCVI. In their study, 48 patients were deemed high risk and were evaluated with DSA. Twenty-one patients were diagnosed with BCVI, for an overall incidence of 1.1%. The analysis found no complications with DSA and validated the widespread use of screening. Despite their screening protocol, 5 of the 26 patients (19.2%) diagnosed with BCVI were only identified on a delayed basis, after onset of neurologic symptoms. One of these patients presented 7 months after the initial injury with massive epistaxis and was found to have a carotid-cavernous sinus fistula. This finding is consistent with other reports that even aggressive screening protocols miss up to 20% of patients with BCVI [14,17,18].

Cothren and the group from Denver [19,20] have worked to refine the screening criteria. In reviewing their series of patients, they found that certain cervical spine fractures were most predictive of BCVI. Their recommendations included limiting the screening criteria to include only fractures of C1 to C3, cervical spine fractures involving the transverse foramen, or cervical subluxation. However, Kopelman and colleagues [21] reviewed their series of patients with BCVI and found that not screening patients with C4-C7 fractures would have led to missing 2 of 15 patients with BCVI. Emmett and colleagues [17] similarly found that lower cervical spine fractures confer equivalent risk of BCVI as higher cervical fractures; in their study 9% of patients who would not have been screened using "limited cervical spine criteria" actually had a BCVI.

In an effort to clarify the best screening criteria, Franz and colleagues [22] recently performed a meta-analysis of diagnostic screening criteria for BCVI. In their meta-analysis they compared associated injuries in 418 patients with documented BCVI with 22,568 non-BCVI patients. Their evaluation of 9 common screening criteria (head injury, basilar skull fracture, cervical spine fracture, cervical abrasion, neurologic deficit, facial fracture, thoracic injury, abdominal injury, and Glasgow Coma Scale <8) found that only cervical spine fracture and thoracic injury were significantly associated with BCVI. This meta-analysis also cautioned against the use of isolated cervical abrasion (or "seat-belt sign") as an indication for screening, as no association between the physical finding and BCVI could be demonstrated.

While it is clearly important to identify risk factors for BCVI and institute aggressive screening protocols, one must be somewhat cautious and remember that the absence of risk factors does not eliminate the possibility of BCVI (Box 1). Regardless of screening criteria used, approximately 20% of patients with confirmed BCVI are not found, based on any of the traditional screening criteria [14,17,18,22].

Screening for BCVI became widespread without a clear understanding of the cost-effectiveness of this approach. Kaye and colleagues [23] performed an analysis of the cost-effectiveness of all screening methods: no screening, screening with ultrasonography, CT angiography (CTA)-based screening, or DSA. The investigators looked at the data from both an institutional and a societal prospective. From an institutional standpoint, they found that no screening was the least costly, but had an 11% associated stroke rate. From a societal standpoint, taking into consideration the significant lifetime costs associated with strokes, CTA was most cost-effective, provided a sensitivity of greater than 93% is associated with the CTA. If the sensitivity is less than 93%, DSA becomes the most cost-effective tool for BCVI screening.

DIAGNOSTIC MODALITIES TO SCREEN FOR BCVI

During the initial phase of aggressive screening for BCVI, DSA was the only available technology capable of reliably detecting these injuries, and it remains the gold standard today. DSA has proved to be highly effective and safe. The

---

Box 1: BCVI screening criteria

Skull base fracture

Cervical spine fracture

LeFort II or III fracture

Neck soft-tissue injury

Horner syndrome

Unexplained neurologic deficit

CTA of the neck positive for an injury or an irregularity

series of patients from Denver shows that 643 patients underwent screening angiography with minimal complications: 2 patients had a puncture-site hematoma and 1 patient (0.1%) developed a stroke after screening DSA [10]. In a large series of patients from Memphis, 764 DSA examinations were performed in 684 patients with a total of 8 (1%) procedure-related complications. Four of these were self-limited puncture-site hematomas. Four patients (0.5%) had major complications. Three patients suffered temporary femoral artery occlusion secondary to the closure device, and underwent successful surgical repair of the femoral artery. One patient had an iatrogenic dissection of a vertebral artery, which was treated with endovascular stenting [24]. Combining these 2 large series of DSA procedures in trauma patients shows that only 5 serious complications occurred in 1407 procedures, making the serious complication rate of DSA in this population approximately 0.36%.

Although DSA is safe, it does remain labor intensive and requires interventional radiology support, which may not be readily available, particularly in smaller hospitals. For these reasons, there has been considerable interest in finding a noninvasive screening test that would be reliable in diagnosing BCVI. Although ultrasonography and magnetic resonance angiography (MRA) technology have both been considered, neither have gained popular support. Ultrasonography is not effective for visualizing the arteries as they travel through the bony carotid canal or the transverse foramina, and therefore would miss many BCVIs [25]. MRA has also been proved to be difficult logistically. Many patients have contraindications to MRA, and early sensitivity of MRA was shown to be only 50% for cervical artery injuries and 47% for vertebral artery injuries, clearly not adequate for an effective screening examination [26].

CTA has gained considerable favor as a screening test for BCVI because of its wide availability, noninvasive nature, and because most of these blunt trauma patients are already going to the CT scanner, allowing for a single trip to diagnose BCVI as well as other major injuries (Box 2). Two early reports with outdated CT scanning technology clearly showed that the early-generation CTAs were inadequate to diagnose BCVI [26,27]. More recent data, based on CTA images obtained with significantly more advanced CT technology, still shows mixed results. However, because of ease of use and widespread availability, CTA is currently the most common method being used to diagnose BCVI. A recent survey of 785 clinicians found that CTA was by far the preferred method to diagnose BCVI, and among the 137 responding trauma surgeons 92.7% of them preferred CTA [28]. Careful review of the data does not support this transition to CTA-based diagnosis of BCVI.

In 2006, Biffl and the Denver group published their experience screening for BCVI with a 16-slice CTA. A total of 331 patients were screened with CTA, 18 of whom were identified as having 20 BCVIs. Fifteen positive CTAs were followed up with DSA; 4 false-positive CTAs (and normal DSAs) were identified. Patients with negative CTA were followed clinically and none developed any neurologic findings of BCVI. Because only the patients with positive CTAs underwent DSA, the true accuracy of CTA cannot be determined based on this study [29].

Box 2: Criteria for obtaining a CTA of the neck during the initial trauma evaluation

Potential head or skull injury
  Loss of consciousness
  Altered mental status
  Periorbital ecchymosis
  Supramastoid ecchymosis
Potential cervical spine fracture or soft-tissue neck injury
  Paralysis with cervical spine level
  Cervical step-off
  Tenderness to palpation
  Soft-tissue injury (seat-belt mark)
Potential LeFort facial fracture
  Midface instability
  Marked external deformity
Potential significant thoracic injury

Berne and colleagues [30] prospectively studied 486 blunt trauma patients at risk for BCVI. Forty-eight patients had abnormal findings on CTA and therefore underwent subsequent DSA. Of the 48 DSAs, only 18 patients were diagnosed with BCVI; there were 30 false-positive CTAs in this series. Positive predictive value was 37.5% and specificity was 94% for CTA in the diagnosis of BCVI. Patients with negative initial CTAs underwent no further imaging but were followed clinically, with no patients developing symptoms during the study. These same investigators reevaluated the role of CTA in the diagnosis of BCVI after changing to a 16-slice scanner. In the second series they followed 435 patients screened for BCVI with CTA, and found injuries in 24 patients for an incidence of 1.2%. The fact that this incidence was higher than the incidence during the era of the 4-slice CT scanner was interpreted as evidence that newer CT technology was appropriate to diagnose BCVI. Patients with negative CTAs were followed clinically, and none were found to deteriorate neurologically, leading to the conclusion that CTA identified all neurologically significant BCVIs [31].

In one of the few studies to strictly evaluate patients who had both CTA and DSA, Eastman and colleagues evaluated 146 patients at risk for BCVI. In this series, 46 BCVIs were diagnosed in 45 patients on CTA. There was one false-negative CTA, but in 45 of 46 cases the results of CTA and DSA were the same. In addition, the 103 patients with negative CTA were evaluated and also found to have negative DSA. This study found the sensitivity of CTA to be 97.7% and the specificity of CTA for BCVI to be 100% [32]. This same group developed a set of BCVI treatment guidelines based on CTA results alone, which were implemented in 2005. Over the next year, they diagnosed 26 patients with BCVI based on CTA and were able to start treatment rapidly. During the era when this group had been using DSA to diagnose BCVI, the average time to diagnosis was 31.2 hours. With the implementation of the CTA-based diagnosis, average time to diagnosis, and treatment, was 2.65 hours. This shorter time to treatment correlated with a significantly decreased stroke rate of 3.8% (compared with 15.2% during the era of catheter-based diagnosis) [33].

However, subsequent reports have been unable to reproduce these outstanding results with CTA. In 2006, Utter and colleagues [34] published their retrospective experience with 16-slice CTA to diagnose BCVI. Based on their protocol, all patients were screened with CTA and DSA was obtained, at the discretion of the clinical service, in certain patients with normal CTAs. Eighty-two of the patients with normal CTAs were further evaluated with DSA, and 7 additional injuries were found (1 minimal luminal irregularity, 3 dissections, 2 pseudoaneurysms, and 1 occlusion). On retrospective review of the initial CTAs, 5 of the 7 could be seen (but were initially missed) on the CTA; however, being able to identify an injury only retrospectively is not reassuring clinically, whereby only real-time interpretations affect patient outcomes. Their conclusion that CTA adequately supplants DSA for the screening of BCVI is difficult to understand in light of the 7 missed injuries.

In another study that followed patients receiving both CTA and DSA for the diagnosis of BCVI, Malhotra and colleagues [35] found that CTA was not accurate for diagnosis or exclusion of BCVI. In this study, 92 patients underwent both CTA and DSA. Sensitivity of CTA was only 74%, specificity 86%, positive predictive value 65%, and negative predictive value 90%. On further review of their data, they found that all the false-negative CTAs were done in the first half of the study, possibly because of a learning curve for radiologists in interpreting these types of images. However, the false-positive rate of CTA did not vary with time and may continue to be a limiting factor in the accuracy of CTA.

Another study of 83 blunt trauma patients evaluated with both DSA and CTA compared whole-body CTA with neck CTA, and failed to find either type of CTA adequate to screen for BCVI. This study was a retrospective review conducted by experienced trauma radiologists in an effort to avoid the possible learning curve seen in other trials; the radiologists had no knowledge of the DSA results. The sensitivities for BCI were low, regardless of CTA type: 69% sensitivity for whole-body CTA and 64% sensitivity for neck CTA. Sensitivities for BVI were slightly better: 74% for whole-body CTA and 68% for neck CTA. Specificities were higher for both: 82% and 94% for BCI, and 91% and 100% for BVI. However, given the significant morbidity and mortality associated with BCVI, the low sensitivities reported in this study make CTA an inadequate screening test [36].

A recent prospective trial shows the need to be cautious before adopting CTA as equivalent to DSA for the diagnosis of BCVI. Goodwin and colleagues [37] screened 158 patients for BCVI and prospectively collected their data. All of the patients received both CTA and DSA. A total of 32 injuries were identified in 27 patients on DSA. CTA reported 16 false-negative and 4 false-positive results. The CTA and DSA results agreed in the other 138 cases. Sensitivity of CTA was calculated to be 41% for BCVI, with specificity of 97%. Both a 16-slice and a 64-slice scanner was used and, though the sensitivity trended toward being higher with the 64-slice machine, there was no statistical difference between the 2 models of CT scanner.

In what is the largest study to date, the Memphis group studied 684 patients at risk for BCVI who underwent both CTA (with a 32-slice scanner) and DSA; direct comparison of the 2 diagnostic modalities shows that CTA is not yet

Table 2
Comparison of reported efficacy of CTA versus DSA

Reference, Year	N	Study design	Findings
Berne et al [30], 2004	486	All pts had CTA, 48 pts with abnormal CTAs then had DSA	18/48 pts had BCVI on DSA 30 false-positive CTAs Sensitivity 100%, specificity 94%, PPV 37.5%, NPV 100%
Biffl et al [29], 2006	331	All pts had CTA, 15 pts with abnormal CTAs then had DSA	4 false-positive CTAs 16/17 injuries graded the same on CTA & DSA
Eastman et al [32], 2006	146	All pts had both CTA & DSA	Sensitivity 97.7%, specificity 100%, PPV 100%, NPV 99.3%
Utter et al [34], 2006	372	All pts had CTA, 82 pts had DSA after normal CTA	DSA found 7 additional injuries in 82 pts, NPV 92%
Malhotra et al [35], 2007	119	All pts had CTA, 92 of the pts also had DSA	Sensitivity 74%, specificity 86%, PPV 65%, NPV 90%
Sliker and Mirvis [25], 2007	108	All pts had both CTA & DSA—whole-body vs neck CTA	Whole-body CTA: BCI: sensitivity 69%, specificity 82% BVI: sensitivity 74%, specificity 91% Neck CTA: BCI: sensitivity 64%, specificity 94% BVI: sensitivity 68%, specificity 100%
Goodwin et al [37], 2009	158	All pts had both CTA & DSA	Sensitivity 41%, specificity 97%
DiCocco et al [13], 2011	684	All pts had both CTA & DSA	Sensitivity 51%, specificity 97% PPV 43%, NPV 98%
Emmett et al [17], 2011	748	All pts had both CTA & DSA	19/117 (16%) pts diagnosed with BCVI had no traditional screening criteria, only an abnormal CTA Adding abnormal CTA findings to traditional DSA screening criteria captures nearly all pts with BCVI

Abbreviations: BCVI, blunt cerebrovascular injury; CTA, computed tomography angiogram; DSA, digital subtraction angiogram; NPV, negative predictive value; PPV, positive predictive value; pts, patients.

adequate to be the diagnostic test of choice for BCVI. In this series, 90 patients had 109 injuries identified. BCVI was diagnosed in 0.5% of the blunt trauma patients and in 13% of the screened patients. Overall sensitivity of CTA was 51%, clearly inadequate for an effective screening test. The specificity, however, was found to be 97%, meaning that injuries, when visualized on CTA, tended to be real. The real problem with CTA in this patient population was that normal CTA does not exclude BCVI any more accurately than would a flip of a coin [24].

A separate study by the group in Memphis addresses the question of what might be the most appropriate role for CTA in the diagnosis of BCVI. CTA does have a high specificity, is widely available, and may help identify a certain subset of injuries. Remembering that the traditional screening criteria for BCVI fail to identify approximately 20% of patients with injuries, the group found that adding abnormal CTA findings to the traditional screening criteria allowed them to accurately identify nearly all patients at risk of BCVI before the development of symptoms. Only 1 patient during the 29-month study period, during which 20,049 blunt trauma patients were evaluated, was identified as needing a DSA for delayed onset of unexplained neurologic findings without any conventional screening criteria or CTA findings. Specifically, 16% (19 of 117 patients) diagnosed with BCVI during this study were screened on the sole indication of abnormal CTA finding; in other words, adding the single screening criteria of abnormal CTA finding increased the yield of screening by 16% [17].

SUMMARY

BCVI remains a potentially devastating consequence of blunt-force trauma. However, over the past decades significant advances have been made in understanding the pathophysiology, risk factors, and natural history of BCVI. Given the initial asymptomatic period, there is time to diagnose and treat these lesions before the onset of neurologic insult. This early recognition and intervention greatly improves morbidity and mortality directly associated with BCVI.

Screening criteria have been identified and reviewed. All patients at risk of BCVI, based on mechanism of injury and risk factors, should be rapidly evaluated for possible injury. It is the authors' current belief that even the newest generation of CT scanners has not been proved to reliably diagnose BCVI. Until further work is done to advance the technology of CTA and prove its equivalence to DSA, there exists too much potential neurologic morbidity and mortality for one to rely on CTA alone (Table 2). Given the variable, and often low, reported sensitivities of CTA, the cost analysis done by Kaye and colleagues [23] would also recommend initial DSA as being cost-effective in avoiding the long-term devastating sequelae of stroke.

At the time of writing the authors recommend that CTA be included in an algorithm to evaluate BCVI, but the current data are too disparate with widely variable reported sensitivities, and the risk of missed injury and stroke too severe, to rely on CTA as the definitive diagnostic or screening test for BCVI. Rather, abnormal CTA findings should be added to the traditional screening criteria to identify patients at risk of BCVI; these patients should be evaluated with DSA for definitive screening. Adding abnormal CTA findings to the traditionally described BCVI screening criteria widens the criteria substantially, allowing identification of almost all of the elusive 20% of patients traditionally not identified with basic screening criteria [17]. In addition, given the high specificity of CTA and the decreased morbidity of BCVI with rapid institution of treatment, the authors recommend beginning a low-dose heparin drip (if there are no contraindications to anticoagulation) based on CTA findings while awaiting the confirmatory DSA.

Despite advances in CTA technology in recent years, DSA currently remains the gold standard for the diagnosis of BCVI. All patients with standard risk factors for BCVI, or abnormal findings on CTA, should undergo DSA as the screening test of choice for BCVI.

References

[1] Fabian TC, Patton JH, Croce MA, et al. Blunt carotid injury: importance of early diagnosis and anticoagulant therapy. Ann Surg 1996;223:513–25.

[2] Crissey MM, Bernstein EF. Delayed presentation of carotid intimal tear following blunt craniocervical trauma. Surgery 1974;75:543–9.

[3] Burlew CC, Biffl WL. Blunt cerebrovascular trauma. Curr Opin Crit Care 2010;16:587–95.

[4] Davis JW, Holbrook TL, Hoyt DB, et al. Blunt carotid artery dissection: incidence, associated injuries, screening, and treatment. J Trauma 1990;30:1514–7.

[5] Biffl WL, Cothren CC, Moore EE, et al. Western trauma association critical decisions in trauma: screening for and treatment of blunt cerebrovascular injuries. J Trauma 2009;67: 1150–3.

[6] Biffl WL, Moore EE, Elliott JP, et al. The devastating potential of blunt vertebral arterial injuries. Ann Surg 2000;231:672–81.

[7] Miller PR, Fabian TC, Bee TK, et al. Blunt cerebrovascular injuries: diagnosis and treatment. J Trauma 2001;51:279–86.

[8] Burlew CC, Biffl WL. Imaging for blunt carotid and vertebral artery injuries. Surg Clin North Am 2011;91:217–31.

[9] Stein DM, Boswell S, Sliker CW, et al. Blunt cerebrovascular injuries: does treatment always matter? J Trauma 2009;66:132–44.

[10] Cothren CC, Moore EE, Biffl WL, et al. Anticoagulation is the gold standard therapy for blunt carotid injuries to reduce stroke rate. Arch Surg 2004;139:540–6.

[11] Biffl WL, Ray CE, Moore EE, et al. Treatment-related outcomes from blunt cerebrovascular injuries - importance of routing follow-up arteriography. Ann Surg 2002;235:699–707.

[12] Edwards NM, Fabian TC, Claridge JA, et al. Antithrombotic therapy and endovascular stents are effective treatment for blunt carotid injuries: results from longterm followup. J Am Coll Surg 2007;204:1007–15.

[13] DiCocco JM, Fabian TC, Emmett KP, et al. Optimal outcomes for patients with blunt cerebrovascular injury (BCVI): tailoring treatment to the lesion. J Am Coll Surg 2011;212:549–59.

[14] Biffl WL, Moore EE, Offner PJ, et al. Optimizing screening for blunt cerebrovascular injuries. Am J Surg 1999;178:517–22.

[15] Berne JD, Norwood SH, McAuley CE, et al. The high morbidity of blunt cerebrovascular injury in an unscreened population: more evidence of the need for mandatory screening protocols. J Am Coll Surg 2001;192:314–21.

[16] Kerwin AJ, Bynoe RP, Murray J, et al. Liberalized screening for blunt carotid and vertebral artery injuries is justified. J Trauma 2001;51:308–14.

[17] Emmett KP, Fabian TC, DiCocco JM, et al. Improving the screening criteria for blunt cerebrovascular injury: the appropriate role for computed tomography angiography. J Trauma 2011;70:1058–65.

[18] Bromberg WJ, Collier BC, Diebel LN, et al. Blunt cerebrovascular injury practice management guidelines: the eastern association for the surgery of trauma. J Trauma 2010;68: 471–7.

[19] Cothren CC, Moore EE, Biffl WL, et al. Cervical spine fracture patterns predictive of blunt vertebral artery injury. J Trauma 2003;55:811–3.

[20] Cothren CC, Moore EE, Ray CE, et al. Cervical spine fracture patterns mandating screening to rule out blunt cerebrovascular injury. Surgery 2007;141:76–82.

[21] Kopelman TR, Leeds S, Berardoni NE, et al. Incidence of blunt cerebrovascular injury in low-risk cervical spine fractures. Am J Surg 2011;202:684–9.

[22] Franz RW, Willette PA, Wood MJ, et al. A systematic review and meta-analysis of diagnostic screening criteria for blunt cerebrovascular injuries. J Am Coll Surg 2012;214:313–27.

[23] Kaye D, Brasel KJ, Neideen T, et al. Screening for blunt cerebrovascular injuries is cost-effective. J Trauma 2011;70:1051–7.

[24] DiCocco JM, Emmett KP, Fabian TC, et al. Blunt cerebrovascular injury screening with 32-channel multidetector computed tomography: more slices still don't cut it. Ann Surg 2011;253:444–50.

[25] Sliker CW, Mirvis SE. Imaging of blunt cerebrovascular injuries. Eur J Radiol 2007;64: 3–14.

[26] Miller PR, Fabian TC, Croce MA, et al. Prospective screening for blunt cerebrovascular injuries. Ann Surg 2002;236:386–95.

[27] Biffl WL, Ray CE, Moore EE, et al. Noninvasive diagnosis of blunt cerebrovascular injuries: a preliminary report. J Trauma 2002;53:850–6.

[28] Harrigan MR, Weinberg JA, Peaks YS, et al. Management of blunt extracranial traumatic cerebrovascular injury: a multidisciplinary survey of current practice. World J Emerg Surg 2011;6:11.

[29] Biffl WL, Egglin T, Benedetto B, et al. Sixteen-slice computed tomographic angiography is a reliable noninvasive screening test for clinically significant blunt cerebrovascular injuries. J Trauma 2006;60:745–52.

[30] Berne JD, Norwood SH, McAuley CE, et al. Helical computed tomographic angiography: an excellent screening test for blunt cerebrovascular injury. J Trauma 2004;57:11–9.

[31] Berne JD, Reuland KS, Villareal DH, et al. Sixteen-slice multi-detector computed tomographic angiography improves the accuracy of screening for blunt cerebrovascular injury. J Trauma 2006;60:1204–10.

[32] Eastman AL, Chason DP, Perez CL, et al. Computed tomographic angiography for the diagnosis of blunt cervical vascular injury: is it ready for primetime? J Trauma 2006;60:925–9.

[33] Eastman AL, Muraliraj V, Sperry JL, et al. CTA-based screening reduces time to diagnosis and stroke rate in blunt cervical vascular injury. J Trauma 2009;67:551–6.

[34] Utter GH, Hollingworth W, Hallam DK, et al. Sixteen-slice CT Angiography in patients with suspected blunt carotid and vertebral artery injuries. J Am Coll Surg 2006;203:838–48.

[35] Malhotra AK, Camacho M, Ivatury RR, et al. Computed tomographic angiography for the diagnosis of blunt carotid/vertebral artery injury: a note of caution. Ann Surg 2007;246: 632–43.

[36] Sliker CW, Shanmuganathan K, Mirvis SE. Diagnosis of blunt cerebrovascular injuries with 16-MDCT: accuracy of whole-body MDCT compared with neck MDCT angiography. Am J Radiol 2008;190:790–9.

[37] Goodwin RB, Beery PR, Dorbish RJ, et al. Computed tomographic angiography versus conventional angiography for the diagnosis of blunt cerebrovascular injury in trauma patients. J Trauma 2009;67:1046–50.

How Important is Glycemic Control During Coronary Artery Bypass?

Harold L. Lazar, MD*

Department of Cardiothoracic Surgery, Boston University School of Medicine, Boston Medical Center, Boston, MA, USA

Keywords
• Glycemic control • Coronary artery bypass graft surgery • Diabetes mellitus

Key Points
• Hyperglycemia is detrimental to the cardiac surgical patient.
• Glycemic control reduces morbidity and mortality in the CABG patient.
• The optimal range for glucose values in the immediate postoperative period is 120–180 mg/dL.

The incidence of diabetes mellitus in patients undergoing coronary artery bypass graft (CABG) surgery continues to increase. Nearly 30% to 40% of all patients undergoing CABG have diabetes mellitus or the metabolic syndrome [1]. Despite improvements in surgical techniques, anesthetic management, myocardial protection, and postoperative care, patients with diabetes mellitus have higher perioperative morbidity and mortality, significantly reduced long-term survival, and less freedom from recurrent episodes of angina [2–5]. Furthermore, nondiabetic patients with perioperative hyperglycemia (>250 mg/dL) also have increased morbidity and mortality following CABG surgery [6,7]. Diabetes mellitus and perioperative hyperglycemia in nondiabetic patients are independent risk factors for short- and long-term mortality following CABG surgery and are used as metrics for risk stratification in national databases [8]. Increased morbidity and mortality in these patients had been attributed to a higher incidence of left ventricular dysfunction, more diffuse coronary and peripheral vascular disease, and renal insufficiency [9]. It was thought that these comorbidities were irreversible, predisposing these patients to worse clinical outcomes and increased medical costs.

In recent years, numerous studies have shown that achieving glycemic control in patients with diabetes mellitus and those with hyperglycemia undergoing CABG surgery decreases perioperative morbidity and mortality,

*Department of Cardiothoracic Surgery, Boston Medical Center, 88 East Newton Street, Boston, MA 02218. E-mail address: harold.lazar@bmc.org

0065-3411/12/$ – see front matter
doi:10.1016/j.yasu.2012.03.007

improves long-term survival, and decreases the incidence of recurrent ischemic events. The management of perioperative hyperglycemia is now a major therapeutic focus in CABG surgery. Performance measurements of glycemic control are now used internally by hospitals for quality improvement, externally as part of national databases for public reporting of operative outcomes, and by third-party payers to establish monetary reimbursement based on quality of care. This article (1) discusses the detrimental effects of hyperglycemia in patients undergoing CABG, (2) reviews the evidence to show the benefits and importance of glycemic control in these patients, and (3) discusses whether more aggressive glycemic control will result in more optimal clinical outcomes and less morbidity than can be achieved with moderate control.

IMPACT OF DIABETES MELLITUS ON OUTCOMES IN PATIENTS UNDERGOING CABG SURGERY

Patients with diabetes mellitus that undergo CABG surgery continue to have inferior short- and long-term survival compared with nondiabetic patients [5]. Insulin-dependent patients with diabetes have been shown to have a significantly longer length of hospital and intensive care unit (ICU) stay and greater total hospital charges than patients with diabetes who are not insulin dependent and nondiabetic patients [10]. Postoperative morbidity, including renal failure and dialysis, stroke, mediastinitis, wound infections, transfusions, and the need for inotropic agents, is increased in all patients with diabetes compared with patients without diabetes [2,4]. Type 2 diabetes requiring insulin or oral agents is associated with an increased risk of death or acute myocardial infarction (MI) after CABG [5]. These patients are more likely to require a repeat revascularization procedure and have a higher incidence of postoperative neurologic complications [11]. Patients with diabetes who are undergoing cardiac procedures have been shown to have a 44% higher risk for rehospitalization for any cause and a 24% higher risk of readmission for cardiac-related issues [12].

The increased incidence of perioperative and long-term morbidity and mortality in cardiac surgical patients with diabetes has had a significant impact on medical costs. Every 50 mg/dL increase in blood glucose in the perioperative period has been associated with a 0.76-day increase in the length of stay, which increased hospital charges by $2824 and hospital costs by $1769 [13]. This finding is of particular concern because the incidence of diabetes mellitus in patients undergoing surgical revascularization has increased by 32% between 1990 and 1999 and continues to increase [14]. The importance of glycemic control in these patients was shown in a study in which intensive management of patients with diabetes with coronary heart disease yielded better outcomes with an estimated cost-effectiveness ratio of approximately $50,000 per life-year added [15].

DETRIMENTAL EFFECTS OF HYPERGLYCEMIA ON THE CARDIOVASCULAR SYSTEM AND ITS REVERSAL WITH INSULIN

The primary energy substrate for the nonischemic myocardium is free fatty acids [16]. However, during periods of ischemia, free fatty acids are detrimental to the myocardium because they increase oxygen consumption, decrease contractility, predispose to arrhythmias, and increase free radicals, which impair endothelial function [17]. Free fatty acids also impair glucose use, which is the preferred energy substrate during periods of myocardial ischemia [16]. Shifting myocardial oxidative metabolism from free fatty acids to glucose is a protective mechanism that allows the ischemic myocardium to more efficiently use limited supplies of oxygen to preserve cellular integrity and ultimately contractility. However, the diabetic myocardium has impaired glucose oxidation caused by impaired glucose transport into the myocyte, altered glucose phosphorylation, and decreased endogenous insulin secretion, all of which contribute to hyperglycemia [18].

Hyperglycemia leads to the formation of advanced glycation end products and its cell surface receptor (RAGE) [19]. Activation of RAGE is directly related to the level of glucose and is associated with an increased inflammatory response and oxidative stress [20]. This increase results in the activation of 3 key proinflammatory transcription factors normally suppressed by insulin: nuclear factor Kappa B (NFKB), activated protein 1 (AP-1), and early growth response 1 (EGR-1) [21]. Hyperglycemia also directly affects pathways responsible for changes in endothelial function, inflammation, and oxidative stress. It alters the polyol pathway leading to the depletion of reduced nicotinamide-adenine dinucleotide phosphate, which is essential for the generation of antioxidants and the cofactor for endothelial nitric oxide synthase [22]. It increases the synthesis of diacylglycerol, which activates the protein kinase-C pathway, which directly results in a decrease in endothelial nitric oxide synthase and increased levels of endothelin-1 [23]. Endothelin-1 is a potent vasoconstrictor and directly impairs myocardial contractility [24]. This altered endothelial function during CABG contributes to postoperative ischemic necrosis and may lead to decreased long-term survival and recurrent ischemic events caused by reduced graft patency. Bioassays from internal mammary artery and saphenous vein grafts taken from patients with diabetes undergoing CABG show decreased nitric oxide activity and increased production of superoxide radicals compared with nondiabetic patients [25–27]. The activation of the protein kinase-C pathway leads to the increased activation of prothrombotic factors, which contribute to vascular thrombosis, and increased levels of metalloproteinases, which make atheromatous plaques more susceptible to rupture. This leads to increased levels of plasminogen activator-1 and adhesion molecules, which contribute to the impaired platelet function seen in patients with diabetes [28,29]. Platelet adhesiveness and hyperaggregability are increased, which predisposes to coronary thrombosis, which ultimately may affect long-term vein graft patency. In summary, hyperglycemia alters metabolic pathways resulting in increased oxidative stress, inflammation, vasoconstriction, and thrombosis, all of which contribute to increased morbidity and mortality during CABG surgery.

In contrast, intravenous (IV) insulin reverses the detrimental effects of hyperglycemia by stimulating myocardial glucose use, suppressing the inflammatory response, and minimizing apoptosis. Insulin enhances myocardial glucose metabolism by facilitating the transport of glucose into the myocyte; augmenting aerobic metabolism by stimulating pyruvate dehydrogenase; and inhibiting the release of free fatty acids, which facilitate glycolytic pathways [30]. Insulin acts as an antiinflammatory agent by suppressing the proinflammatory transcription factors, NFKB, EGR-1, and AP-1 [21]. It reduces C-reactive protein and inflammatory mediators, such as interleukin 6, tumor necrosis factor alpha, intracellular adhesion molecule (ICAM)-1, and E-selectin [31,32]. Insulin upregulates the L-arginine nitric oxide pathway, thus, promoting vasodilatation and minimizing endothelial dysfunction [18]. It improves platelet function by decreasing plasminogen activator (PA)-1 and increasing prostacyclin release [28]. Experimental studies have shown that insulin also reduces apoptosis by increasing nitric oxide levels via a P13-kinase–dependent pathway [33,34].

IV infusions of insulin after CABG surgery have been shown to decrease levels of free fatty acids and increase myocardial uptake of glucose [35]. Insulin added to cardioplegic solutions in patients undergoing CABG enhances aerobic metabolism on reperfusion and improves left ventricular stroke work index [36]. Low-dose infusions of insulin in obese patients significantly decreased levels of reactive oxygen species, adhesion molecules, and C-reactive protein [21]. These pleiotropic properties of insulin on the cellular and molecular level decrease oxidative stress and the inflammatory response, which result in decreased morbidity and mortality in patients with diabetes and in nondiabetic patients with perioperative hyperglycemia.

DETRIMENTAL EFFECTS OF HYPERGLYCEMIA IN THE PERIOPERATIVE PERIOD

Several clinical studies have documented the detrimental effects of hyperglycemia in both patients with diabetes and nondiabetic patients undergoing CABG surgery. Doenst and coworkers [37] retrospectively reviewed the effects of hyperglycemia on the clinical outcomes of 6280 patients undergoing cardiac surgery procedures (4701 nondiabetic patients, 1579 patients with diabetes). There were no established protocols for treating hyperglycemia during surgery in these patients. Intermittent boluses of insulin were administered when serum glucose levels exceeded 270 mg/dL. Patients with higher peak glucose levels (>360 mg/dL) on cardiopulmonary bypass had an increased incidence of preoperative risk factors, including a reduced ejection fraction, congestive heart failure, cardiogenic shock, renal failure, previous cardiac surgery, and were more likely to have required urgent surgery. Higher glucose levels during surgery were an independent predictor of mortality in both patients with diabetes and nondiabetic patients, regardless of the type of procedure performed, and was unrelated to CBP or cross-clamp times. Mortality was 3 times higher in patients with hyperglycemia. Fish and coworkers reviewed the importance of blood glucose levels in the intraoperative and immediate postoperative period to predict morbidity in 200 consecutive patients undergoing CABG [38]. In this series, 31% of patients were known to have diabetes mellitus and 21% were suspected to have diabetes because of an HbA1c level greater than 6.0%. They found that a postoperative serum glucose level greater than 250 mg/dL was associated with a 10-fold increase in complications. A glucose level of less than 200 mg/dL in the immediate postoperative ICU period was associated with a 13% incidence of complications. A serum glucose greater than 200 mg/dL but less than 250 mg/dL had a 36% incidence of complications; if the glucose level exceeded 250 mg/dL, the risk was 63%. There was no correlation between the incidence of complications and the preoperative HbA1c level. Only the immediate postoperative ICU serum glucose was a significant predictor of total length of hospital stay. For every 30 mg/dL increase in serum glucose, there was a 1-day increase in the length of stay. Forty percent of the complications were cardiac related and 21% were related to infectious causes. Similar findings were reported by McAlister and coworkers [39] in a retrospective study of 291 patients undergoing CABG surgery over a 1-year period. The average serum glucose on the first postoperative day predicted the development of an adverse outcome. Patients whose average serum glucose level was in the highest quartile had a significantly higher risk of adverse outcomes than those with glucose levels in the lowest quartile. In a recent, large, multicenter observational study involving 5050 patients undergoing CABG, a postoperative blood glucose greater than or equal to 250 mg/dL was associated with increased mortality in nondiabetic patients [6]. In a retrospective observational study of 409 cardiac surgical patients, Gandhi and coworkers [40] also reported on the detrimental effects of elevated intraoperative glucose levels. Intraoperative hyperglycemia was an independent risk factor for perioperative complications, including death. For every 20 mg/dL increase in serum glucose greater than 100 mg/dL during surgery, there was a 34% increase in the incidence of postoperative complications. Abnormal glucose values before surgery may also be predictive of decreased survival following surgery. Anderson and coworkers [41] studied the effect of impaired fasting blood glucose levels before surgery in a group of 1375 patients undergoing CABG. Patients with impaired fasting glucose had a 1-year mortality, which was twice as great as patients with normal fasting values and equal to that of patients who were suspected or known to have diabetes mellitus. Imran and coworkers [42] noted that admission blood glucose levels were associated with increased morbidity following CABG. Fluctuations and variability in intraoperative and postoperative blood glucose levels have also been associated with increased mortality and morbidity following cardiac surgery [43].

These studies strongly suggest that impaired fasting glucose levels before surgery and persistently elevated glucose levels during and immediately following cardiac surgery are predictive of increased perioperative morbidity and mortality in both patients with diabetes and nondiabetic patients.

GLYCEMIC CONTROL IMPROVES OUTCOMES IN PATIENTS UNDERGOING CABG SURGERY

Although it had been established that hyperglycemia was associated with adverse outcomes in patients undergoing CABG, data were still necessary to prove that lowering glucose levels with insulin would decrease morbidity and mortality in these patients.

INSULIN AS A COMPONENT OF GLUCOSE-INSULIN-POTASSIUM SOLUTIONS

The earliest use of insulin to treat coronary artery disease was as a component of glucose-insulin-potassium (GIK) solutions. During periods of myocardial ischemia, exogenous glucose is the major substrate for myocardial energy metabolism [16]. Hence, it was hypothesized that a solution containing high concentrations of glucose combined with insulin would act to enhance myocardial glucose uptake and limit myocardial injury. In 1965, Sodi-Pollares and colleagues [44] used GIK in patients with acutely infarcted myocardium and found that it limited electrocardiographic changes. However, other trials failed to show a survival benefit in patients with acute MIs [45]. These studies were performed before percutaneous transluminal coronary angioplasty, stenting, and CABG surgery. The emergence of these new technologies prompted a renewed interest in using GIK in patients with ischemic heart disease. In an experimental study in a porcine model simulating surgical revascularization of acutely ischemic myocardium, Lazar and coworkers [46] found that hearts treated with GIK had less myocardial tissue acidosis, better preservation of regional wall motion, and the lowest area of tissue necrosis. These favorable results led to a clinical trial in nondiabetic patients undergoing urgent CABG in which no attempt was made to control serum glucose levels [47]. GIK patients had significantly higher mean postoperative glucose levels (240 mg/dL vs 145 mg/dL; $P<.02$). Despite these higher glucose values, the GIK-treated patients had higher postoperative cardiac indices, required less inotropic support, had less weight gain, spent less time on the ventilator, had a lower incidence of atrial fibrillation, and shorter stays in the ICU and hospital. This study was completed in 1996 when the incidence of diabetes in patients undergoing CABG was only 5% to 10%. A more recent study by Quinn and coworkers [48] looked at the use of GIK in an era when diabetes compromises nearly 40% of all patients undergoing CABG. In this study, 280 nondiabetic patients undergoing isolated CABG surgery were prospectively randomized to receive either D5W or GIK. Supplemental boluses of IV insulin were used to keep serum glucose less than or equal to 270 mg/dL. GIK treated patients had significantly higher cardiac indices, a lower incidence of low cardiac output syndrome, less need for inotropic support and less biochemical and electrocardiographic evidence of myocardial injury. Similar to the results reported by Lazar and coworkers, these beneficial results occurred despite the fact that GIK patients had higher serum glucose values.

Nevertheless, there was still concern about using GIK during cardiac surgery because of the potential for hyperglycemia in patients who have undiagnosed diabetes mellitus. Koskenkari and coworkers [49] addressed this issue in 49 patients with diabetes undergoing cardiac surgery. Patients were prospectively randomized to a GIK group with supplemental IV insulin to maintain serum glucose between 108 and 180 mg/dL and an intermittent IV insulin group targeted to maintain serum glucose less than 180 mg/dL. The infusions were started at the time of surgery and continued for 16 hours in the ICU. The GIK patients achieved lower mean postoperative glucose levels (150 mg/dL vs 190 mg/dL; $P<.01$), had lower lactate and free fatty acid levels, and required less inotropic support. The study provided further evidence that continuous insulin infusions are superior to intermittent insulin boluses in achieving lower glucose levels and that using supplemental insulin avoids the hyperglycemia that may be associated with GIK therapy.

FAVORABLE EFFECTS OF INSULIN INFUSIONS IN PATIENTS UNDERGOING CABG

Patients known to have diabetes mellitus were excluded from GIK trials. However, evidence was accumulating that GIK infusions might also have a beneficial effect in patients with diabetes with acutely ischemic myocardium.

The Diabetes Mellitus, Insulin, Glucose Infusion in Acute Myocardial Infarction trial involved 620 patients with an acute MI who were prospectively randomized to receive an IV GIK infusion followed by multidose subcutaneous insulin injections [50]. Patients treated with GIK had a 30% reduction in mortality after 1 year. These favorable effects persisted for a mean of 3.5 years [51]. Based on these findings, Lazar and coworkers [52] sought to determine whether using a modified GIK solution with more insulin and less glucose designed to maintain a serum glucose less than 180 mg/dL would limit ischemic damage in patients with diabetes undergoing CABG. In this trial involving 141 patients with diabetes undergoing isolated CABG surgery, patients were prospectively randomized to receive either GIK (500 mL D5W plus 80 units regular insulin plus 40 mEq KCl) to keep serum glucose between 120 and 180 mg/dL or sliding-scale insulin coverage to maintain glucose less than 250 mg/dL. The GIK was started on anesthetic induction and continued for 12 hours in the ICU. GIK-treated patients achieved significantly better glycemic control immediately before cardiopulmonary bypass (169 mg/dL vs 209 mg/dL; $P<.0001$) and the following 12 hours in the ICU (134 mg/dL vs 266 mg/dL; $P<.0001$). Serum lactate levels were also significantly lower in the GIK-treated patients at 6 and 12 hours. This finding was reflected in significantly lower free fatty acid levels at 6 hours in the ICU in the GIK-treated patients. Although these favorable changes in myocardial metabolism did not result in any difference in mortality (0% for each group), they were reflected in a decrease in postoperative morbidity and improved long-term survival. Patients treated with tight glycemic control had significantly higher cardiac indices and less need for inotropic support and pacing. GIK-treated patients gained less weight and spent less time on the ventilator. Tighter glycemic control also resulted in a lower incidence of infections (0% vs 13%; $P = .01$) and atrial fibrillation (15% vs 60%; $P = .007$). This all contributed to a shorter hospital length of stay (6.5 days vs 9.2 days; $P = .0003$). Following 5 years, Kaplan-Meier curves showed a significant survival advantage ($P = .04$) for patients receiving tight glycemic control. They had a significantly lower incidence of recurrent ischemia, wound infections, and were able to maintain a lower angina class. Lazar and coworkers concluded that tight glycemic control (120–180 mg/dL) during surgery and for 12 hours in the ICU improved postoperative outcomes and enhanced long-term survival in patients with diabetes undergoing CABG.

Furnary and coworkers [53] reported one of the earliest studies that examined the effects of tight glycemic control during cardiac surgery. The study involved

3554 patients undergoing CABG surgery from 1987 to 2001. Patients were divided into 3 groups based on the year of surgery, the method of glycemic control, and the targeted glucose level. From 1987 to 1991, patients received subcutaneous insulin given every 4 hours to keep serum glucose less than 200 mg/dL. From 1991 to 1998, a continuous insulin infusion was used to keep serum glucose to within 150 to 200 mg/dL. From 1999 to 2001, the Portland protocol was instituted, which used a continuous insulin drip to keep serum glucose between 100 and 150 mg/dL. Continuous insulin infusions resulted in significantly lower mean glucose levels than could be obtained with intermittent subcutaneous insulin therapy. The perioperative mortality in patients with diabetes undergoing CABG was decreased by 50% after 1992 (4.5% vs 1.9%; $P<.001$) when continuous insulin protocols were instituted and was similar to that for nondiabetic patients undergoing CABG. There was also a significant decrease in the incidence of deep sternal wound infections ($P<.001$). The study showed that continuous insulin infusions resulted in more optimal control of perioperative glucose values, which contributed to improved clinical outcomes.

Furnary and coworkers [54] expanded their original series to include an additional 1980 patients managed with the Portland protocol from 2001 to 2005. They introduced a new method to assess glycemic control called 3-BG. This method consisted of the average of all glucose values obtained on the day of surgery and the first and second postoperative days. An increase in 3-BG was an independent predictor of perioperative mortality ($<.001$). Although the significant association between hyperglycemia and mortality was no longer apparent after the second postoperative day, it remained a significant independent risk factor for mortality, as long as the patient remained in the ICU. Changes in 3-BG were also associated with postoperative morbidity. A mean 3-BG greater than 175 mg/dL was associated with a significant increase in deep sternal wound infections and hospital length of stay. Length of stay was independently increased for every 64 mg/dL increase in 3-BG. Increased 3-BG also independently increased the risk of blood transfusions, new onset atrial fibrillation, and low cardiac output syndrome. Based on their findings, Furnary and coworkers [54] recommended that all cardiac surgical patients with diabetes receive a continuous insulin infusion starting in the operating room and continuing for 48 hours following surgery. Furthermore, they advised continuing the insulin infusion as long as the patient required ICU care.

Previous studies have shown that patients with a mean glucose greater than 200 mg/dL in the postoperative period have an increased risk for postoperative wound infections [55]. Kerr and coworkers [56] demonstrated the importance of glycemic control in lowering sternal wound infections. In 1585 patients with diabetes undergoing CABG, the incidence of sternal wound infections increased from 1.3% in patients with mean glucose values of 100 to 150 mg/dL to 6.7% in patients with levels of 250 to 300 mg/dL. In a retrospective study involving patients with diabetes undergoing CABG, Hruska and coworkers [57] found that a continuous insulin infusion maintaining glucose levels between 120 and 160 mg/dL significantly decreased the incidence of sternal wound infections compared with intermittent subcutaneous injections. Similar to the data from Lazar and Furnary, the institution of continuous insulin infusions resulted in a significant decrease in wound infections, such that there was no difference in sternal infections between patients with diabetes and nondiabetic patients. In a prospective randomized study in cardiac surgical patients with diabetes, Rassias and coworkers [58] provided further insight into the mechanism for the favorable effect of insulin infusions on wound infections. Patients receiving a continuous insulin infusion had significantly lower glucose levels intraoperatively and in the immediate postoperative ICU period compared with patients treated with an intermittent sliding-scale protocol. As a result, neutrophil phagocytic activity decreased only 75% of the baseline in the continuous insulin-infusion group compared with 47% in the patients treated with intermittent insulin boluses. This study strongly suggested that continuous insulin infusions resulting in tight glycemic control improve phagocytic function in the neutrophils of patients with diabetic undergoing cardiac surgery. This mechanism may be responsible for the reduced incidence of wound infections seen in these patients.

The importance of tight glycemic control in patients undergoing CABG surgery was also demonstrated in a study by Van den Berghe and coworkers [59] involving 1548 ventilated patients admitted to a surgical ICU. In this prospective randomized study, 62% of the patients had undergone cardiac surgery and only 13% had a prior history of diabetes. During their ICU stay, patients were randomized to a conventional therapeutic group whereby insulin was administered only if serum glucose exceeded 250 mg/dL to maintain a target goal of 180 to 200 mg/dL and an intensive group that received a continuous insulin infusion to maintain glucose levels between 80 and 110 mg/dL. In the patient cohort, which included general surgery patients, intensive insulin therapy resulted in a significant reduction in mortality (10% vs 20%, $P = .005$) exclusively in those patients requiring 5 or more days of ICU care with multiorgan failure and sepsis. Similarly, cardiac surgical mortality was only reduced in those patients requiring 3 or more days of ICU care. These patients also had a significant reduction in renal failure and the need for blood transfusions. The overall hospital mortality for patients requiring 3 or more days of ICU care was reduced from 22% to 8% ($P<.05$). Hospital mortality for all cardiac surgical patients regardless of their ICU stay was reduced from 5.1% to 2.1% ($P<.05$). In their study, Van den Berghe and coworkers [59] demonstrated that tight glycemic control was beneficial for cardiac surgical patients requiring 3 or more days of ICU care, especially in ventilated patients and those with multisystem failure. Similar to Furnary and coworkers, their data show that maintaining insulin infusions for the duration of the ICU stay in all cardiac surgical patients contributes to improved survival [53,54]. They also demonstrated that it is the degree of glycemic control achieved rather than the quantity of insulin administered, which resulted in decreased mortality in patients with multiorgan dysfunction. In their series, intensive glycemic control had no effect on morbidity and mortality in those patients spending 3 days or less in the ICU. In a further attempt to identify those patients who might benefit the most from tight glycemic control, D'Alessandro and coworkers [60] sought to correlate the effect of tight glycemic control with expected EuroScore outcomes in patients with diabetes undergoing CABG. Three hundred patients with diabetes undergoing CABG surgery from January 2003 to June 2004 receiving tight glycemic control were matched with 300 patients with diabetes undergoing CABG treated from March 2001 to September 2002, when insulin protocols were not present, using propensity-based analyses. Tight glycemic control was achieved with intermittent subcutaneous insulin infusions during surgery to maintain serum glucose between 150 and 200 mg/dL. In the ICU, the insulin infusion was titrated to keep serum glucose less than 150 mg/dL. The baseline EuroScore risk profiles were similar in both groups, as were preoperative mean blood glucose levels. However, blood glucose levels following surgery and on postoperative days 1 and 2 were significantly lower in the tight glycemic group, resulting in an observed mortality in the tight glycemic group that was significantly lower than expected (1.3% vs 4.3%; $P = .01$). This finding was especially lower in the higher-risk cohort (EuroScore >4; 2.5% vs 8.0%; $P = .03$). In contrast, there was no difference between observed and expected mortality in the group without tight glycemic control (4.0% vs 3.9% for the group; 8.3% vs 7.6% in patients with a EuroScore >4). These findings strongly suggest that patients with diabetes with the highest risk tend to benefit the most from tight glycemic control.

IS TIGHT GLYCEMIC CONTROL NECESSARY IN NONDIABETIC PATIENTS UNDERGOING CABG?

Butterworth and coworkers [61] studied the effects of tight glycemic control in 381 nondiabetic patients undergoing isolated CABG surgery. In this prospective randomized trial, one group received an insulin infusion when intraoperative glucose levels exceeded 100 mg/dL. The other group received no insulin coverage. The primary outcome was the incidence of new neurologic, neuro-ophthalmologic, or neurobehavioral deficits and neurologic-related deaths. Intraoperative glucose levels were significantly lower in the patients that received an insulin infusion; however, there was no difference between the incidences of neurologic complications between the groups. Furthermore, there was no difference in operative mortality, need for inotropic support, or length of hospital stay between the groups despite the fact that patients without intraoperative insulin had glucose levels greater than or equal to 200 mg/dL. Butterworth concluded that in nondiabetic patients, intraoperative tight glycemic control failed to improve short- or long-term clinical outcomes. Gandhi and coworkers [62] looked at the effects of intensive intraoperative insulin therapy in 400 elective patients undergoing CABG. Patients were prospectively randomized to a continuous insulin group to maintain serum glucose between 80 and 100 mg/dL or a conventional group targeted to keep serum glucose less than 200 mg/dL using intermittent boluses of IV insulin. The incidence of diabetes was 20% in both groups. There was no difference in the primary outcome between the groups, which consisted of the composite incidence of death, sternal wound infections, prolonged ventilation, cardiac arrhythmias, strokes, and renal failure within 30 days of surgery. There was also no difference in ICU or hospital stay between the groups. Patients receiving aggressive glycemic control in the operating room had significantly lower mean intraoperative glucose levels (114 mg/dL vs 157 mg/dL; $P<.01$), but there was no difference in glucose levels 24 hours following surgery (103 mg/dL vs 104 mg/dL). There was a tendency for more deaths and strokes in the intensive insulin group. The study was limited in that it included both patients with diabetes and nondiabetic patients. Both groups received intensive insulin therapy in the immediate postoperative period so that a clear distinction between tight glycemic control versus intermittent insulin therapy could not be made. Furthermore, in both studies, the average postoperative serum glucose 24 hours following surgery was less than 180 mg/dL in the group that did not receive a continuous insulin infusion. So in fact, these patients actually achieved the same degree of glycemic control as seen in patients with diabetes who received continuous insulin therapy. This finding suggests that tight glycemic control might also be beneficial in nondiabetic patients during CABG surgery. Further clarification of the role of glycemic control in nondiabetic patients was provided by Szekely and coworkers [6] in their large (550 patients) multicenter series of patients undergoing primary CABG surgery. In this trial, early (48 hours) postoperative maximum glucose levels greater than or equal to 250 mg/dL were associated with increased in-hospital mortality in nondiabetic but not diabetic patients. However, only 25% of nondiabetic patients were treated with a perioperative insulin infusion compared with 84.4% of the patients with diabetes. Study protocols were not used to control the level of serum glucose in this series.

A growing number of patients undergoing CABG surgery may have abnormal glucose tolerance, metabolic syndrome, or early diabetes that remains undetected before surgery. Elevated blood glucose levels in the perioperative period in these nondiabetic patients have been attributed to stress hyperglycemia. However, this patient cohort most likely suffers from either diabetes or abnormal glucose metabolism, has reduced ejection fractions and more unstable disease, and would benefit from maintaining serum glucose levels less than or equal to 180 mg/dL. All patients with diabetes and those at risk for diabetes with abnormal preoperative glucose levels should have an HbA1c level before surgery to help guide their perioperative glucose management.

CURRENT GUIDELINES FOR GLYCEMIC CONTROL DURING CARDIAC SURGERY

Based on these studies, the current recommendations of the Society of Thoracic Surgery regarding blood glucose management during adult cardiac surgery is as follows [63]:

1. All patients with diabetes undergoing cardiac surgical procedures should receive an insulin infusion in the operating room and for at least 24 hours postoperatively to maintain serum glucose levels less than or equal to 180 mg/dL (class I; level of evidence B).

2. An HbA1c level should be obtained before surgery in patients with diabetes or those patients at risk for postoperative hyperglycemia to characterize the level of postoperative glycemic control (class I; level of evidence C).
3. Glucose levels greater than 180 mg/dL that occur in patients without diabetes only during cardiopulmonary bypass may be treated initially with a single intermittent dose of IV insulin as long as levels remain less than or equal to 180 mg/dL. However, in those patients with persistently elevated glucose (>180 mg/dL) after cardiopulmonary bypass, a continuous insulin drip should be instituted (class I; level of evidence B).
4. Patients with and without diabetes with persistently elevated serum glucose (>180 mg/dL) should receive IV insulin infusions to maintain serum glucose less than 180 mg/dL for the duration of their ICU care (class I; level of evidence A).
5. All patients who require 3 or more days in the ICU because of ventilatory dependency or require the need for inotropes, an intra-aortic balloon pump or left ventricular assist support, antiarrhythmics, dialysis, or continuous veno-venous hemofiltration should have a continuous insulin infusion to keep blood glucose less than or equal to 150 mg/dL regardless of their diabetic status (class I; level of evidence B).

WHAT IS THE OPTIMAL GOAL FOR PERIOPERATIVE GLYCEMIC CONTROL: IS TOO AGGRESSIVE DETRIMENTAL?

Based on data from studies cited in this article, there is now a general consensus that tight glycemic control improves the outcomes in both patients with diabetes and patients without diabetes undergoing CABG surgery. However, the optimal target for perioperative blood glucose levels is unknown. Although studies have shown that maintaining serum glucose levels less than 180 mg/dL reduces morbidity and mortality in patients undergoing CABG, the effects of more aggressive control on clinical endpoints is less clearly defined. Studies involving medical ICU patients failed to show any improvement in mortality with more aggressive glycemic control and had to be discontinued because of a significant increase in hypoglycemic episodes [64,65]. In the study by Van den Berghe and coworkers [59], in which blood glucose levels were kept between 80 and 100 mg/dL, cardiac surgical mortality was only reduced in those patients who received more than 3 days of ICU care and in patients with multiorgan failure and sepsis. Aggressive glycemic control had no effect on morbidity and mortality in those CABG patients spending less than 3 days in the ICU, which represents most patients in most practices. Recent trials in both ICU and non-ICU and surgical and nonsurgical patients have raised concerns that more aggressive glycemic control may actually increase mortality [64,66–69]. To determine the effects of more aggressive glycemic control in patients with diabetes during CABG surgery, Lazar and coworkers [70] prospectively randomized patients either to an aggressive (90–120 mg/dL) or moderate (120–180 mg/dL) protocol. There was no difference in the incidence of 30-day mortality, MI, neurologic events, deep sternal infections, or atrial fibrillation between the groups. Patients with aggressive control had a higher incidence of hypoglycemic events, but this did not result in any clinical sequelae. Hence, more aggressive glycemic control did not result in any significant improvement in clinical outcomes that could not be achieved with more moderate control. These results were consistent with a study by Bhamidipati and coworkers [71] that showed that achieving moderate glycemic control (120–179 mg/dL) in patients with diabetes undergoing CABG was associated with the least amount of morbidity and mortality. The American College of Physicians now recommends achieving a more moderate glucose level of 140 to 200 mg/dL in surgical and medical ICU patients [72].

There are several explanations for why more aggressive protocols to achieve glycemic control failed to enhance clinical outcomes. Many patients were already receiving optimal cardiovascular prevention with statins, angiotensin-converting enzyme inhibitors, aspirin, and weight-reduction programs. Therefore, the added benefit of more aggressive glucose control may not have been as significant in these patients. Furthermore, moderate control has already been shown to significantly improve clinical outcomes in CABG patients, which may be difficult to improve on with a more aggressive protocol. Although more aggressive control did not improve short-term outcomes, it did lower markers of inflammation, such as free fatty acids [70]. It is conceivable that this reduction in the inflammatory response may result in improved long-term outcomes by enhancing vein graft patency. This area will be the subject of future studies to determine the most optimal level of glycemic control in patients undergoing CABG.

SUMMARY

In summary, poor perioperative glycemic control in patients undergoing CABG is associated with increased morbidity and mortality. Maintaining serum glucose less than or equal to 180 mg/dL in patients with diabetes during CABG reduces morbidity and mortality, lowers the incidence of wound infections, reduces hospital length of stay, and enhances long-term survival. In nondiabetic patients undergoing CABG surgery, maintaining serum glucose less than 180 mg/dL has also resulted in improved perioperative outcomes. More aggressive glycemic control (80–120 mg/dL) provides no added improvement in CABG patients with less than or equal to 3 days of ICU care in the absence of ventilatory support or multiorgan failure.

Although the precise value for achieving glycemic control in the perioperative period is the subject of much debate, the benefits of perioperative glycemic control with continuous insulin infusions in patients undergoing CABG is no longer debatable.

References
[1] SMART Study Group. Prevalence of the metabolic syndrome in patients with coronary heart disease, peripheral arterial disease, or abdominal aortic aneurysm. Atherosclerosis 2004;173(2):363–9.
[2] Szabo Z, Sakanson E, Svedjeholm R. Early postoperative outcome and medium-term survival in 540 diabetic and 2,239 non-diabetic patients undergoing coronary artery bypass grafting. Ann Thorac Surg 2002;74:712–9.

[3] Cohen Y, Raz I, Merin G, et al. Comparison of factors associated with 30-day mortality after coronary artery bypass grafting in patients with versus without diabetes mellitus. Am J Cardiol 1998;81:7–11.

[4] Carson JL, Scholz PM, Chen AY, et al. Diabetes mellitus increases short-term mortality and morbidity in patients undergoing coronary artery bypass graft surgery. J Am Coll Cardiol 2002;40:418–23.

[5] Alserium T, Hammar N, Nordquist T, et al. Risk of death or acute myocardial infarction 10 years after coronary artery bypass surgery in relation to type of diabetes. Am Heart J 2006;152(3):599–605.

[6] Szekely A, Levin J, Miao Y, et al. Impact of hyperglycemia on perioperative mortality after coronary artery bypass graft surgery. J Thorac Cardiovasc Surg 2011;142:430–7.

[7] Ascione R, Rogers CA, Rajakaruna C, et al. Inadequate blood glucose control is associated with in-hospital mortality and morbidity in diabetic and non-diabetic patients undergoing cardiac surgery. Circulation 2008;118:113–23.

[8] Roques F, Nashef SA, Michel P, et al. Risk factors and outcome in European cardiac surgery: analysis of the EuroScore multi-national database of 19,030 patients. Eur J Cardiothorac Surg 1999;15:816–22.

[9] Jacoby R, Nesto R. Acute myocardial infarction in the diabetic patient: pathophysiology, clinical course and prognosis. J Am Coll Cardiol 1992;20:736–44.

[10] Steward RD, Lahey SJ, Levitsky S, et al. Clinical and economic impact of diabetes following coronary artery bypass. J Surg Res 1998;76(2):124–30.

[11] Herlitz J, Wognesen GB, Emanvelsson H, et al. Mortality and morbidity in diabetic and non-diabetic patients during a 2-year period after coronary artery bypass grafting. Diabetes Care 1996;19(7):698–703.

[12] Whang W, Bigger JT Jr. Diabetes and outcomes of coronary artery bypass graft surgery in patients with severe left ventricular dysfunction: results from the CABG Patch Trial database. The CABG Patch Trial Investigators and Coordinators. J Am Coll Cardiol 2000;36(4): 1166–72.

[13] Estrada CA, Young JA, Nifong LW, et al. Outcomes and perioperative hyperglycemia in patients with or without diabetes mellitus undergoing coronary artery bypass grafting. Ann Thorac Surg 2003;75(5):1392–9.

[14] Ferguson TF Jr, Hammill BG, Peterson ED, et al. For the STS National Database Committee. A decade of change – risk profiles and outcomes for isolated coronary artery bypass grafting procedures, 1990-1999: a report from the STS National Database Committee and the Duke Clinical Research Institute. Ann Thorac Surg 2002;73:480–90.

[15] Hlatky MA, Melson KA, Boothroyd DB. Bypass Angioplasty Revascularization Investigation 2 Diabetes (BARI 2D) Trial Investigators. Economic evaluation of alternative strategies to treat patients with diabetes mellitus and coronary artery disease. Am J Cardiol 2006;97(12A):59G–65G.

[16] Opie LH. Effects of regional ischemia on metabolism of glucose and fatty acids. Relative rates of aerobic and anaerobic energy production during myocardial infarction and comparison with effects of anoxia. Circ Res 1976;38:152–74.

[17] Liv Q, Docherty J, Rendell JC, et al. High levels of fatty acids delay the recovery of intracellular pH and cardiac efficiency in post-ischemic hearts by inhibiting glucose oxidation. J Am Coll Cardiol 2002;39:718–25.

[18] Sowers JR, Epstein M. Diabetes mellitus and associated hypertension, vascular disease, and nephropathy. Hypertension 1995;26:869–79.

[19] Schmidt AM, Yan SD, Wautier JL, et al. Activation of receptor for advanced glycation endpoints: a mechanism for chronic vascular dysfunction in diabetic vasculopathy and atherosclerosis. Circ Res 1999;84:489–97.

[20] Viassara H. Recent progress in advanced glycation end-products and diabetic complications. Diabetes 1997;46:519–25.

[21] Dandona P, Aljada A, Mohanty P, et al. Insulin inhibits intranuclear nuclear factor Kappa B and stimulates 1 Kappa B in mononuclear cells in obese subjects: evidence for anti-inflammatory effect. J Clin Endocrinol Metab 2001;86:3257–65.

[22] Guerci B, Bohme P, Kearney-Schwartz A, et al. Endothelial dysfunction and type-2 diabetes. Diabetes Metab 2001;27:436–47.

[23] Park JY, Takahara N, Gabriele A, et al. Induction of endothelin-1 expression by glucose. An effect on protein kinase-C activation. Diabetes 2001;49:1239–48.

[24] Verma S, Maitland A, Weisel RD, et al. Hyperglycemia exaggerates ischemia-reperfusion-induced cardiomyocyte injury: reversal with endothelium antagonism. J Thorac Cardiovasc Surg 2002;123:1120–4.

[25] Lazar HL, Joseph L, San Mateo C, et al. Expression of inducible nitric oxide synthase in conduits used in patients with diabetes mellitus undergoing coronary revascularization. J Card Surg 2010;25:120–6.

[26] Pompilio G, Rossoni G, Alamanni F, et al. Comparison of endothelium-dependent vasoactivity of internal mammary arteries from hypertensive, hypercholesterolemic, and diabetic patients. Ann Thorac Surg 2001;72:1290–7.

[27] Guzik TS, Mussa S, Gastaldi D, et al. Mechanisms of increased vascular superoxide production in human diabetes mellitus: role of NAD(1)H oxidase and endothelial nitric oxide synthase. Circulation 2001;105:1656–62.

[28] Davi G, Catalan I, Averna M. Thromboxane biosynthesis and platelet function in type II diabetes mellitus. N Engl J Med 1990;322:1769–74.

[29] Marfella R, Esposito K, Gionata R, et al. Circulating adhesion molecules in humans: role of hyperglycemia and hyperinsulinemia. Circulation 2000;101:2247–51.

[30] Suzuka K, Kono T. Evidence that insulin causes translocation of glucose transport activity to the plasma membrane from intracellular storage site. Proc Natl Acad Sci U S A 1980;77:2542–7.

[31] Jeschke MG, Klein D, Javch KW. Insulin attenuates the systemic inflammatory in endotoxemic rats. Endocrinology 2004;145:4084–93.

[32] Langovche L, Vanhorebeek I, Vlaselaers D, et al. Intensive insulin therapy protects the endothelium of critically ill patients. J Clin Invest 2005;115:1177–86.

[33] Johassen AK, Sack MN, Ejos OD, et al. Myocardial protection by insulin at reperfusion requires early administration and is mediated via AKT and p70s6 kinase cell-survival signaling. Circ Res 2001;89:1191–8.

[34] Gao F, Gao E, Yue EL, et al. Nitric oxide mediates the antiapoptotic effect of insulin in myocardial ischemia-reperfusion: the roles of P13-kinase, AKT, and endothelial nitric oxide synthase phosphorylation. Circulation 2002;105:1497–502.

[35] Svensson S, Svedjeholm R, Ekroth R. Trauma metabolism of the heart: uptake of substrates and effects of insulin early after cardiac operations. J Thorac Cardiovasc Surg 1990;99:1063–73.

[36] Rao V, Merante F, Weisel RD, et al. Insulin stimulates pyruvate dehydrogenase and protects human ventricular cardiomyocytes from simulated ischemia. J Thorac Cardiovasc Surg 1998;116:485–94.

[37] Doenst T, Wiseysundera D, Karkouti K, et al. Hyperglycemia during cardiopulmonary bypass is an independent risk factor for mortality in patients undergoing cardiac surgery. J Thorac Cardiovasc Surg 2005;130:1140–50.

[38] Fish LH, Weaver TW, Moore AL, et al. Value of postoperative blood glucose in predicting complications and length of stay after coronary artery bypass grafting. Am J Cardiol 2003;92:74–6.

[39] McAlister FA, Man J, Bistritz L, et al. Diabetes and coronary artery bypass surgery. Diabetes Care 2003;26:1518–24.

[40] Gandhi GY, Nuttall GA, Abel MD, et al. Intraoperative hyperglycemia and perioperative outcomes in cardiac surgery patients. Mayo Clin Proc 2005;80:862–6.

[41] Anderson RE, Klerdal K, Ivert T. Fasting blood glucose and mortality after coronary artery bypass graft surgery. Eur Heart J 2005;26:1513–8.

[42] Imran SA, Ransom TB, Bluth KR, et al. Impact of admission serum glucose level on in-hospital outcomes following coronary artery bypass grafting surgery. Can J Cardiol 2010;26:151–4.

[43] Duncan AE, Abd-Elsayed A, Maheshwari A, et al. Role of intraoperative and postoperative blood glucose concentrations in predicting outcomes after cardiac surgery. Anesthesiology 2010;112:860–71.

[44] Sodi-Pollares D, Testelli MD, Fisleder BL, et al. Effects of an intravenous infusion of a potassium-glucose-insulin solution on the electrocardiographic signs of myocardial infarction. Am J Cardiol 1965;5:166–81.

[45] Medical Research Council Working Party. Potassium, glucose, and insulin treatment for acute myocardial infarction. Lancet 1968;2:1355–60.

[46] Lazar HL, Zhang X, Rivers S, et al. Limiting ischemic myocardial damage using glucose-insulin-potassium solutions. Ann Thorac Surg 1995;60:411–6.

[47] Lazar HL, Philippides G, Fitzgerald C, et al. Glucose-insulin-potassium solutions enhance recovery after urgent coronary artery bypass grafting. J Thorac Cardiovasc Surg 1997;113:354–62.

[48] Quinn DW, Pagano D, Bonser RS, et al. Improved myocardial protection during coronary artery surgery with glucose-insulin-potassium: a randomized controlled trial. J Thorac Cardiovasc Surg 2006;131:34–42.

[49] Koskenkark JK, Kaukoranta PK, Kivilvoma KT, et al. Metabolic and hemodynamic effects of high-dose insulin treatment in aortic valve and coronary surgery. Ann Thorac Surg 2005;80:511–7.

[50] Malmberg K, Ryden L, Efendic S, et al. Randomized trial of insulin-glucose infusion followed by subcutaneous insulin treatment in diabetic patients with acute myocardial infarction (DIGAMI Study): effects on mortality at 1 year. J Am Coll Cardiol 1995;26:57–65.

[51] DIGAMI Study Group. Prospective, randomized study of intensive insulin treatment on long-term survival after acute myocardial infarction in patients with diabetes mellitus. BMJ 1997;314:1512–5.

[52] Lazar HL, Chipkin SR, Fitzgerald CA, et al. Tight glycemic control in diabetic coronary artery bypass graft patients improves perioperative outcomes and decreases recurrent ischemic events. Circulation 2004;109:1497–502.

[53] Furnary AP, Gao G, Grunkemeier GL, et al. Continuous insulin infusion reduces mortality in patients with diabetes undergoing coronary artery bypass grafting. J Thorac Cardiovasc Surg 2003;125:1007–21.

[54] Furnary A, Wu Y, Bookin S. Effect of hyperglycemia and continuous intravenous insulin infusions on outcomes of cardiac surgical procedures: the Portland diabetic project. Endocr Pract 2004;10(Suppl 2):21–33.

[55] Golden SH, Peart-Vigilance C, Kao WH, et al. Perioperative glycemic control and the risk of infectious complications in a cohort of adults with diabetes. Diabetes Care 1999;22:1408–14.

[56] Kerr K, Furnary A, Grunkemeier G, et al. Glucose control lowers the risk of wound infections in diabetics after open heart operations. Ann Thorac Surg 1997;63:356–61.

[57] Hruska LA, Smith JM, Hendy MP, et al. Continuous insulin infusion reduces infectious complications in diabetes following coronary surgery. J Card Surg 2005;20:402–7.

[58] Rassias AJ, Marrin CA, Arruda J, et al. Insulin infusion improves neutrophil function in diabetic cardiac surgery patients. Anesth Analg 1999;88:1011–6.

[59] Van den Berghe G, Wouters P, Weekers F, et al. Intensive insulin therapy in critically ill patients. N Engl J Med 2001;345:1359–67.

[60] D'Allessandro C, Leprince P, Golmard JL, et al. Strict glycemic control reduces EuroScore expected mortality in diabetic patients undergoing myocardial revascularization. J Thorac Cardiovasc Surg 2007;134:29–37.

[61] Butterworth J, Wagenknecht LE, Legault C, et al. Attempted control of hyperglycemia during cardiopulmonary bypass fails to improve neurologic or neurobehavioral outcomes in patients without diabetes mellitus undergoing coronary artery bypass grafting. J Thorac Cardiovasc Surg 2005;130:1319–25.

[62] Gandhi GY, Nuttall GA, Abel ND, et al. Intensive intraoperative insulin therapy versus conventional glucose management during cardiac surgery. Ann Intern Med 2007;146: 233–42.

[63] Lazar HL, McDonnell M, Chipkin S, et al. The Society of Thoracic Surgeons practice guideline series: blood glucose management during adult cardiac surgery. Ann Thorac Surg 2009;87:663–9.

[64] NICE-SUGAR Study Investigators, Finfer S, Chittock DR, Su SY, et al. Intensive versus conventional glucose control in critically ill patients. N Engl J Med 2009;360:1283–97.

[65] Preiser JC, Devos P. Clinical experience with tight glucose control by intensive insulin therapy. Crit Care Med 2007;35:S503–7.

[66] Action to Control Cardiovascular Risk in Diabetes Study Group, Gerstein HC, Miller ME, Byinton RP, et al. Effects of intensive glucose lowering in type 2 diabetes. N Engl J Med 2008;358:2545–59.

[67] The UK Prospective Diabetes Study (UKPDS) Group. Effect of intensive blood-glucose control with metformin on complications in overweight patients with type 2 diabetes (UKPDS 34). Lancet 1993;352:854–65.

[68] Advance Collaborative Group, Patel A, MacMahond A, Chalmers J, et al. Intensive blood glucose control and vascular outcomes in patients with type 2 diabetes. N Engl J Med 2008;358:2560–72.

[69] Zoungas S, Patel A, Chalmers J, et al, The ADVANCE Collaborative Group. Severe hypoglycemia and risks of vascular events and death. N Engl J Med 2010;363:1410–6.

[70] Lazar HL, McDonnell M, Chipkin S, et al. Effects of aggressive versus moderate glycemic control on clinical outcomes in diabetic coronary artery bypass graft patients. Ann Surg 2011;254(3):458–64.

[71] Bhamidipati CM, LaPar DJ, Stukenborg GJ, et al. Superiority of moderate control of hyperglycemia to tight control in patients undergoing coronary artery bypass grafting. J Thorac Cardiovasc Surg 2010;141:1–9.

[72] Qaseem A, Humphrey LL, Chou R, et al. For the Clinical Guidelines Committee of the American College of Physicians. Use of intensive insulin therapy for the management of glycemic control in hospitalized patients. A clinical practice guideline fro American College of Physicians. Ann Intern Med 2011;154:260–7.

Capillary Leak Syndrome in Trauma
What is it and What are the Consequences?

Deborah M. Stein, MD, MPH[a,b,*], Thomas M. Scalea, MD[a,b]

[a]University of Maryland School of Medicine, 22 South Greene Street, Baltimore, MD 21201, USA;
[b]R Adams Cowley Shock Trauma Center, 22 South Greene Street, Baltimore, MD 21201, USA

Keywords
- Capillary leak syndrome • Traumatic injury • Compartment syndrome
- Systemic inflammation

Key Points
- TICS is a complex multifactorial disease in the traumatically injured patient.
- The mainstay of therapy for TICS is prevention and attenuation of its effects.
- Newer resuscitation strategies and prompt are currently the best available strategies to combat TICS.

INTRODUCTION

Largely considered a component of the systemic inflammatory response syndrome (SIRS), capillary leak syndrome (CLS) is poorly defined. Described as increased endovascular or microvascular permeability, CLS is known to occur in a variety of disease states. Although most widely reported in the setting of sepsis and septic shock, following traumatic injury CLS is also frequently seen. There are several features of traumatic disease that allow the injured patient to be uniquely susceptible to CLS. Inflammation plays a prominent role in the sequela of both systemic injury and organ-specific injury and is central to the development of trauma-induced capillary leak syndrome (TICS). Large-volume crystalloid administration, a mainstay of resuscitation strategies following trauma, also contributes significantly to the development of TICS. In addition, hypoproteinemia caused by systemic catabolic states following tissue injury plays a significant role in the development and worsening of capillary leak and tissue edema.

Direct tissue destruction due to dynamic forces applied across tissues directly causes local tissue edema and increased capillary permeability, precipitating more widespread systemic inflammation and amplifying the SIRS response to

*Corresponding author. R Adams Cowley Shock Trauma Center, 22 South Greene Street, Baltimore, MD 21201. E-mail address: dstein@umm.edu

0065-3411/12/$ – see front matter
doi:10.1016/j.yasu.2012.03.008

injury. Postcapillary hypertension due to direct lymphatic or venous injury may cause localized CLSs in affected areas. These more localized edematous states then subsequently also worsen the overall TICS due to the systemic response to local injury. CLS causes organ dysfunction and failure, which contributes to both morbidity and mortality after critical injury. Although no specific therapy is widely used to combat the effects of capillary leak, there are strategies that may be used to minimize its occurrence and attenuate its effects once it occurs. These strategies include hemostatic resuscitation and more goal-directed therapies following severe trauma. This review focuses on the development of TICS and the strategies that may be used to combat its effects following trauma.

EPIDEMIOLOGY

The leading cause of death following injury is traumatic brain injury (TBI), followed by acute hemorrhage [1]. Deaths from these diseases typically occur within the first hours to days after injury. For those who survive these acute insults, sepsis and the attendant multiple organ dysfunction syndrome (MODS) and multiple organ failure (MOF) are the leading causes of death and typically occur at approximately 2 weeks after injury. MODS and MOF account for more than 10% of injury-related deaths, [1] and mortality following the development of MODS and MOF is as high as 70% [2,3]. Following trauma, CLS plays an integral role in the development of organ dysfunction not only as part of a systemic inflammatory process but also as a direct result of both the traumatic injury itself and the treatments applied to combat its effects.

TICS is poorly described in the literature. In unpublished data from the authors' institution, the authors found TICS in as many as 21% of injured patients admitted to the intensive care unit (ICU) [4]. Once TICS occurs, mortality rate is exceptionally high, with a 10-fold increase in the risk of death. In patients with the most severe form of the disease, as defined by a serum albumin level of up to 1 mg/dL, mortality rate was 70%. Failure of albumin levels to improve over a period of 72 hours after admission resulted in a 91% positive predictive value for death. One study which used the levels of microalbuminuria to define CLS, found that levels of microalbuminuria also predicted mortality in critically ill trauma, burn, and surgical patients in adjusted analysis [5]. Because of the lack of any consensus as to the definition of TICS, population-based incidence rates following traumatic injury are currently unavailable.

DIAGNOSIS

There is currently no established definition of CLS in the setting of trauma or other disease processes. CLS has been described in several diseases aside from trauma, namely sepsis [6] and burns [7,8]. An idiopathic version called systemic capillary leak syndrome or Clarkson disease also exists [9,10]. Positive fluid balance/edema is listed as one of the suggested criteria for the definition of sepsis in a consensus conference [11], but as a syndrome that is largely considered part of the SIRS/sepsis continuum. One review article describes "... increased microvascular permeability and capillary leakage which, in turn, result in interstitial fluid accumulation, loss of protein and tissue oedema" [6]. Another defines capillary leak as "… the excess loss of fluid alone or in conjunction with protein into the interstitial and, ultimately, the lymphatic spaces, resulting in edema formation" [12]. Other definitions include: "non-cardiogenic generalized edema and haemodynamic instability" [13] or ">3% increase of body weight within 24 hours, combined with generalized oedema" [14]. Given the lack of consensus definition, the diagnosis of TICS is largely based on clinical acumen at the bedside. The general approach is "I know it when I see it."

There have been attempts to define CLS, however, in the setting of a variety of causative disease processes. In the series from the authors' institution, TICS was defined by severe hypoalbuminemia (albumin levels <2.0 mg/dL). Severe TICS was defined as an albumin level of up to 1 mg/dL [4]. Another study used microalbuminuria, defined as the urine albumin to creatinine ratio (ACR), to predict mortality in critically ill patients with CLS [5]. In this study, patients with a higher ACR had higher mortality rates in adjusted analysis. Other studies have also used microalbuminuria to detect CLS [5,15,16]. Albumin-to-globulin ratios were used in another study of patients with burns to grade the severity of the capillary leak and associate it with mortality [17]. Other studies have demonstrated an association between hypoproteinemia and increased pulmonary vascular permeability [18] emphasizing the importance of serum protein levels and CLS.

PATHOPHYSIOLOGY AND ETIOLOGY OF TICS

In the normal state, there is an exquisite balance of fluid and proteins between the capillary beds and the interstitium. The forces that govern the movement of fluid into and out of the capillaries is governed by the Starling equation [19,20]:

$$J_v = K_f([P_c - P_i] - \sigma[\pi_c - \pi_i])$$

where J_v is the net fluid movement between compartments, K_f is the capillary filtration coefficient, P_c is the capillary hydrostatic pressure, P_i is the interstitial hydrostatic pressure, σ is the reflection coefficient, π_c is the capillary colloid oncotic pressure, and π_i is the interstitial colloid oncotic pressure. The fluid is then removed from the interstitium and returned to the intravascular space by lymphatic flow. In addition to the diffusive forces that govern the movement of fluid, substances such as small proteins pass through the capillary basement membrane through intracellular vesicles and intercellular clefts [6,12,21]. The normal capillary physiology and regulation of extravascular fluid balance are expertly described in a review article by Fishel and colleagues [12].

As a result of the conditions mentioned above, any disorder that causes an increase in capillary or decrease in interstitial hydrostatic pressure or a decrease in capillary or increase in interstitial oncotic pressure results in an efflux of fluid out of the capillaries and into the extravascular tissue space. In addition, alterations in the permeability of the capillary basement membrane also allows substances to enter the interstitial space.

Inflammation

Any discussion of CLS is intimately tied to systemic inflammation following injury and hemorrhagic shock. These events have been extensively described elsewhere and involve several biochemical processes and pathways [22–24]. Briefly, following trauma there is an acute proinflammatory response that involves the release of a variety of cytokines and chemokines, namely Interleukin (IL) -1, IL-2, IL-6, and tumor necrosis factor (TNF) [22,25–28]. These substances are released largely in response to the activation of toll-like receptors (TLR) by pathogen-associated molecular patterns, which are expressed by bacteria in the setting of sepsis [25,29,30] or the newly recognized endogenous damage-associated molecular patterns [31].

Following trauma, the initiating events that signal the release of inflammatory mediators are less well described but are linked to activation of lymphocytes by the acute phase reactants that are released because of injury [22,32] or activation of TLRs by endogenous proteins, the so-called *sterile inflammation* [33]. This response is thought to be a primarily adaptive response to injury because it initiates hemostasis and tissue repair [22]. Several elegant experiments have demonstrated that interleukins directly lower the levels of interstitial fluid pressure [34–36]. In addition, IL-1 and TNF have been demonstrated to directly increase capillary permeability [12,37–40]. IL-2 has been used therapeutically to treat various forms of metastatic disease, but the use of IL-2 has been limited by the edema that occurs with administration because of an increase in capillary permeability [12], which is thought to be because of the activation of neutrophils causing endothelial cell damage [41,42] through a nitric oxide (NO)-mediated pathway [43,44].

Following injury, activation of complement pathways also occurs. Complement components C3a and C5a are well-known neutrophil attractants [22]. These neutrophils then release free oxygen radicals that are toxic to endothelial cells causing alterations in vascular permeability in the capillary bed [12,45,46]. This process is likely to occur through NO-mediated pathways, which may promote apoptosis of the endothelial cells in response to certain stimuli, such as lipopolysaccharides [38,47,48]. Histamine and bradykinin released from mast cells in areas of local tissue injury may act in a paracrine fashion to alter local tissue permeability and amplify the systemic response [22].

All these pathways and biochemical processes occur to a varying degree following severe trauma. Due to either increased permeability or altered hydrostatic or oncotic pressure, capillary leak occurs, which contributes to the impairment of tissue perfusion and oxygenation [29]. Similar to other inflammation-mediated events, such as formation of microthrombi, reduced red cell deformability [49], microvascular shunting [50], mitochondrial dysfunction [51], and vasodilatation [38], capillary leak promotes the development of organ dysfunction and subsequent failure [52].

Fluid administration

One of the mainstays of treatment of shock after injury is restoration of intravascular fluid status, which is accomplished with the administration of large volumes of blood products in the setting of hemorrhagic shock and/or crystalloid administration to combat vasodilatory-induced decreases in circulatory blood volume. The American College of Surgeon's Advanced Trauma Life Support Course recommends 1 to 2 L of warmed crystalloid infusion for any patient presenting with signs or symptoms of hypovolemia [53]. In the prehospital environment, crystalloid infusion is used for any patient with suspicion of significant injury. Restoration of blood volume is important in the setting of hypotension and hypoperfusion because splanchnic circulation is severely impaired, which may additionally lead to organ dysfunction because of the initiation of an SIRS response [54]. Hemorrhagic shock in and of itself induces inflammation as well [55].

Although fluid administration is necessary to restore circulating blood volume, it may also lead to increases in tissue edema, which is largely mediated by an increase in capillary hydrostatic pressure. When tissue edema occurs in the setting of increased capillary permeability, capillary leak ensues leading to organ dysfunction, which has been well-described in the lung in which perivascular edema from volume administration causes a decrease in oxygenation diffusion and subsequent hypoxia [54]. High volumes of crystalloid administration have been associated with not only respiratory insufficiency but also compartment syndromes, gastrointestinal dysfunction, and cardiac dysfunction from increases in tissue edema [55,56]. Crystalloid solutions, namely Ringer lactate solution, have also been associated with direct induction of the inflammatory response through increased expression of adhesion molecules [57] and induction of apoptosis [58,59] among other mechanisms [55]. In addition, crystalloid administration induces a highly dilutional state whereby fluid that is intrinsically rich in proteins is replaced by fluid with very low oncotic pressure further exacerbating capillary leak.

Aggressive fluid resuscitation is still advocated for the patient with SIRS and sepsis to restore organ perfusion and prevent further systemic inflammation [2,23,60]. Although this process may worsen capillary leak, the risks are outweighed by the benefits of restoring organ perfusion. Colloid solutions do not seem to be much better. Although associated with less of a direct induction of inflammation [56], in the setting of SIRS and altered capillary membrane permeability, colloid solutions, whether hetastarch-based or albumin, lead to increased edema because of the larger molecular weight substances going into the interstitium leading to increased oncotic pressure in the interstitial space and worsening of edema [6,12].

Catabolism

Trauma can induce a profound hypoproteinemic state [56]. Patients with tissue injury are, by definition, catabolic in the early stages after injury [61,62]. In one study, trauma was associated with a 13% loss of body protein stores [63]. Following injury, there is a recognized shift in hepatic protein synthesis from albumin to acute phase reactants and immune mediators [64,65] causing an overall reduction in protein production to maintain plasma and subsequently, capillary oncotic pressure. To provide adequate protein to vital organs, amino acids are actively extracted from the bloodstream as part of the response to injury [66]. As predicted by the Starling equation, this hypoproteinemia will lead to an efflux of fluid out of the capillaries and into the interstitial space causing tissue edema. Once MODS and MOF develop after trauma, the catabolic response is markedly amplified resulting in worsening of the edematous states [2].

Direct tissue injury

Tissue edema and capillary leak occurs in the area of tissue injury. Direct tissue destruction that occurs as a result of both direct energy transfer and indirect shearing injury causes local tissue edema and increased capillary permeability. This is seen in virtually all tissues of the body and features preeminently in secondary insults following neurologic injury and the development of compartment syndromes following injury. This direct local injury then induces systemic effects, largely through activation of the immune system and initiation of a systemic inflammatory response [67]. Classic examples of this phenomenon are seen in the setting of isolated TBI [68,69] and isolated femur fractures [70–72], which induce powerful systemic inflammation.

Postcapillary hypertension

In addition to the alterations in oncotic and hydrostatic pressures, given the role of the lymphatic system in overall regulation of tissue fluid, any disruption in the lymphatic system causes increases in tissue edema. Disruption of lymphatics occurs frequently after injury due to either primary soft tissue injury or surgical exposures for repairs of injuries. In addition, with the advent of damage control techniques, venous ligation as a lifesaving measure is being more routinely applied [73–75]. This technique can result in venous hypertension, leading to increased tissue edema and postcapillary hypertension. Postcapillary hypertension if severe and left untreated, compartment syndrome can result. These localized insults can similarly have systemic effects through induction of a systemic inflammatory response.

ORGAN-SPECIFIC EFFECTS OF TICS

Abdominal compartment syndrome

The classic example of organ injury following TICS is the development of abdominal compartment syndrome (ACS). ACS was first described in the 1980s and is currently defined as a sustained intraabdominal pressure of greater than 20 mm Hg with evidence of new organ dysfunction or failure [76]. The incidence is reported to be as high as 36% following traumatic injury [77]. The pathophysiology of the development of ACS following trauma has been described in numerous publications and has been the focus of intense investigation over the years. ACS is the quintessential TICS-related disease (Fig. 1). Capillary leak from systemic inflammation resulting from shock and aggressive fluid resuscitation leads to marked changes in abdominal wall compliance, splanchnic and retroperitoneal edema, and increases in the level of intraluminal and extraluminal fluid. This process leads to increased intraabdominal pressure, which results in

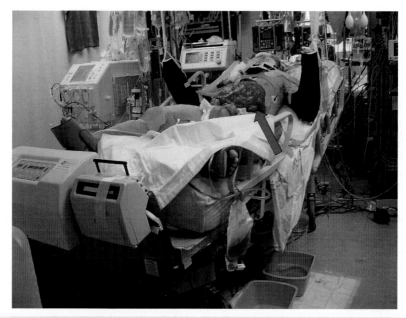

Fig. 1. A patient after polytrauma with obvious ACS due to TICS. Bowel edema is obvious in the eviscerated bowel (*arrow*) as is the overall edematous state of the patient.

direct organ compression and hypoperfusion. This leads to organ dysfunction, which subsequently worsens the capillary leak process by inducing further systemic inflammatory response [67]. If left untreated, renal and respiratory failure occur, and ultimately intestinal ischemia, leading to death [78,79].

Lung injury

The lung is considered to be the most susceptible organ to the effects of systemic edema and inflammation [2]. Large-volume fluid resuscitation with crystalloid solution has been associated with the development of pulmonary edema and inflammation [55,80–82]. This inflammatory process in the lung further exacerbates the systemic inflammatory response [83]. Decreases in plasma proteins, such as albumin and transferrin correspond to increased pulmonary vascular permeability as measured by the pulmonary leak index [18], and direct endothelial cell injury is seen in autopsy biopsy results of patients who died from acute respiratory distress syndrome (ARDS) [84]. Whether it is the decrease in plasma oncotic pressure associated with hypoproteinemia or capillary leak from endothelial cellular dysfunction, the lung is particularly prone to the deleterious effects of tissue edema. Using microalbuminuria as a marker for TICS, as measured by the albumin excretion rate, one study has demonstrated an association with development of ARDS in patients with trauma [15]. When ARDS occurs following trauma, it is historically associated with a 50% mortality rate [83,85]. Despite advances in lung protective strategies and improvement in mortality rates, there is still an unacceptably high morbidity rate in patients with ARDS [85,86].

Neurologic injury

The mainstay of treatment of TBI is mitigation of secondary insults such as cerebral edema. When forces are applied across the brain tissue, through either impact or impulsive loading, primary injury to neurons occurs, which is, at present, not modifiable or treatable. The secondary insults that occur following TBI involve an exceptionally complex interplay of numerous factors and substances resulting in cerebral edema and ultimately ischemia [87,88]. These secondary insults are targeted in our current therapies. Cerebral edema following TBI is governed by some of the same mechanisms that contribute to CLS. TNF-α, for example, is also thought to play a key role in blood-brain barrier dysfunction following TBI, which is one of the key pathologic mechanisms that allows the influx of fluid into the brain [89]. Excitotoxic mediators and free-radical formation also play a key role. TICS also plays a significant role in the development of cerebral edema as part of a spectrum of disease termed multiple compartment syndrome [90]. Secondary insults such as cerebral edema contribute significantly to outcome [91–93], and if left untreated, cerebral edema can be fatal following TBI and even with treatment leads to death from herniation in the most severe cases.

TREATMENT

At present, there is no specific treatment for TICS once it develops. The mainstay of therapy once the syndrome develops is to address the underlying cause. Source control following sepsis is clearly of utmost importance in the sepsis-induced forms of the disease. For TICS, treating hemorrhagic shock with blood products and surgical hemostasis, fracture fixation, and craniotomy for evacuation of mass lesions following TBI are examples of obvious first-line therapies. None of these therapies directly addresses the treatment of TICS.

There have been a huge number of experimental treatments that have been studied to attenuate the inflammatory response and subsequent capillary leak following sepsis, burns, and trauma. In experimental models of CLS, antibodies to inflammatory mediators such as IL-1 and IL-6 have been demonstrated to reduce capillary leak [7] similar to C1 inhibitors [46], all without successful transition to clinical trials. There have been several clinical trials of therapies targeting various inflammatory pathways, which include antiendotoxin therapies and antagonists/antibodies to a variety of cytokines and other mediators of inflammation [12,94–100]. Corticosteroids have also been trialed because of the overall reduction in systemic inflammation and inhibition of NO-induced vasodilatation [12,101,102]. All of these therapies have been largely unsuccessful. The one exception is the use of drotrecogin alfa (activated), which is a recombinant human activated protein C. Drotrecogin alfa was initially demonstrated in clinical trails to improve mortality in patients with severe sepsis [103]. Recently; however, drotrecogin alfa was voluntarily withdrawn from the market by the manufacturer after additional studies failed to demonstrate clinical efficacy.

PREVENTION

Given the lack of success of clinical trials in ameliorating the effects of CLS, research has begun to focus on the prevention of the development. Large-volume fluid administration contributes to the development of systemic capillary leak and edema. As a mainstay of treatment of shock states for years, aggressive resuscitation with crystalloid was initially shown to be associated with improved outcomes in patients with sepsis and traumatic injury [104]. Subsequent work has refuted the concept that supranormal resuscitation is beneficial [105], and it is now accepted that more judicious administration of fluid to injured patients may be beneficial [106,107]. It is still, however, not clear how much or what type of fluid is optimal.

The debate over volume administration to patients in shock is emphasized by the extensive body of literature on what type of fluid administration is better in critically ill patients: colloid or crystalloid? Hypertonic fluid or isotonic fluid? These debates remain largely unsettled and are beyond the scope of this discussion. The authors refer the reader to several excellent reviews of the topic [55,57]. Although each has potential risks and benefits, all fluids do help restore tissue perfusion but also subject the patient to the risk of TICS. One interesting and unique strategy that addresses this issue was emphasized in a recent study. Cai and colleagues [108] demonstrated that antiinflammatory resuscitation with ethyl pyruvate attenuated the inflammatory response when added to a resuscitative fluid regimen. Although this work is still early and not ready for clinical trials, it presents a novel approach to more directly address the inflammatory state following hemorrhagic shock.

There are a few newer concepts that are particularly applicable to the prevention of TICS that deserve special mention: hemostatic resuscitation and goal-directed resuscitation.

Hemostatic resuscitation

There is a large and ever-evolving body of literature that addresses the concept of hemostatic resuscitation and the potential beneficial effects on survival following traumatic injury. The concept has 2 main components. The first is an old concept, originally described by Cannon and colleagues in 1918 [109] and then revisited by Shaftan [110] that discussed the risk of "popping the clot" with elevation of blood pressure before surgical hemostasis. Based on the results of several animal studies, a randomized prospective trial in the prehospital environment was conducted, which demonstrated that patients with penetrating torso trauma have improved survival if fluid resuscitation is delayed until operative intervention [111]. The results of this trial were confirmed by others [112,113]. This resulted in an evolution in trauma care that suggested that hypotensive resuscitation may be beneficial in selected patient populations [107], which led to an overall recommendation that more judicious use of crystalloid is preferable, which may result in a reduction of the overall incidence of TICS.

The second concept came to the forefront of the trauma literature during the early phases of the Iraq and Afghanistan conflicts. This is the concept of what has come to be colloquially called 1-to-1 resuscitation. This strategy is founded on the principle that patients who are bleeding need replacement with whole blood, or as close to whole blood as can be achieved in the civilian setting. This led to the groundbreaking work by military researchers that suggested that blood product replacement should occur in ratios comparable to whole blood [114,115]. Other studies have demonstrated that crystalloid restriction and large-volume blood product replacement are associated with improved survival following hemorrhagic shock [106,116,117].

Goal-directed resuscitation
The concept of early goal-Directed Therapy in patients with sepsis was first proven effective in the landmark study by Rivers and colleagues [118] published in the *New England Journal of Medicine* in 2001. The endpoints of resuscitation that were used in this study were similar to the endpoints that intensivists had been using for years in the ICU. The application of goal-directed therapy early in the course of sepsis and septic shock has been touted as the main reason for success of this resuscitative approach [119]. Improvements in organ dysfunction in patients treated with this approach are largely thought to be the result of a modulation of the inflammatory response. Using this philosophy of early goal-directed therapy toward the resuscitation of the injured patient may also prove beneficial, but this research is still relatively early in its evolution and has yet to be verified in a major multicenter clinical trial.

One strategy for goal-directed resuscitation in patients with acute hemorrhage has been promulgated primarily in Europe but is now catching the attention of trauma surgeons in the United States. The uses of viscoelastic point-of-care hemostatic assays (VHA) that can be used to target specific coagulation and/or fibrinolytic defects as a tool to guide blood product and procoagulant product administration have been described in several studies with favorable results [120]. Rotation thromboelastometry-guided therapy specifically uses the values obtained (ie, clot formation time, maximum clot firmness, and clot amplitude.) to guide specific product administration, such as fibrinogen concentrate in patients with low maximum clot firmness [121]. Use of these parameters has also been used to predict the need for massive transfusion [122,123] and, in at least 1 study, patients managed with VHA-directed therapy as opposed to standard coagulation test had significantly lower 30-day mortality [124]. A recent *Cochrane Database Review* of 9 trials concluded that, although the use of VHA seems to decrease hemorrhage, there was no evidence of improvement in morbidity or mortality rates [125].

SUMMARY
TICS is a complex disease that is clearly multifactorial in the traumatically injured patient (Fig. 2). Although systemic inflammation that occurs directly as a result of injury plays the most prominent role, the local tissue and organ

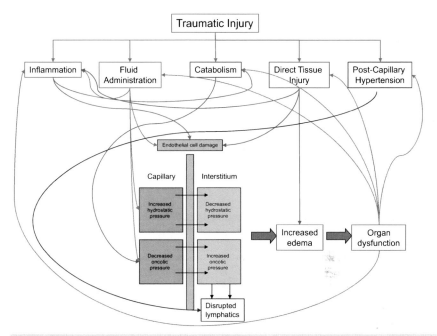

Fig. 2. Schema of the causative factors in TICS. (*Black arrows* are the normal flow of fluid. Colors denote specific pathologic pathways.)

injury effects of trauma not only cause local capillary leak and edema but also further amplify the SIRS response. High volume fluid administration and hypoproteinemic states further exacerbate the problem. All of this leads to organ dysfunction and failure, which is the third leading cause of death following injury. Strategies to treat TICS and attenuate its effects once it occurs by targeting inflammatory pathways have been wholly unsuccessful. The mainstay of therapy for TICS is prevention and minimization of its lethal effects. Newer resuscitation strategies such as hemostatic resuscitation and early goal-directed therapies are currently the best available strategies to combat TICS. Whether these result in better outcomes remains to be seen and the authors anxiously await the results of well-designed prospective trials.

References

[1] Dutton RP, Stansbury LG, Leone S, et al. Trauma mortality in mature trauma systems: are we doing better? An analysis of trauma mortality patterns, 1997–2008. J Trauma 2010;9(3): 620–6.

[2] Deitch EA, Goodman ER. Prevention of multiple organ failure. Surg Clin North Am 1999;79(6):1471–88.

[3] Baue AE. MOF/MODS, SIRS: an update. Shock 1996;6:1–5.

[4] Bochicchio G, Ilahi O, Bochicchio K, et al. Traumatic induced capillary leak syndrome is highly predictive of mortality [abstract 6]. In: Programs and abstracts of the 131st Annual Meeting of the American Surgical Association. Boca Raton (FL), April 14–16, 2011. p. 53.

[5] Gosling P, Brudney S, McGrath L, et al. Mortality prediction at admission to intensive care: a comparison of microalbuminuria with acute physiology scores after 24 hours. Crit Care Med 2003;31(1):98–103.

[6] Marx G. Fluid therapy in sepsis with capillary leakage. Eur J Anaesthesiol 2003;20: 429–42.

[7] Ravage ZB, Gomez HF, Czermak BJ, et al. Mediators of microvascular injury in dermal burn wounds. Inflammation 1998;22:619–29.

[8] Infanger M, Schmidt O, Kossmehl P, et al. Vascular endothelial growth factor serum level is strongly enhanced after burn injury and correlated with local and general tissue edema. Burns 2004;30:305–11.

[9] Clarkson B, Thompson D, Horwith M, et al. Cyclical edema and shock due to increased capillary permeability. Am J Med 1960;29:193–216.

[10] Gousseff M, Arnaud L, Lambert M, et al. The systemic capillary leak syndrome: a case series of 28 patients from a European registry. Ann Intern Med 2011;154:464–71.

[11] Levy MM, Fink MP, Marshall JC, et al. 2001 SCCM/ESICM/ACCP/ATS/SIS International sepsis definitions conference. Crit Care Med 2006;32:421–7.

[12] Fishel RS, Are C, Barbul A. Vessel injury and capillary leak. Crit Care Med 2003;31(8): S502–11.

[13] Seghaye MC, Grabitz RG, Duchateau J, et al. Inflammatory reaction and capillary leak syndrome related to cardiopulmonary bypass in neonates undergoing cardiac operations. J Thorac Cardiovasc Surg 1996;112:687–97.

[14] Nurnberger W, Michelmann I, Petrik K, et al. Activity of C1 esterase inhibitor in patients with vascular leak syndrome after bone marrow transplantation. Ann Hematol 1993;67:17–21.

[15] Pallister I, Gosling P, Alpar K, et al. Prediction of post traumatic adult respiratory distress syndrome by albumin excretion eight hours after admission. J Trauma 1997;42:1056–61.

[16] Smith CT, Gosling P, Sanghera K, et al. Microproteinuria predicts the severity of systemic effects of reperfusion injury following infra renal aortic aneurysm surgery. Ann Vasc Surg 1994;8:1–5.

[17] Pallister I, Dent C, Wise CC, et al. Early post-traumatic acute respiratory distress syndrome and albumin excretion rate: a prospective evaluation of a 'point-of-care' predictive test. Injury 2001;32:177–81.

[18] Aman J, van der Heijden M, van Lingen A, et al. Plasma protein levels are markers of pulmonary vascular permeability and degree of lung injury in critically ill patients with or at risk for acute lung injury/acute respiratory distress syndrome. Crit Care Med 2011;39(1): 89–97.

[19] Starling E. On the absorption of fluids from the connective tissue spaces. J Physiol 1896;19:312–26.

[20] Michel CC. Starling: the formulation of his hypothesis of microvascular fluid exchange and its significance after 100 years. Exp Physiol 1997;82:1–30.

[21] Michel CC, Curry FE. Microvascular permeability. Physiol Rev 1999;79:703–61.

[22] Lenz A, Franklin GA, Cheadle WG. Systemic inflammation after trauma. Injury 2007;38: 1336–45.

[23] Keel M, Trentz O. Pathophysiology of polytrauma. Injury 2005;36:691–709.

[24] Heirholzer C, Billiar TR. Molecular mechanisms in the early phase of hemorrhagic shock. Langenbecks Arch Surg 2001;386:302–8.

[25] Herzum I, Renz I. Inflammatory markers in SIRS, sepsis and septic shock. Curr Med Chem 2008;15:581–7.

[26] Faist E, Wichmann MW. Immunology in the severely injured. Chirurg 1997;68:1066–70.

[27] Moore FA, Moore EE. Evolving concepts in the pathogenesis of post injury multiple organ failure. Surg Clin North Am 1995;75:257–77.

[28] Polk HC Jr, George CD, Wellhausen SR, et al. A systematic study of host defense processes in badly injured patients. Ann Surg 1986;204:282–99.

[29] Gustot T. Multiple organ failure in sepsis: prognosis and role of systemic inflammatory response. Curr Opin Crit Care 2011;17:153–9.

[30] Mackey D, McFall AJ. MAMPs and MIMPs: proposed classifications for inducers of innate immunity. Mol Microbiol 2006;61:1365–71.

[31] Gill R, Ruan X, Menzel CL, et al. Systemic inflammation and liver injury following hemorrhagic shock and peripheral tissue trauma involve functional TLR9 signaling on bone marrow-derived cells and parenchymal cells. Shock 2011;35(2):164–70.

[32] Miller AC, Rashis RM, Elamin EM. The T in trauma: the helper T-cell response and the role of immunomodulation in trauma and burn patients. J Trauma 2007;63:1407–17.

[33] Mollen KP, Anand RJ, Tsung A, et al. Emerging paradigm: toll-like receptor 4-sentinel for the detection of tissue damage. Shock 2006;26(5):430–7.

[34] Nedrebø T, Berg A, Reed RK. Effect of tumor necrosis factor-alpha, IL-beta, and IL-6 on interstitial fluid pressure in rat skin. Am J Physiol 1999;277:H1857–62.

[35] Hynes RO. Integrins: versatility, modulation and signaling in cell adhesion. Cell 1992;69: 11–25.

[36] Tingström A, Heldin C, Rubin K. Regulation of fibroblast mediated collagen gel contraction by platelet derived growth factor, interleukin-1α and transforming growth factor-1. J Cell Sci 1992;102:315–22.

[37] Nootcboom A, vander Linden CJ, Hendriks T. Tumor necrosis factor-α and interleukin-1β mediate endothelial permeability induced by lipopolysaccharide-stimulated whole blood. Crit Care Med 2002;30:2063–8.

[38] Matsuda N, Hattori Y. Vascular biology in sepsis: pathophysiological and therapeutic significance of vascular dysfunction. J Smooth Muscle Res 2007;43(4):117–37.

[39] Goldblum SE, Ding X, Campbell-Washington J. TNF-α induces endothelial cell F-actin depolymerization, new actin synthesis, and barrier dysfunction. Am J Physiol 1993;264: C894–905.

[40] Ferro T, Neumann P, Gertzberg N, et al. Protein kinase C-α mediates endothelial barrier dysfunction induced by TNF-α. Am J Physiol 2000;278:L1107–17.

[41] Carey PD, Wakefield CH, Guilbu PJ. Neutrophil activation, vascular leak toxicity, and cytolysis during interleukin-2 infusion in human cancer. Surgery 1997;122:918–26.

[42] Lentsch AB, Miller FN, Edwards MJ. Mechanisms of leukocyte-mediated tissue injury induced by interleukin-2. Cancer Immunol Immunother 1999;47:243–8.

[43] Orucevic A, Lala PK. Role of nitric oxide in IL-2 therapy-induced capillary leak syndrome. Cancer Metastasis Rev 1986;17:127–42.

[44] Samlowski WE, Kondapanemi M, Tharkar S, et al. Endothelial nitric oxide synthase is a key mediator of interleukin-2-induced hypotension and vascular leak syndrome. J Immunother 2011;34(5):419–27.

[45] Hugli TE. Biochemistry and biology of anaphylatoxins. Complement 1986;3:111–27.

[46] Radke A, Mottaghy K, Goldmann C, et al. C1 inhibitor prevents capillary leakage after thermal trauma. Crit Care Med 2000;28:3224–32.

[47] Rockey DC, Chung JJ. Regulation of inducible nitric oxide synthase in hepatic sinusoidal endothelial cells. Am J Physiol 1996;271:G260–7.

[48] Higaki A, Ninomiya H, Sjai M, et al. Protective effect of neurotropin against lipopolysaccharide-induced hypotension and lethality linked to suppression of inducible nitric oxide synthase induction. Jpn J Pharmacol 2001;86:329–35.

[49] Piagnerelli M, Boudjeltia KZ, Brochee D, et al. Alterations of red blood cell shape and sialic acid membrane content in septic patients. Crit Care Med 2003;31:2156–62.

[50] De Backer D, Creteur J, Preiser JC, et al. Microvascular blood flow is altered in patients with sepsis. Am J Respir Crit Care Med 2002;166:98–104.

[51] Brealey D, Brand M, Hargreaves I, et al. Association between mitochondrial dysfunction and severity and outcome of septic shock. Lancet 2002;360:219–23.

[52] Gustot T, Durand F, Lebrec D, et al. Severe sepsis in cirrhosis. Hepatology 2009;50: 2022–33.

[53] Advanced trauma life support for doctors. 8th edition. Chicago: American College of Surgeons; 1997.

[54] Kreimeier U. Pathophysiology of fluid imbalance. Crit Care 2000;4(Suppl 2):S3–7.

[55] Santry HP, Alam HB. Fluid resuscitation: past, present, and the future. Shock 2010;33(3): 229–41.

[56] Cotton BA, Guy JS, Morris JA Jr, et al. The cellular, metabolic, and systemic consequences of aggressive fluid resuscitation strategies. Shock 2006;26(2):115–21.

[57] Alam HB, Sun L, Ruff P, et al. E- and P- selectin expression depends on the resuscitation fluid used in hemorrhaged rats. J Surg Res 2000;94:145–52.

[58] Deb S, Martin B, Sun L, et al. Resuscitation with lactated Ringer's solution in rats with hemorrhagic shock induces immediate apoptosis. J Trauma 1999;46:582–8.

[59] Deb S, Sun L, Martin B, et al. Lactated Ringer's solution and hetastarch but not plasma resuscitation after rat hemorrhagic shock is associated with immediate lung apoptosis by the up-regulation of the bax protein. J Trauma 2000;49:47–53.

[60] Dellinger RP, Levy MM, Carlet JM, et al. Surviving Sepsis Campaign: international guidelines for management of severe sepsis and septic shock. Crit Care Med 2008;36: 296–327 [published correction appears in Crit Care Med 2008; 36:1394–1396].

[61] Wilmore DW. Metabolic response to severe surgical illness: overview. World J Surg 2000;24:705–11.

[62] Blackburn GL. Metabolic considerations in management of surgical patients. Surg Clin North Am 2011;91:467–80.

[63] Plank LD, Hill GL. Sequential metabolic changes following induction of systemic inflammatory response in patients with severe sepsis or major blunt trauma. World J Surg 2000;24: 630–8.

[64] Shaw JHF, Wolfe RR. An integrated analysis of glucose, fat, and protein metabolism in severely traumatized patients. Studies in the basal state and the response to total parenteral nutrition. Ann Surg 1989;209:63–72.

[65] McClave SA, Martindale RG, Vanek VW, et al. Guidelines for the provision and assessment of nutrition support therapy in the adult critically ill patient: Society of Critical Care Medicine (SCCM) and American Society for Parenteral and Enteral Nutrition (ASPEN). JPEN J Parenter Enteral Nutr 2009;33:277–316.

[66] Wilmore DW, Goodwin CW, Aulick LH, et al. Effect of injury and infection on visceral metabolism and circulation. Ann Surg 1980;192:491.

[67] Rezende-Neto JB, Moore EE, Melo de Andrade MV, et al. Systematic inflammatory response secondary to abdominal compartment syndrome: stage for multiple organ failure. J Trauma 2002;53:1121–8.

[68] Stein DM, Lindell A, Murdock KR, et al. Relationship of serum and CSF biomarkers to intracranial hypertension and cerebral hypoperfusion following severe traumatic brain injury. J Trauma 2011;70(5):1096–103.

[69] Lu J, Goh SJ, Tng PY, et al. Systemic inflammatory response following acute traumatic brain injury. Front Biosci 2009;14:3795–813.

[70] Sears BW, Volkmer D, Yong S, et al. Correlation of measurable serum markers of inflammation with lung levels following bilateral femur fracture in a rat model. J Inflamm Res 2010;3: 105–14.

[71] Pape HC, Griensven MV, Hildebrand FF, et al. Systemic inflammatory response after extremity or truncal fracture operations. J Trauma 2008;65(6):1379–84.

[72] Kobbe P, Vodovotz Y, Kaczorowski DJ, et al. The role of fracture-associated soft tissue injury in the induction of systemic inflammation and remote organ dysfunction after bilateral femur fracture. J Orthop Trauma 2008;22(6):385–90.

[73] Aucar JA, Hirshberg A. Damage control for vascular injuries. Surg Clin North Am 1997;77(4):853–62.

[74] Pourmoghadam KK, Fogler RJ, Shaftan GW. Ligation: an alternative for control of exsanguination in major vascular injuries. J Trauma 1997;43:126–30.

[75] Pappas PJ, Haser PB, Teehan EP, et al. Outcome of complex venous reconstructions in patients with trauma. J Vasc Surg 1997;25(2):398–404.
[76] Malbrain ML, Cheatham ML, Kirkpatrick, et al. Results from the international conference on experts on intra-abdominal compartment syndrome. I. Definitions. Intensive Care Med 2006;32:1722–32.
[77] Rizoli S, Mamtani A, Scarpelini S. Abdominal compartment syndrome in trauma resuscitation. Curr Opin Anaesthesiol 2010;23:251–7.
[78] Raeburn CD, Moore EE, Biffl WL, et al. The abdominal compartment syndrome is a morbid complication of post-injury damage control surgery. Am J Surg 2001;182:542–6.
[79] Balogh Z, McKinley BA, Cancour CS, et al. Secondary abdominal compartment syndrome is an elusive early complication of traumatic shock resuscitation. Am J Surg 2002;184: 538–42.
[80] Demling RH. The pathogenesis of respiratory failure after trauma and sepsis. Surg Clin North Am 1980;60:1373–90.
[81] Layon J, Dincan D, Gallagher TJ, et al. Hypertonic saline as a resuscitation solution in hemorrhagic shock: effects on extra vascular lung water and cardiopulmonary function. Anesth Analg 1987;66:154–8.
[82] Rackow EC, Weil MH, Macneil AR, et al. Effects of crystalloid and colloid fluids on extravascular lung water in hypoproteinemic dogs. J Appl Physiol 1987;62:2421–5.
[83] Bhatia M, Moochhala S. Role of inflammatory mediators in the pathophysiology of acute respiratory distress syndrome. J Pathol 2004;202:145–6.
[84] Meyrick B. Pathology of the adult respiratory distress syndrome. Crit Care Clin 1986;2: 405–25.
[85] Rocco TR Jr, Reinert SE, Cioffi W, et al. A 9 year, single-institution, retrospective review of death rate and prognostic factors in adult respiratory distress syndrome. Ann Surg 2001;233(3):414–22.
[86] Martin M, Salim A, Murray J, et al. The decreasing incidence and mortality of acute respiratory distress syndrome after injury: a 5-year observational study. J Trauma 2005;59(5): 1107–13.
[87] Kennedy CS, Moffatt M. Acute traumatic brain injury in children: exploring the cutting edge in understanding, therapy, and research. Clin Pediatr Emerg Med 2004;5(4):224–38.
[88] Vos PE, Lamers KJB, Hendriks JCM, et al. Glial and neuronal proteins in serum predict outcome after severe traumatic brain injury. Neurology 2004;62(8):1303–10.
[89] Maier B, Lehnert M, Laurer HL, et al. Delayed elevation of soluble tumor necrosis factor receptors P75 and P55 in cerebrospinal fluid and plasma after traumatic brain injury. Shock 2006;26:122–7.
[90] Scalea TM, Bochicchio GV, Habashi N, et al. Increased intra-abdominal, intrathoracic, and intracranial pressure after severe brain injury: multiple compartment syndrome. J Trauma 2007;62:647–56.
[91] Miller JD, Sweet RC, Narayan R, et al. Early insults to the injured brain. JAMA 1978;240: 439–42.
[92] Signorini DF, Andrews PJ, Jones PA, et al. Adding insult to injury: the prognostic value of early secondary insults to survival after traumatic brain injury. J Neurol Neurosurg Psychiatry 1999;66:26–31.
[93] Chambers IR, Treadwell L, Mendelow AD. The cause and incidence of secondary insults in severely head-injured adults and children. Br J Neurosurg 2000;14:424–31.
[94] Zeigler EJ, Fisher CJ, Sprung CL, et al. Treatment of gram-negative bacteremia and septic shock with HA-1A human monoclonal antibody against andotoxin: a randomized double blind, placebo-controlled trial. The HA-1A sepsis study group. N Engl J Med 1991;324: 429–36.
[95] Abraham E, Wunderink R, Silverman H, et al. Efficacy and safety of monoclonal antibody to human tumor necrosis factor alpha in patients with sepsis syndrome. JAMA 1995;273: 934–41.

[96] Cohen J, Cartlet J. INTERSEPT: an international, multicenter, placebo controlled trial of monoclonal antibody to human tumor necrosis factor-alpha in patients with sepsis. Crit Care Med 1996;24:1431–40.

[97] Abraham E, Angueto A, Guiterrez G, et al. Double blind randomized controlled trial of monoclonal antibody to human tumor necrosis factor in treatment of septic shock. Lancet 1998;351:929–33.

[98] Opal SM, Fisher CJ, Dhainaut JF, et al. Confirmatory interleukin-1 receptor antagonist trial in severe sepsis: a phase III randomized double-blind, placebo-controlled, multicenter trial. Crit Care Med 1997;25:1115–24.

[99] Dhainaut JF, Tenaillon A, Le TY, et al. Platelet-activating factor receptor antagonist BN 52021 in the treatment of severe sepsis: a randomized, double-blind, placebo-controlled, multicenter clinical trial. Crit Care Med 1994;22:1720–8.

[100] Dhainaut JF, Tenaillon A, Hemmer M. Confirming phase III clinical trial to study the efficacy of a PAF antagonist, BN 52021, in reducing mortality in patients with severe gram-negative sepsis. Am J Respir Crit Care Med 1995;151:A447.

[101] Cronin L, Cook DJ, Carlet J. Corticosteroids treatment for sepsis: a critical appraisal and meta-analysis of the literature. Crit Care Med 1995;23:1430–9.

[102] Lefering R, Neuberger EA. Steroid controversy in sepsis and septic shock: a meta-analysis. Crit Care Med 1995;23:1294–303.

[103] Bernard GR, Vincent JL, Laterre PF, et al. Efficacy and safety of recombinant human activated protein C for severe sepsis. N Engl J Med 2001;344:699–709.

[104] Shoemaker WC, Appel PL, Kram HB, et al. Prospective trial of supranormal values of survivors as therapeutic goals in high-risk surgical patients. Chest 1988;94:1176–86.

[105] Ronco JJ, Phang PT, Walley KR, et al. Oxygen consumption is independent of changes in oxygen delivery in severe adult respiratory syndrome. Am Rev Respir Dis 1993;143:25–31.

[106] Shaz BH, Dente CJ, MacLeod JB, et al. Increased number of coagulation products in relationship to red blood cell products transfused improves mortality in trauma patients. Transfusion 2010;50:493–500.

[107] Beekley AC. Damage control resuscitation: a sensible approach to the exsanguinating surgical patient. Crit Care Med 2008;36(7):S267–74.

[108] Cai B, Dietch EA, Grande D, et al. Anti-inflammatory resuscitation improves survival in hemorrhage with trauma. J Trauma 2009;66:1632–40.

[109] Cannon W, Fraser J, Cowell E. The preventative treatment of wound shock. JAMA 1918;70:618.

[110] Shaftan GW, Chiu CJ, Dennis C, et al. Fundamentals of physiologic control of arterial hemorrhage. Surgery 1965;58:851–6.

[111] Bickell WH, Wall NJ, Pepe PE, et al. Immediate versus delayed fluid resuscitation for hypotensive patients with torso injuries. N Engl J Med 1994;331:1105–9.

[112] Hambly PR, Dutton RP. Excess mortality associated with the use of a rapid infusion system at a level 1 trauma center. Resuscitation 1996;31:127–33.

[113] Dutton RP, Mackenzie CF, Scalea TM. Hypotensive resuscitation during active hemorrhage: impact on in-hospital mortality. J Trauma 2002;56:1141–6.

[114] Borgman MA, Spinella PC, Perkins JG, et al. The ratio of blood products transfused affects mortality in patients receiving massive transfusions at a combat support hospital. J Trauma 2007;63:805–13.

[115] Holcomb JB, Hess JR. Early massive trauma transfusion: state of the art. J Trauma 2006;60:S1–2.

[116] Zink KA, Sambisavin CN, Holcomb JB, et al. A high ratio of plasma and platelets to packed red blood cells in the first 6h of massive transfusion improves outcomes in a large multicenter study. Am J Surg 2009;197:565–70.

[117] Holcomb JB, Wade CE, Michalek JE, et al. Increased plasma and platelet to red blood cell ratios improves outcome in 466 massively transfused civilian trauma patients. Ann Surg 2008;248:447–58.

[118] Rivers E, Nguyen B, Havstad, et al. Early goal-directed therapy in the treatment of severe sepsis and septic shock. N Engl J Med 2001;345:1368–77.

[119] Otero RM, Nguyen HB, Huang DT, et al. Early goal-directed therapy in severe sepsis and septic shock revisited: concepts, controversies, and contemporary findings. Chest 2006;130:1579–95.

[120] Johansson PI, Stissing T, Bochsen L, et al. Thrombelastography and tromboelastometry in assessing coagulopathy in trauma. Scand J Trauma Resusc Emerg Med 2009;17:45.

[121] Schöchl H, Nienaber U, Hofer G, et al. Goal-directed coagulation management of major trauma patients using thromboelastometry (ROTEM)-guided administration of fibrinogen concentrate and prothrombin complex concentrate. Crit Care 2010;14(2):R55.

[122] Leemann H, Lustenberger T, Talving P, et al. The role of rotation thromboelastometry in early prediction of massive transfusion. J Trauma 2010;69(6):1403–8.

[123] Schöchl H, Cotton B, Inaba K, et al. FIBTEM provides early prediction of massive transfusion in trauma. Crit Care 2011;15(6):R265.

[124] Johansson PI, Stensballe J. Effect of haemostatic control resuscitation on mortality in massively bleeding patients: a before and after study. Vox Sang 2009;96:111–8.

[125] Afshari A, Wikkelso A, Brok J, et al. Thrombelastography (TEG) or thromboelastometry (ROTEM) to monitor haemotherapy versus usual care in patients with massive transfusion. Cochrane Database Syst Rev 2011;3:CD007871.

Morbidity and Effectiveness of Laparoscopic Sleeve Gastrectomy, Adjustable Gastric Band, and Gastric Bypass for Morbid Obesity

Timothy D. Jackson, MD, MPH[a,b],
Matthew M. Hutter, MD, MPH[a,c,*]

[a]The Codman Center for Clinical Effectiveness in Surgery, Massachusetts General Hospital, Boston, MA, USA; [b]Department of Surgery, University of Toronto, University Health Network, 399 Bathurst Street, 8MP-322, Toronto, Ontario, Canada M5T 2S8; [c]Division of General and Gastrointestinal Surgery, Department of Surgery, Massachusetts General Hospital, 15 Parkman Street WACC 460, Boston, MA 02114, USA

Keywords
• Morbid obesity • Bariatric surgery • Sleeve gastrectomy • Adjustable gastric band
• Gastric bypass • Outcomes • Comparative effectiveness

Key Points
• Laparoscopic sleeve gastrectomy (LSG), laparoscopic adjustable gastric band (LAGB) and laparoscopic Roux-en-Y gastric bypass are all considered acceptable contemporary surgical options for the treatment of morbid obesity.
• Recent quality improvement efforts have significantly reduced the morbidity and mortality associated with modern bariatric surgical procedures.
• LRYGB appears to be most effective although is associated with more risk when compared to both LAGB and LSG.
• LSG is positioned between the LRYGB and LABG in associated morbidity and effectiveness although long-term outcome data is lacking.

OBESITY AS A SURGICAL DISEASE

Obesity continues to be a leading public health concern [1]. Current data indicate that 34.4% of the United States population has class I obesity (body mass index [BMI] >30 kg/m^2) and 6% has class III obesity (BMI >40 kg/m^2) [2]. Obesity is associated with many comorbidities that significantly decrease life expectancy

*Corresponding author. Division of General and Gastrointestinal Surgery, Department of Surgery, Massachusetts General Hospital, 15 Parkman Street WACC 460, Boston, MA 02114. E-mail address: mhutter@partners.org

0065-3411/12/$ – see front matter
doi:10.1016/j.yasu.2012.05.002

[3]. Estimates suggest that obesity accounts for up to 15% of all deaths annually in the United States and will soon emerge as the single leading cause of preventable death in the developed world [4].

Surgery remains the only effective treatment modality for morbid obesity, resulting in long-term weight loss and sustained improvement in weight-related comorbidities [5]. At present, there are limited pharmacologic therapies, and medically supervised diets have yielded only modest results [6,7]. Results from the Swedish Obesity Subjects (SOS) study, a large prospective cohort study with more than 10 years of follow-up, showed bariatric surgery to be associated with long-term weight loss and decreased overall mortality [8]. There have been significant improvements in the safety of bariatric procedures in recent years [9], and bariatric surgery has repeatedly been shown to be a cost-effective intervention [10–12]. Eligibility for bariatric procedures continues to be determined by the National Institutes of Health (NIH) criteria [13] from 1991 in which surgery is indicated for patients with a BMI of 40 kg/m^2 or greater, or a BMI of 35 kg/m^2 or greater with significant weight-related comorbidities.

Examination of current trends in bariatric surgery shows 3 options emerging as the surgical procedures of choice: the laparoscopic sleeve gastrectomy (LSG), laparoscopic adjustable gastric band (LAGB), and laparoscopic Roux-en-Y gastric bypass (LRYGB) [14]. This article provides a current summary of recent available outcomes data on the LSG, LAGB, and LRYGB.

CONTEMPORARY SURGICAL OPTIONS

Contemporary surgical options for morbid obesity include the LSG, LAGB, and LRYGB. At present, greater than 90% of bariatric surgical procedures are performed via a laparoscopic approach [14], and this is thought to be an important factor in recent improved outcomes [15].

LSG

The LSG involves excision of the lateral aspect of the stomach to create a lesser curve–based gastric tube (Fig. 1). This procedure was initially performed as part of the biliopancreatic diversion with duodenal switch [16] and later as the first step in staged procedures for the superobese [17–19]. Since its description laparoscopically [20], sleeve gastrectomy has been gaining popularity as a stand-alone procedure despite the lack of long-term outcomes data [21,22]. It is currently being performed for 7.8% of primary bariatric operations, according to the American College of Surgeons (ACS) Bariatric Surgery Center Network (BSCN) data [23]. At present, the LSG is not a reimbursable procedure by the Centers for Medicare and Medicaid Services (CMS) but is covered by several insurers [24].

LAGB

The LAGB was initially described in 1993 but was not approved for use in the United States until 2001 [25]. This procedure involves placement of an adjustable gastric band around the cardia of the stomach via the pars flaccida connected with tubing to a subcutaneous port implanted on the rectus fascia (Fig. 2). The degree of restriction is titrated with fills through the subcutaneous

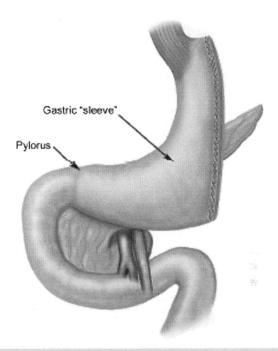

Fig. 1. Sleeve gastrectomy. (*From* Jones DB, Maithel SK, Schneider BE. Atlas of minimally invasive surgery. Woodbury, CT: Ciné-Med, 2006. Copyright © Ciné-Med Inc; with permission.)

port. The LAGB is potentially a fairly noninvasive surgical option and its popularity in North America has been increasing [26]. It is currently being performed for 46% of primary bariatric operations, according to ACS-BSCN data [23]. In Europe and Australia, where there is longer clinical experience with this procedure, the number of LAGB procedures is declining [14].

LRYGB
The modern gastric bypass reported by Mason and colleagues [27] was first described via a laparoscopic approach in 1994 [28] and had overtaken the open procedures by 2004 [29]. This procedure involves making a small gastric pouch (typically 30 cm^3), which is connected to a Roux limb of 75 to 150 cm (Fig. 3). It is currently being performed for 44% of primary bariatric operations, according to ACS-BSCN data [23]. The LRYGB has the most long-term data and is thought to represent the current gold standard against which other bariatric procedures are benchmarked.

QUALITY IMPROVEMENT IN BARIATRIC SURGERY
Improvements in outcomes after bariatric surgical procedures have been achieved in the past decade and have played an important role in defining LSG, LAGB, and LRYGB as the modern surgical procedures of choice.

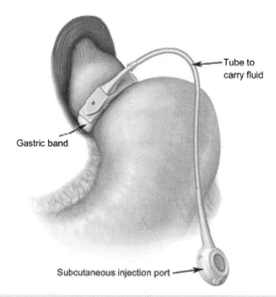

Fig. 2. Laparoscopic adjustable gastric band. (*From* Jones DB, Maithel SK, Schneider BE. Atlas of minimally invasive surgery. Woodbury, CT: Cine-Med, 2006. Copyright © Ciné-Med Inc; with permission.)

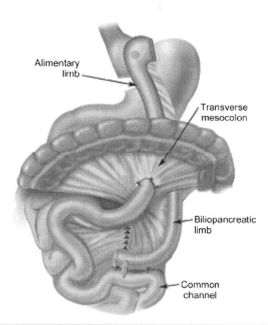

Fig. 3. Laparoscopic Roux-en-Y gastric bypass. (*From* Jones DB, Maithel SK, Schneider BE. Atlas of minimally invasive surgery. Woodbury, CT: Cine-Med, 2006. Copyright © Ciné-Med Inc; with permission.)

Early reports of poor outcomes after bariatric surgery raised significant concerns about the safety and quality of care [30]. Thirty-day mortalities from administrative claims data were estimated to be as high as 2% [30]. In response, CMS announced in November 2005 that it would no longer cover bariatric procedures. To address these and other concerns about access to safe surgical care, 2 large national surgical associations independently developed accreditation programs in bariatric surgery: the American Society of Bariatric and Metabolic Surgeons (ASMBS) [31] and the ACS [32]. Both accreditation programs require centers performing bariatric surgery to meet established standards of care and have appropriate facilities, organization, and trained personnel. In February 2006, CMS announced that bariatric surgery would be reimbursed only when performed within centers accredited by either the ASMBS or the ACS [24]. LSG, LAGB, and LRYGB are all considered acceptable surgical options for the purposes of accreditation.

Reporting of outcomes data is a mandatory requirement for accreditation as a center for bariatric surgery. The ACS has established the BSCN [33] Data Collection Program and the ASMBS has developed the Bariatric Outcomes Longitudinal Database (BOLD) [34]. The ACS-BSCN database was built on the success and methodological rigor of the National Surgical Quality Improvement Program (NSQIP). Information from both prospective databases is playing an important role in ensuring quality of bariatric surgical care delivery and is helping to better define the real-world outcomes for LSG, LAGB, and LRYGB.

In addition to the introduction of accreditation in bariatric surgery, the widespread adoption of laparoscopic techniques, the increased clinical experience, and the development of fellowship training programs have also contributed to the reduced mortality and morbidity associated with these procedures.

MORTALITY

With recent quality improvement successes in bariatric surgery, the mortality associated with LSG, LAGB, and LRYGB has decreased significantly. Current mortalities for all patients are 15 to 20 times lower than the previously widely reported 2% mortality found in high-risk populations (see later discussion). The highest mortality has been associated with the LRYGB. In the first Longitudinal Assessment of Bariatric Surgery (LABS-1) study [35], a large NIH-funded multi-institutional prospective cohort study with 10 centers and 4776 patients, the 30-day mortality for Roux-en-Y gastric bypass (RYGB) was 0.2% compared with 0% in the LAGB group. The open RYGB (ORYGB) group had a 10-fold higher 30-day mortality at 2.1%. A subsequent analysis of all early mortalities within the LABS study cohort revealed that the recognized complications of anastomotic leak, cardiac events, and pulmonary complications accounted for most of the deaths [36].

Data from multiple large prospective cohorts of patients having bariatric surgery has allowed for an estimate of mortality outside of the study setting. An initial report from the NSQIP data showed a similar 30-day mortality for patients undergoing LAGB and LRYGB (0.09% vs 0.14%) in a sample of 4756 patients between 2005 and 2006 [37]. The baseline data from ASMBS-BOLD reports 30-day mortality of 0.09% and 90-day mortality of 0.11%, although the data were not stratified by procedure type [34].

Recent data from the Michigan Bariatric Surgery Collaborative (MBSC), which consists of 29 hospitals and 25,469 patients throughout Michigan, reported early mortality after LSG, LAGB, and LRYGB as 0.1%, 0.04%, and 0.1% respectively [38]. Data from the ACS-BSCN reports 0.11%, 0.05%, and 0.14% for 30-day mortality after LSG, LAGB, and LRYGB with data from 28,616 patients at 109 centers from across the United States (Table 1). Within the same cohort, 1-year mortality was reported at 0.21%, 0.08%, and 0.34% for LSG, LAGB, and LRYGB respectively. Considering these recent data, mortality is consistently low among all 3 procedures, with the LSG and LRYGB having higher rates than LAGB.

MORBIDITY

With mortality low across all procedure types, and because LSG, LAGB, and LRYGB are all considered to be safe options for the treatment of morbid obesity, increasing emphasis is being placed on their associated morbidity. Each procedure has unique risk profiles that continue to be better defined as more data become available.

The LSG has a 30-day morbidity of 5.61% reported in the first results from the ACS-BSCN; lower than LRYGB at 5.91% but significantly higher than LAGB at 1.44% (see Table 1) [23]. Readmission rates within 30 days after surgery followed a similar trend (LSG 5.40%, LAGB 1.71%, LRYGB 6.47%), as did the need for reoperation/intervention (LSG 2.97%, LAGB 0.92%, LRYGB 5.02%) [23]. Initial data from the MBSC also shows that the LSG is positioned between the LRYGB and LAGB in rates of postoperative complications. The number of patients experiencing more than 1 serious complication was 2.3% in LSG, 0.9% in LAGB, and 3.3% in LRYGB [38]. Similar findings are emerging from the ASMBS-BOLD data: the percentage of patients experiencing 1 or more complication was 10.84% in LSG, 4.62% in LAGB, and 14.87% in RYGB [34].

Although LSG was excluded from the analysis, in the LABS-1 study, the investigators also showed higher morbidity associated with LRYGB compared

Table 1
Morbidity and mortality associated with LRYGB, LSG, and LAGB from the ACS-BSCN dataset

	LRYGB	LSG	LAGB
30-d mortality (%)	0.14	0.11	0.05
1-y mortality (%)	0.34	0.21	0.08
30-d morbidity (%)	5.91	5.61	1.44
30-d readmission (%)	6.47	5.40	1.71
30-d reoperation/intervention(%)	5.02	2.97	0.92

Data from Hutter MM, Schirmer BD, Jones DB, et al. First report from the American College of Surgeons Bariatric Surgery Center Network: laparoscopic sleeve gastrectomy has morbidity and effectiveness positioned between the band and the bypass. Ann Surg 2011;254(3):410–20 [discussion: 420–2].

with LAGB. The LABS-1 composite end point (death, deep vein thrombosis [DVT]/PE, reintervention/reoperation, and failure to be discharged from hospital within 30 days) was 1.0% in the patients having LAGB compared with 4.8% in the LRYGB group [30].

Conversion to open rate was lowest in LSG at 0.1%, LAGB was 0.25%, and highest in LRYGB at 1.43% in the ACS-BSCN data [23].

Evaluation of anastomotic or staple line leaks reveals similar low rates in both LSG and LRYGB. This complication does not occur in the LAGB because there are no anastomoses or staple lines to dehisce. The MBSC reported a higher leak rate associated with LSG at 1% compared with 0.8% with LRYGB [38]. A similar low leak rate was found in the ACS-BSCN dataset: 0.74% for LSG and 0.78% for LRYGB. These recent leak rates are lower than typically reported in previous literature. In a meta-analysis of LSG with 36 studies and data from 2570 patients, the leak rate was determined to be 2.7% in patients undergoing LSG as a primary procedure [21]. Similarly, leaks after LRYGB have been reported at 1.5% [39] and 2.1% [40] in recent large case series. Although the leak rates of LSG and LRYGB are similar, managing leaks after LSG may represent a more challenging clinical problem [41,42].

Bleeding is a rare early complication that can occur after any bariatric procedure. Major bleeding, as defined by transfusion of more than 4 units of blood, occurred in 0.3% of patients having LSG, 0.04% in LAGB, and 0.7% in LRYGB in the MBSC data [38]. Minor bleeding was reported at 0.7%, 0.1%, and 2.0% for LSG, LAGB, and LRYGB respectively [38]. In the ACS-BSCN cohort, bleeding events occurred in 0.64% after LSG, 0.05% after LAGB, and 1.11% after LRYGB [23]. LSG is between LAGB and LRYGB in bleeding risk.

Medical complications can be an important source of morbidity during the postoperative period. The rates of venous thromboembolic (VTE) events seem to be similar in LSG and LRYGB and lower in LAGB. In the MBSC, VTE rates were 0.4% for both LSG and LRYGB and 0.1% for LAGB [38]. Rates of DVT were 0.11% for LSG, 0.03% for LAGB, and 0.14% for LRYGB from ACS-BSCN data [23]. Incidence of pulmonary embolism was also low and followed a similar trend in that study. Slightly higher rates of VTE were reported for LAGB (0.3%) and LRYGB (0.4%) in the LABS-1 study [35]. Cardiac events are typically rare after bariatric procedures. LRYGB seems to have the greatest associated cardiac risk, with cardiac events occurring in 0.1% [38] and 0.09% [23] of patients in the MBSC and ACS-BSCN databases respectively. In LAGB and LSG, cardiac events were rarer. Pulmonary complications such as pneumonia also occur with more frequency in LRYGB compared with LSG and are lowest in LAGB.

Later complications such as stricture, marginal ulcers, bowel obstructions, and nutritional deficiencies tend to occur more frequently after LRYGB compared with LSG and are infrequent after LAGB. In the ACS-BSCN cohort, strictures occurred in 1.42% of patients having LRYGB, 0.42% in LSG, and 0.13% LAGB [23]. Similarly, in the MBSC data, strictures developed in 1.8% of patients after LRYGB, 0.7% after LSG, and no strictures were reported in patients having LAGB [38]. Marginal ulcers occur with variable frequency after LRYGB, with reported incidences ranging from 0.6% to 16% in previous studies [43], depending on how and when they were identified. The 30-day marginal ulcer rate in the ACS-BSCN database was 0.47% [23]. Although most marginal ulcers respond well to medical therapy, some patients require surgical revision; 9% in a recent case series [43]. Another complication unique to LRYGB is the risk of developing internal hernias. Estimates of the incidence of internal hernias range from 0.5% to 9% in the literature [44]. Lack of long-term follow-up data after LRYGB makes lifetime risk difficult to estimate. If not recognized and treated early, the consequences of internal hernias can be devastating. Although any patient can develop nutritional deficiencies after a bariatric procedure, the risk is more pronounced in patients who have had LRYGB given its malabsorptive and restrictive mechanism of action. If patients are not monitored and do not take appropriate supplementation, they can develop micronutrient deficiencies associated with significant morbidity [45]. The potential for patients to develop strictures, marginal ulcers, internal hernias, and micronutrient deficiencies after LRGYB adds to the longer-term morbidity associated with this procedure.

Although early complications are rare with the LAGB, there exists considerable controversy about rates of long-term complications and failure. Within the ACS-BSCN data, 0.11% of patients having LAGB experienced early complications [23]. Similar findings were present in the MBSC, which showed that only 0.4% of patients having LAGB developed an early band complication requiring reoperation such as slippage, obstruction, gastric or esophageal perforation, and port site infection [38]. This low early morbidity associated with the LAGB has established this procedure as the lowest-risk surgical option, although longer-term data are calling this notion into question. A recent case series from Belgium with 12 years of follow-up showed that 39% of patients experienced major complications, 28% developed band erosion, 17% were converted to LRGYB, and only 51% of patients had their band in place at the end of the follow-up period [46]. Although the findings were dramatic, the study had significant limitations because it consisted of only 151 patients, was from a single surgeon, and had only 54.3% follow-up. Another recent small case series from Chile supports these findings, reporting a surgical failure rate greater than 40% and 24.1% reoperation rate in patients having LAGB after 5 years of follow-up [47]. A recent meta-analysis of 19 studies reports lower surgical failure rates, with rates of erosion and slippage of 1.03% and 4.93% after an average follow-up of more than 6 years [48]. Data from the University Health System Consortium Clinical Database with 10,151 patients undergoing LAGB showed even more favorable results, with a 0.76% band revision rate and 0.87% band explantation rate over the 3-year study period [49]. Changes in surgical technique, band devices, increased clinical experience, and process of care between early LAGB procedures and current LAGB procedures are being put forward to reconcile the large discrepancies in morbidity associated with LAGB in the current literature [50]. Longer-term data will continue to better define the morbidity associated with LAGB and allow a more complete estimate of risk.

At present, there is a paucity of medium-term to long-term data on the morbidity associated with the LSG. Studies with follow-up beyond 5 years are scarce, and needed to better define the risks of LSG compared with LRYGB and LAGB.

COMPARATIVE EFFECTIVENESS

LSG, LAGB, and LRYGB have variable results in achieving sustained weight loss and resolution of weight-related comorbidities. Short-term studies suggest that the sleeve lies between the bypass, which has greater weight loss and reduction in weight-related comorbidities, and the band, which seems to have a lesser impact.

Reduction in weight

LRYGB has consistently been shown to be the more effective procedure in achieving and sustaining reduction in weight compared with the LSG and LAGB. As highlighted in the first report form the ACS-BSCN data, the LRYGB resulted in average reduction in BMI of 15.34 kg/m^2 at 12 months compared with 11.87 kg/m^2 in the LSG group and 7.05 kg/m^2 in the LAGB group (Table 2) [23]. The follow-up at 12 months in this study was approximately 70%. Beyond 1 year, it seems that all procedures can result in sustained weight loss. A recent meta-analysis reported sustained weight loss in patients having both LAGB and LRYGB up to 3 years [51]. In patients having LAGB, mean percent excess body weight loss (%EBWL) was 42.6% at 1 year (data from 15 studies), 50.3% at 2 years (12 studies), and 55.2% at 3 years (9 studies). For patients having LRYGB, %EBWL was 61.5% at 1 year (10 studies), 69.7% at 2 years (5 studies), and 71.2% at 3 years (2 studies). In an updated meta-analysis, Buchwald and colleagues [52] also showed sustained weight in patients having both LAGB and LRYGB. LRYGB was found to result in a BMI reduction of 16 kg/m^2 (22 studies, 2757 patients) and %EBWL of 63.3%, whereas LAGB resulted in a reduction in BMI of 9.63 kg/m^2 (66 studies,

Table 2
Effectiveness of LRYGB, LSG, and LRYGB at 1 year from the ACS-BSCN [23]. Reduction in BMI and percentage with improvement or resolution of select weighted related comorbidities. Estimates are limited by small numbers at time of follow-up

	LRYGB	LSG	LAGB
Reduction in BMI (kg/m^2)	15.34	11.87	7.05
Diabetes (%)	83	55	44
Hypertension (%)	79	68	44
Hyperlipidemia (%)	66	35	33
Obstructive sleep apnea (%)	66	62	38
Gastroesophageal reflux disease (%)	70	50	64

6128 patients) and %EBWL of 43.9% beyond 2 years. There is a paucity of data beyond 5 years with appropriate follow-up. A recent case series of 242 patients undergoing LRYGB with 19% follow-up at 10 years showed a mean %EBWL of 57% [53]. A case series of 151 patients having LAGB with 54.3% follow-up at 12 years reported a mean %EBWL of 42.8% [46]. Fewer data are available on the longer-term weight loss outcomes in LSG, although a cross-sectional review of patients undergoing LSG showed a sustained reduction in BMI of 11.1 kg/m^2 at 5 years [22].

To summarize the available data, the LRGYB results in the most weight loss in the short term, followed by the LSG, whereas the LAGB seems to be the least effective option. Medium-term data suggest that the LSG, LAGB, and LRYGB all seem to provide sustained weight loss, although overall data are limited (and almost absent for the LSG). Long-term weight loss outcomes are still needed, and the percentage of patients followed up remains a challenge for most cohort studies.

Reduction in weight-related comorbidities

LSG, LAGB, and LRYGB all result in significant improvement in the comorbidities associated with obesity. These comorbidities include diabetes, hypertension, hyperlipidemia, obstructive sleep apnea (OSA), and gastroesophageal reflux disease (GERD). The extent to which these comorbidities improve is correlated with weight loss; the LRYGB tends to perform better than the LAGB and LSG, with the LSG being more effective that the LAGB.

Multiple studies have shown the effectiveness of these procedures in the treatment of diabetes. An analysis of 19 studies with 11,175 patients, follow-up greater than 2 years reporting diabetes-specific end points after bariatric surgery showed that diabetes resolved in 78% of patients and improved in 87% [52]. In these studies, LRYGB was more effective than LAGB with 70.9% resolution beyond 2 years compared with 58.3% in the patients having LAGB. This trend was shown in the ASC-BSCN data and placed the LSG between the LRYGB and LAGB: at 1 year, 83% of patients who underwent LRYGB had resolution or improvement in their diabetes compared with 55% of patients having LSG and 44% of patients having LAGB (see Table 2) [23]. The enhanced ability for LRYGB to improve diabetes compared with LSG and LAGB may be related to additional metabolic effects induced by intestinal bypass independently of weight loss alone [54].

Hypertension, hyperlipidemia, GERD, and OSA also all reliably improve after bariatric surgery, with LRYGB having the greatest treatment effect. In the ASC-BSCN data, the LSG consistently performed better than the LAGB but not as well as the LRYGB (see Table 2). The 1 exception was GERD, which improved or resolved in 50% who received the LSG, compared with 70% in patients having LRYGB and 64% in the LAGB group [23]. From the available literature, it seems that LRYGB results in both the most weight loss and resolution of weight-related comorbidities. LSG is positioned between the LAGB and the LRYGB, although long-term data are lacking.

TOWARD OPTIMIZING OUTCOMES

Remarkable progress has been made in recent years in improving patient safety and quality of care in bariatric surgery. The introduction of accreditation and mandatory reporting of outcomes has created a wealth of clinically rich data to better inform clinicians of the real-world morbidity and effectiveness associated with different surgical options. The LSG, LAGB, and LRYGB have emerged as the contemporary procedures of choice for the treatment of morbid obesity. Although there are ample data supporting the short-term safety of these procedures, the lack of long-term data limits the ability of clinicians to fully understand their effectiveness. Obesity is a chronic disease that requires lifelong treatment and monitoring. Efforts to improve follow-up after bariatric procedures are needed to ensure that potential late morbidity is reduced. Subsequent data from sources such as the ACS-BSCN, ASMBS-BOLD, MBSC, and the LABS consortium will better define long-term effectiveness and risks associated with these procedures. Furthermore, these data may inform future policy decisions on issues such as coverage determinations and the expansion of current surgical indications.

An improved understanding of the risk/benefit profile associated with each procedure type has the potential to improve the matching of patient to procedure type. The development of risk/benefit assessment tools derived from current outcomes data may better inform the procedure selection process for both patients and providers. Additional data collection evaluating more patient-centered outcomes and quality of life will help to better define the overall impact of these procedures in the treatment of morbid obesity.

SUMMARY

LSG, LAGB, and LRYGB are all safe and effective modern surgical options for the treatment of morbid obesity. Recent quality improvement successes in bariatric surgical care delivery have resulted in low mortality and morbidity after these procedures. All seem to result in sustained weight loss and improvement in weight-related comorbidities, although appropriate long-term outcomes data for all procedure types are needed. The LRYGB seems to be associated with the most risk but offers the most benefit, whereas the LAGB seems to have the lowest risk and to be least effective. The LSG seems to be positioned between the LRYGB and LAGB in associated morbidity and effectiveness in short-term and medium-term studies. Because the LSG has only recently been performed, there are currently no data about its long-term effectiveness. A better understanding of the unique risk/benefit profile associated with each procedure type will better inform patient selection and has the potential to further optimize outcomes.

References

[1] WHO. Obesity: preventing and managing the global epidemic. World Health Organ Tech Rep Ser 2000;894:1–253.
[2] Shields M, Carroll M, Odgen C. Adult obesity prevalence in Canada and the United States. NCHS Data Brief 2011;56:1–8 [in French].
[3] Fontaine KR, Redden DT, Wang C, et al. Years of life lost due to obesity. JAMA 2003;289(2):187–93.

[4] Stewart ST, Cutler DM, Rosen AB. Forecasting the effects of obesity and smoking on U.S. life expectancy. N Engl J Med 2009;361(23):2252–60.

[5] Buchwald H, Avidor Y, Braunwald E, et al. Bariatric surgery: a systematic review and meta-analysis. JAMA 2004;292(14):1724–37.

[6] Appel LJ, Clark JM, Yeh HC, et al. Comparative effectiveness of weight-loss interventions in clinical practice. N Engl J Med 2011;365(21):1959–68.

[7] Wadden TA, Volger S, Sarwer DB, et al. A two-year randomized trial of obesity treatment in primary care practice. N Engl J Med 2011;365(21):1969–79.

[8] Sjostrom L, Narbro K, Sjostrom CD, et al. Effects of bariatric surgery on mortality in Swedish obese subjects. N Engl J Med 2007;357(8):741–52.

[9] Encinosa WE, Bernard DM, Du D, et al. Recent improvements in bariatric surgery outcomes. Med Care 2009;47(5):531–5.

[10] Picot J, Jones J, Colquitt JL, et al. The clinical effectiveness and cost-effectiveness of bariatric (weight loss) surgery for obesity: a systematic review and economic evaluation. Health Technol Assess 2009;13(41):1–190, 215–357, iii–iv.

[11] Cremieux PY, Ghosh A, Yang HE, et al. Return on investment for bariatric surgery. Am J Manag Care 2008;14(11):e5–6.

[12] Sampalis JS, Liberman M, Auger S, et al. The impact of weight reduction surgery on health-care costs in morbidly obese patients. Obes Surg 2004;14(7):939–47.

[13] NIH. Gastrointestinal surgery for severe obesity. 1991. Available at: http://consensus.nih.gov/1991/1991gisurgeryobesity084html.htm. Accessed November 27, 2011.

[14] Buchwald H, Oien DM. Metabolic/bariatric surgery worldwide 2008. Obes Surg 2009;19(12):1605–11.

[15] Reoch J, Mottillo S, Shimony A, et al. Safety of laparoscopic vs open bariatric surgery: a systematic review and meta-analysis. Arch Surg 2011;146(11):1314–22.

[16] Hess DS, Hess DW. Biliopancreatic diversion with a duodenal switch. Obes Surg 1998;8(3):267–82.

[17] Almogy G, Crookes PF, Anthone GJ. Longitudinal gastrectomy as a treatment for the high-risk super-obese patient. Obes Surg 2004;14(4):492–7.

[18] Hamoui N, Anthone GJ, Kaufman HS, et al. Sleeve gastrectomy in the high-risk patient. Obes Surg 2006;16(11):1445–9.

[19] Cottam D, Qureshi FG, Mattar SG, et al. Laparoscopic sleeve gastrectomy as an initial weight-loss procedure for high-risk patients with morbid obesity. Surg Endosc 2006;20(6):859–63.

[20] Ren CJ, Patterson E, Gagner M. Early results of laparoscopic biliopancreatic diversion with duodenal switch: a case series of 40 consecutive patients. Obes Surg 2000;10(6):514–23 [discussion: 524].

[21] Brethauer SA, Hammel JP, Schauer PR. Systematic review of sleeve gastrectomy as staging and primary bariatric procedure. Surg Obes Relat Dis 2009;5(4):469–75.

[22] Strain GW, Saif T, Gagner M, et al. Cross-sectional review of effects of laparoscopic sleeve gastrectomy at 1, 3, and 5 years. Surg Obes Relat Dis 2011;7(6):714–9.

[23] Hutter MM, Schirmer BD, Jones DB, et al. First report from the American College of Surgeons Bariatric Surgery Center Network: laparoscopic sleeve gastrectomy has morbidity and effectiveness positioned between the band and the bypass. Ann Surg 2011;254(3):410–20 [discussion: 420–2].

[24] CMS. Decision memo for bariatric surgery for the treatment of morbid obesity. Available at: http://www.cms.gov/medicare-coverage-database/details/ncd-details.aspx?NCDId=57&ncdver=3&bc=AgAAgAAAAAAA&. Accessed November 27, 2011.

[25] Belachew M, Zimmermann JM. Evolution of a paradigm for laparoscopic adjustable gastric banding. Am J Surg 2002;184(6B):21S–5S.

[26] Hinojosa MW, Varela JE, Parikh D, et al. National trends in use and outcome of laparoscopic adjustable gastric banding. Surg Obes Relat Dis 2009;5(2):150–5.

[27] Mason EE, Printen KJ, Blommers TJ, et al. Gastric bypass in morbid obesity. Am J Clin Nutr 1980;33(Suppl 2):395–405.

[28] Wittgrove AC, Clark GW, Tremblay LJ. Laparoscopic gastric bypass, Roux-en-Y: preliminary report of five cases. Obes Surg 1994;4(4):353–7.
[29] Nguyen NT, Root J, Zainabadi K, et al. Accelerated growth of bariatric surgery with the introduction of minimally invasive surgery. Arch Surg 2005;140(12):1198–202 [discussion: 1203].
[30] Flum DR, Salem L, Elrod JA, et al. Early mortality among Medicare beneficiaries undergoing bariatric surgical procedures. JAMA 2005;294(15):1903–8.
[31] ASMBS-BSCOE. The American Society of Metabolic and Bariatric Surgery - Bariatric Surgery Center of Excellence. 2011. Available at: http://www.surgicalreview.org/. Accessed November 27, 2011.
[32] ACS-BSCN. American College of Surgeons Bariatric Surgery Center Network. 2011. Available at: http://www.acsbscn.org. Accessed November 27, 2011.
[33] Schirmer B, Jones DB. The American College Of Surgeons Bariatric Surgery Center Network: establishing standards. Bull Am Coll Surg 2007;92(8):21–7.
[34] DeMaria EJ, Pate V, Warthen M, et al. Baseline data from American Society for Metabolic and Bariatric Surgery-designated Bariatric Surgery Centers of Excellence using the Bariatric Outcomes Longitudinal Database. Surg Obes Relat Dis 2010;6(4):347–55.
[35] Flum DR, Belle SH, King WC, et al. Perioperative safety in the longitudinal assessment of bariatric surgery. N Engl J Med 2009;361(5):445–54.
[36] Smith MD, Patterson E, Wahed AS, et al. Thirty-day mortality after bariatric surgery: independently adjudicated causes of death in the longitudinal assessment of bariatric surgery. Obes Surg 2011;21(11):1687–92.
[37] Lancaster RT, Hutter MM. Bands and bypasses: 30-day morbidity and mortality of bariatric surgical procedures as assessed by prospective, multi-center, risk-adjusted ACS-NSQIP data. Surg Endosc 2008;22(12):2554–63.
[38] Finks JF, Kole KL, Yenumula PR, et al. Predicting risk for serious complications with bariatric surgery: results from the Michigan Bariatric Surgery Collaborative. Ann Surg 2011;254(4):633–40.
[39] Durak E, Inabnet WB, Schrope B, et al. Incidence and management of enteric leaks after gastric bypass for morbid obesity during a 10-year period. Surg Obes Relat Dis 2008;4(3):389–93.
[40] Gonzalez R, Sarr MG, Smith CD, et al. Diagnosis and contemporary management of anastomotic leaks after gastric bypass for obesity. J Am Coll Surg 2007;204(1):47–55.
[41] Tan JT, Kariyawasam S, Wijeratne T, et al. Diagnosis and management of gastric leaks after laparoscopic sleeve gastrectomy for morbid obesity. Obes Surg 2010;20(4):403–9.
[42] Csendes A, Braghetto I, Leon P, et al. Management of leaks after laparoscopic sleeve gastrectomy in patients with obesity. J Gastrointest Surg 2010;14(9):1343–8.
[43] Azagury DE, Abu Dayyeh BK, Greenwalt IT, et al. Marginal ulceration after Roux-en-Y gastric bypass surgery: characteristics, risk factors, treatment, and outcomes. Endoscopy 2011;43(11):950–4.
[44] O'Rourke RW. Management strategies for internal hernia after gastric bypass. J Gastrointest Surg 2011;15(6):1049–54.
[45] Kaplan LM. Gastrointestinal management of the bariatric surgery patient. Gastroenterol Clin North Am 2005;34(1):105–25.
[46] Himpens J, Cadiere GB, Bazi M, et al. Long-term outcomes of laparoscopic adjustable gastric banding. Arch Surg 2011;146(7):802–7.
[47] Boza C, Gamboa C, Perez G, et al. Laparoscopic adjustable gastric banding (LAGB): surgical results and 5-year follow-up. Surg Endosc 2011;25(1):292–7.
[48] Singhal R, Bryant C, Kitchen M, et al. Band slippage and erosion after laparoscopic gastric banding: a meta-analysis. Surg Endosc 2010;24(12):2980–6.
[49] Nguyen NT, Hohmann S, Nguyen XM, et al. Outcome of laparoscopic adjustable gastric banding and prevalence of band revision and explantation at academic centers: 2007-2009. Surg Obes Relat Dis 2011. [Epub ahead of print].

[50] O'Brien P. Comment on: outcome of laparoscopic adjustable gastric banding and the prevalence of band revision and explantation at academic centers: 2007-2009. Surg Obes Relat Dis 2011. [Epub ahead of print].

[51] Garb J, Welch G, Zagarins S, et al. Bariatric surgery for the treatment of morbid obesity: a meta-analysis of weight loss outcomes for laparoscopic adjustable gastric banding and laparoscopic gastric bypass. Obes Surg 2009;19(10):1447–55.

[52] Buchwald H, Estok R, Fahrbach K, et al. Weight and type 2 diabetes after bariatric surgery: systematic review and meta-analysis. Am J Med 2009;122(3):248–56, e245.

[53] Higa K, Ho T, Tercero F, et al. Laparoscopic Roux-en-Y gastric bypass: 10-year follow-up. Surg Obes Relat Dis 2011;7(4):516–25.

[54] Ikramuddin S, Buchwald H. How bariatric and metabolic operations control metabolic syndrome. Br J Surg 2011;98(10):1339–41.

Are Cancer Trials Valid and Useful for the General Surgeon and Surgical Oncologist?

Waddah B. Al-Refaie, MD*, Selwyn M. Vickers, MD

Department of Surgery, Surgical Outcomes Research Center, University of Minnesota and Minneapolis VAMC, MMC# 195, 420 Delaware Street Southeast, Minneapolis, MN 55455, USA

Keywords
- Caner trials • General surgeons • Surgical oncologist • External validity
- Applicability

Key Points
- Cancer trials represent a rigorous and clear approach to test whether an intervention or treatment will alter the outcomes of individuals with cancer in an experimental manner that is beyond the level of observational studies. As such, they remain useful and valid to the day to day practice of general surgeons and surgical oncologist.
- However, the short comings of current cancer clinical trials need to be recognized, especially when less than 1% of adults persons with cancer participate in cancer clinical trials, thus leaving the generalizability of these trials to patients and their surgeons in the real world setting an open question.
- Moving forward, physicians, payers, professional societies, advocates, the NCI, and other stakeholders need to develop broader cancer trials to benefit the millions of patients with cancer in the US.

CANCER CLINICAL TRIALS AND THEIR IMPORTANCE TO ALL STAKEHOLDERS

Well-designed and properly executed randomized clinical trials (RCTs) remain powerful investigational tools to assess the efficacy of cancer treatments in improving the survival and quality of life of persons with cancer. RCTs are critical to the everyday practice of cancer care among surgeons because they provide high-quality evidence to guide treatment recommendations for the patient who has cancer in real-world settings. However, achieving these goals

Supported by the Enhancing Minority Participation in Clinical Trials (EMPaCT) of the National Institute on Minority Health and Health Disparities and 2008 VFW Award.

*Corresponding author. E-mail address: alref003@umn.edu

0065-3411/12/$ – see front matter
doi:10.1016/j.yasu.2012.05.001

Published by Elsevier Inc.

also requires wide-scale adoption and dissemination of trial results into day-to-day clinical practice [1,2]. As such, the traction and engagement of stakeholders remains crucial. These stakeholders include patients with cancer, clinicians, the National Cancer Institute (NCI), payers, regulators, professional societies, policy makers, and patient advocates [1,2].

In addition to their impact on patients with cancer, the extent to which these cancer trials benefit other stakeholders is important for several reasons. First, results from properly conducted, adequately sampled, and well-stratified cancer trials create an environment of highly streamlined, research-driven treatment guidelines, thus encouraging stakeholders to better adhere to research-based treatment recommendations to increase accrual of subjects to newly introduced clinical protocols. Second, when applicable to the practice of clinicians, trials also engage more surgeons to participate and enroll their patients as subjects in cancer trials. Third, high-caliber cancer trials incentivize professional societies, policy makers, and payers to support this strong level of evidence, thus discouraging them from supporting practices in which unnecessary (and perhaps underinvestigated) therapies are administered [1,2].

WHY ARE CLINICAL TRIALS UNIQUE TO PERSONS WITH CANCER?

Cancer trials provide a rigorous and clear approach to testing whether an intervention/treatment will alter (or not alter) the outcomes of individuals with cancer in an experimental manner beyond the level of observational studies. The impact of a treatment or intervention on a designated end point is compared with a control group with a premise to minimize bias and confounding [1,2]. As such, cancer trials are particularly important to persons who have, or are at risk of, cancer because of many key points. First, adequately powered and well-stratified cancer trials are designed to improve the survivorship of persons with cancer. Second, clinical trials also measure whether these oncologic interventions improve the quality of life of their enrollees in the setting of anticipated survival benefit [3–7]. Third, the results of cancer trials allow surgeons and other clinicians to better understand the natural history and biology of various cancer sites, especially when interventions (or lack of them) are interposed [8]. Fourth, cancer trials also provide their enrollees opportunities to access research-driven hospitals and cancer centers, to participate in treatment decisions, and to be closely followed up. Fifth, high-caliber clinical trials will guide and streamline oncologic treatment decisions, thus leading to effective, but resource-conserving, clinical practice, rather than maximally tolerated treatment.

Because of the changing profile of cancer in the United States, cancer trials are timely and particularly important to persons who have, or are at risk of developing, cancer and their surgeons. First, cancer is a leading cause of death in the United States, second to heart disease. Second, the overall demographics of persons with cancer in the United States are evolving. For example, more than 60% of solid organ malignant tumors are diagnosed in persons older than 65 years, with an estimated 85% of all cancer deaths attributed to this elderly population. Twenty percent of the US population is projected to be 65 years or older by 2030. In addition, more than one-third of the US population is a minority population [1,9,10]. Third, the escalating cost of cancer care, in the background of limited resources, challenges health care stakeholders to reconsider the benefits/toxicity ratio of oncologic treatments weighed against the body of evidence from which these treatment recommendations stem. A large proportion of the National Comprehensive Cancer Network's clinical practice guidelines were recently found to stem from a lower level of evidence. Because of these reasons, and others, cancer trials are strategically positioned as a catalyst in transforming new knowledge into measurable and tangible benefits, thus guiding surgeons and other providers who care for patients with cancer [11].

WIDE-SCALE DISSEMINATION AND ADOPTION: EXPECTATIONS VERSUS CHALLENGES

In most cancer trials, subjects are carefully selected based on strict functional and diagnostic criteria, with enormous resources and time expended from concept to completion of cancer trials. Wide-scale adoption and dissemination of trial results into day-to-day clinical practice are critically required. However, the adoption and implementation of such interventions vary significantly and depend on several factors, including the clinician, the facility, the cancer site, and the applicability of these trials to the cohort of people in the community.

Several factors challenge the dissemination and adoption of cancer clinical trial results to surgeons. These factors include cancer (as a disease), the study design, treatment, and clinician-related and hospital-related factors.

In contrast with other conditions (eg, diabetes or coronary artery disease), cancer presents several investigational and therapeutic challenges that influence the conduct of clinical trials and the applicability of their results. First, as a disease, cancer typically involves a wide spectrum of disease sites from least common (eg, retroperitoneal sarcomas) to most common (eg, breast, colon, and lung cancers). Furthermore, the biologic nature of these varied disease sites produces varied survival outcomes from highly lethal (eg, pancreatic cancer) to a more favorable prognosis (eg, early-stage breast cancer). Second, cancer is diagnosed in many populations of different ages, ethnic and racial cohorts, and geographic locations. Third, the nature of multidisciplinary cancer care adds additional layers of complexity to the logistic and process of cancer trials [12,13]. For example, comparing the impact of agent X versus Y with or without radiotherapy after oncologic resection of cancer site Z is a more complex trial design from an interpretation standpoint than when coronary stent placement versus vein graft bypass are tested in persons with coronary artery disease. Furthermore, multidisciplinary cancer care also adds to the cost of cancer clinical trials [12,13]. For example, the cost estimate of nonclinical activities of a 12-month long, randomized, placebo-controlled chemotherapeutic trial approached $4000 per subject after excluding overheads in 2002.

Issues regarding the design of cancer clinical trials are also (and perhaps equally) important to the dissemination and adoption of cancer clinical trials; specifically the eligibility criteria and limitations of cancer trials of oncologic treatments:

- The eligibility criteria of cancer trials

Because of the possibility of oncologic interventions subjecting the enrollees to potential harm, and the need for close follow-up, many cancer trials have stringent inclusion and generous exclusion criteria. Thus, older persons, those with comorbidities, and persons with suboptimal health insurance coverage are either excluded or underenrolled in such trials. Although several trials no longer use older age as a precluding criterion for enrollment, the close ties between older age, comorbidities, frailty, and tolerability to oncologic treatments are likely reasons for their underenrollment. In addition, the close relationship between nonwhite race, suboptimal insurance status, and comorbidities tends to preclude those persons from participating in cancer trials. As a result of the tight eligibility criteria, surgeons and clinicians are faced with the challenges that the results of cancer trials are not necessarily applicable to their day-to-day practice outside the highly controlled cancer trial environment [14].

- The limitations of cancer trials involving cancer therapy

Lancet Oncology recently commissioned a report by national and international stakeholders on delivering affordable cancer care in high-income countries. In this comprehensive report, the limitations of trials involving cancer therapy were recognized as a reason for the lack of suitable clinical research to drive affordable cancer care in high-income countries given the high cost of cancer care in those countries, including $124 billion dollars spent on cancer care in the United States in 2010 [12,13]. Specifically, clinical trials depend heavily on statistical significance between the experimental and control intervention, with less attention paid to the clinical importance of the treatment effects. In this report, national and international experts questioned the results of the National Cancer Institute of Canada PA.3 study, which showed a significant benefit in overall survival, with a median gain of 0.33 months for erlotinib plus gemcitabine compared with gemcitabine alone as first-line treatment of advanced pancreatic cancer. Furthermore, stakeholders have also recognized the use of surrogate end points such as disease-free survival and progression-free survival as another limitation, especially when these surrogates were not necessarily associated with accurate estimates of the cost-effectiveness of new therapy, of quality of life measures, and of overall survival [14].

The type of oncologic intervention and the degree of its invasiveness play a role in its adoption and dissemination in the community. Surgical trials have typically been difficult to perform, especially when the control arm receives a lesser degree of intervention (ie, placebo). For example, laparoscopic colectomy for colon cancer has become an acceptable and safe alternative to the traditional open approach. This acceptance stemmed from 4 large randomized trials (Barcelona, Clinical Outcomes of Surgical Therapy [COST], Colon Carcinoma Open or Laparoscopic Resection [COLOR], Conventional versus Laparoscopic-Assisted Surgery in Patients with Colorectal Cancer [CLASSIC]) that showed the noninferiority of laparoscopic colectomy in overall survival, disease-free survival, and overall and local recurrences [15]. From a surgeon's standpoint, complex minimally invasive procedures can be performed in varied settings and by surgeons with diverse training, despite their procedure volume. Despite these findings, the adoption of laparoscopic colectomy is shown to be slow because of factors including learning curve, adapting hospital and clinician's perceptions, and bias [15].

Other factors, such as patient demographics, their cancer sites, type of treatment they undergo, the facility where they receive their treatments, and the preferences and perceptions of the treating clinician, also play an important role in promoting or slowing the adoption of cancer trial results. Despite their relative contribution to the burden of cancer overall, nonwhite persons, older persons, those who are underinsured or uninsured, those with nonbreast malignancies, and persons treated at community hospitals are less likely to enroll in cancer trials. As a result, the dissemination of results of cancer trials of these cohorts of persons with cancer and the ability to generalize those results to a real-world setting remain open questions. All of the factors and issues mentioned previously complicate the dissemination and adoption of well-designed adequately powered cancer trials [14].

PARTICIPATION IN CANCER CLINICAL TRIALS

Physician engagement plays a critical role in informing and enrolling persons with cancer in cancer clinical trials. Given the critical role surgery plays in the treatment of most malignant solid organ tumors, surgeons are important stakeholders in the process of cancer clinical trials. However, studies including a recent survey showed that surgeons were less likely to participate in cancer trials compared with other medical specialties, especially in those with early-stage cancer, in whose care surgeons are typically involved. Although these patients have greater opportunities for successful treatment compared with patient who have late-stage cancer, they may lack physician engagement to inform and enroll this group of patients in cancer clinical trials. A recent survey showed that many physicians who practiced at a Community Clinical Oncology Program or NCI cancer center did not participate in cancer trials. Specifically, surgeons were 5 times less likely to enroll or refer patients to cancer trials than medical or radiation oncologists.

Previous literature has shed light on reasons for the lack of engagement from patients' and surgeons' perspectives. From a patient's perspective, reasons including distrust, lack of understanding of the premise of clinical trials, and dislike of the random allocation concept have led to their underenrollment in cancer trials. From a surgeon's perspective, several reasons have been identified, including lack of infrastructure, resources, time commitment, and incentives to enroll and participate in clinical trials. Other reasons include a surgeon's personal bias toward one treatment rather than the other; loss of patients to competing health systems; perception of, and experience with, clinical trials, especially with articulating the concept, design, and equipoise in the oncologic literature.

CANCER TRIALS VERSUS THE REAL-WORLD IN THE UNITED STATES

Progress has been made by several cancer clinical trials in improving the survivorship and quality of life of persons with cancer in the United States. To date, many cancer trials have led to practice-changing results that have been offered to patients with cancer in various disease sites in diverse practice settings. Landmark trials by Cancer and Leukemia Group B (CALGB), SWOG, American College of Surgeon Oncology Group (ACOSOG), and North Central Cancer Treatment Group (NCCTG) have incrementally provided clinicians with valuable results to help oncologic treatment decisions in breast, gastrointestinal and lung cancer, to name just a few [3–7]. Recently, results from the ACOSOG Z0011 and Z9001 trials provided important contributions to the knowledge of breast cancer and gastrointestinal stromal tumors.

Despite these accomplishments, overall underenrollment in cancer trials in the United States remains a significant problem [16–18]. Most RCT enrollees have few or no comorbidities, and are often white, more financially secure, and younger than those who do not participate in trials [2,16–21]. In contrast, nonparticipants often have multiple comorbidities (regardless of their treating hospitals), are older, more often from a minority group, and often live on lower incomes with (for now) no or inadequate health insurance [16–18]. At the request of the Director of the NCI, the Institute of Medicine has recently assessed the current state of cancer clinical trials in the US [22]. Despite the accolades of the cancer cooperative group programs, the Institute of Medicine (IOM) report indicated that the status of cancer clinical trials in the United States is approaching a state of crisis. This report predicted that the current status of cancer trials is unable to sustain large-scale clinical trials to benefit the millions of patients with cancer.

We found that less than 1% of 244,528 patients were enrolled in cancer trials in the State of California [10]. Black patients were less likely than white patients to enroll in trials (0.48% vs 0.67%, $P<.05$). On multivariable analysis, older persons (>65 years), those with early-stage cancer, and those with lung or gastrointestinal cancers were less likely to be enrolled in cancer trials. For non-breast cancer protocols, female gender also predicted lack of enrollment. Black and uninsured patients showed trends toward underenrollment. These results suggest that, in addition to low accrual rates to cancer protocols overall, vast underrepresentation by age, cancer stage, and site continue to exist. The ability to generalize these trials to a real-world perspective remains an open question [1,10].

EFFORTS TO ENHANCE APPLICABILITY OF CANCER TRIALS TO REAL-WORLD SETTINGS

Comparative effectiveness research

Despite the achievements in biomedical science, clinicians are still confronted with the lack of a clear treatment decision that best fits their patients in day-to-day oncology practice, including general surgery and surgical oncology. As such, comparative effectiveness research (CER) is designed to facilitate treatment decisions by providing a body of research-based evidence outlining the effectiveness, benefits, and harms of different treatment options. The evidence is generated from research studies that compare drugs, medical devices, tests, surgeries, or ways to deliver health care from existing or new lines or research. As such, CER represent a shift from investigator-driven research to a stakeholder-driven, investigational approach including clinical trials [23].

The American Recovery and Reinvestment Act (ARRA) contains $1.1 billion for CER. CER compares treatments and strategies to improve health. This information is an essential tool that clinicians and patients use to decide on the best treatment.

Research on the implementation gap between efficacy versus effectiveness of cancer trials

Given the widening gap between the efficacy of cancer clinical trials versus its effectiveness in a real-world setting, the ability of practicing surgeons to generalize cancer trials deserves further assessment. Using several datasets representative of clinical practice, The University of Minnesota Surgical Outcomes Research Center (http://www.surg.umn.edu/research/msow/home.html) has been actively seeking a better understanding of the patterns of, and source of variation in, the implementation of guideline-recommended cancer care of various solid cancer sites in the United States. Specifically, we have assessed the association between treatment guidelines that are typically (and ideally) based on level 1 evidence on a growing population of the United States. Special populations include older persons (>65 years), ethnic/racial minorities, the underinsured/uninsured, those with comorbidities, and women. Special populations are a unique cohort of persons with cancer who typically receive cancer care that deviates from recommended care because of underlying circumstances, prompting unanimous interest among NCI-sponsored groups in these persons to ensure their enrollment in cancer trials. Among these groups, we consistently found that older age, nonwhite race/ethnicity, and suboptimal insurance status are powerful predictors of nonadherence to guideline-recommended cancer care in the United States.

Colon cancer represents the third most common cancer worldwide. In an era of limited resources, understanding trends and potential benefits of adjuvant chemotherapy in the elderly is an important tool that aids clinicians in day-to-day practice and decision making. To date, level I evidence supporting adjuvant chemotherapy in stage III colon cancer has a limited ability to be generalized to practice involving patients older than 75 years, because most randomized trials underrepresent persons 75 years of age or older. The ability to generalize these results to a growing elderly population remains unknown. The definitive step to elucidating these previously mentioned relationships (older age and chemotherapy) will be the initiation of phase II and III studies in these patients, which will be an important step toward providing patients with effective and resource-conserving, rather than maximally tolerated, treatments (Abraham and colleagues, unpublished data, presented at 2011 Academic Surgical Congress).

Pancreatic cancer continues to be a formidable challenge, mainly because of its poor biologic features. Although 80% of pancreas cancers are diagnosed in patients 60 years of age or older, the applicability of pancreas cancer trial results to older persons is, arguably, limited. Older age is associated with higher rates of underlying comorbidities, declining performance status, and an increased probability of complications after major cancer surgeries [1]. Pancreaticoduodenectomy, a major oncologic procedure associated with up to 40% morbidity and 50% readmission rates, can be a major undertaking in older persons, even those with good performance status. Thus, adjuvant therapy, which may have been well tolerated by younger patients in clinical trials,

Table 1
Guideline-recommended care among special populations across select cancer sites (older persons, nonwhite, underinsured vs insured)

Selected disease site parameters	>65 y vs <65 y	Nonwhite vs white	Underinsured/ uninsured vs insured
Colon cancer			
Cancer burden distribution	55%–60%	<25%	<10%
Receipt of adjuvant chemotherapy for stage III	Up to 24× less likely	1.2× less likely	1.6× less likely
Refusal of adjuvant therapy	Up to 20× more likely	1.2× more likely	2× more likely
Gastric cancer			
Cancer burden distribution	60%	<22%	8%
Adequate lymph evaluation	1.6× less likely	—	—
Receipt of adjuvant therapy for stage Ib–IVO	5× less likely	—	—
Pancreas cancer			
Cancer burden distribution	60%	<25%	8%
Undergoing pancreatectomy for cancer	Less likely	Less likely	Less likely
Adjuvant therapy after pancreatectomy	5× less likely	1.3× less likely	—
Extremity soft tissue sarcoma			
Cancer burden distribution	30%	<27%	—
Receipt of sarcoma-directed surgery	2× less likely	Less likely	—
Receipt of adjuvant therapy radiotherapy for T2 or high-grade tumors	Twice less likely	Less likely	—
Limb amputation for sarcoma	No association	Twice as likely	—

delivered after major cancer resection may not be endured in older persons. Furthermore, comorbidities as competing causes of mortality can assume a large role in determining the survival in older patients, and the benefit of the adjuvant therapy may thus be diluted. The associations between age, race, and insurance with pancreatic cancer care (Table 1) highlight 2 important (and perhaps unanswered) questions. First, given the underrepresentation of older persons in cancer clinical trials [17], how far can the results of pancreas cancer therapy trials be generalized to the expanding population of older persons in the United States? Second, and in light of emerging evidence to support neo-adjuvant or perioperative systemic chemotherapy (without radiotherapy) in the setting of margin-negative pancreatectomy, is omitting adjuvant radiotherapy, with its known toxicities and financial burden, a reasonable option in older populations? This is particularly important because these results (see Table 1) suggest that most elders do not necessarily receive adjuvant therapies, weighed against the mixed body of scientific evidence on adjuvant radiotherapy after pancreatic cancer surgery. Without further investigations, these questions will remain unanswered.

As for gastric cancer, findings from Table 1 also question the effectiveness of the INT-0116 trial to these expanding populations of older persons in the community. In light of these findings, along with emerging evidence to support perioperative or postoperative systemic chemotherapy (without radiotherapy [RT]), will omitting adjuvant RT, with its known toxicities and financial burden in the setting of adequate surgery and lymphadenectomy, be a reasonable option in older populations? Again, without further investigations, these questions remain speculative [9,24].

The underappreciated impact of hospital attributes on cancer clinical trials

Hospital type plays an important role in the delivery of cancer care and the conduct of cancer clinical trials [25]. At this juncture, most clinical cancer trials are conducted at high-volume hospitals (HVH) or academic centers where adequate support and infrastructure exist [26]. Furthermore, worse operative outcomes have been associated with low-volume hospitals (LVH) following complex cancer surgery. Few regional studies identify racial/ethnic minorities and the underinsured as more likely to receive their cancer surgery at an LVH. Identifying which patient factors significantly contribute to receiving cancer surgery at LVH needs further investigation, because these patients are currently excluded from the benefits of HVH, including participation in clinical trials and improved survival. Whether patient-related factors affect this association remains unknown [24,27]. In addition, inadequate access has contributed to widespread racial disparities in cancer care in the United States.

The University of Minnesota Surgical Outcomes Research Center examined 2 important questions that are relevant to the conduct of cancer clinical trials. Using the 2003 to 2008 National Inpatient Sample (NIS), we identified 59,841 patients who underwent cancer surgeries for lung, esophagus, and pancreas tumors (accepted by Journal of The American College of Surgeons). We found that 38.4% received their cancer surgery at LVH. Multivariate analyses continued to show that nonwhite race, suboptimal insurance status, and comorbidities predicted receipt of cancer surgery at LVH across all 3 procedures. These results provide additional insights into the volume-outcomes relationship. Because of the profound underenrollment of persons in cancer trials overall, persons at LVH represent a population who are often excluded from cancer clinical trials in the United States. To overcome some of these barriers and broaden the applicability of cancer clinical trials, our results should stimulate future policy and programs such as patient and physician navigators to enhance accrual of patients from LVH to centers of cancer clinical trials [28].

Because of the influence of inadequate access caused by widespread racial disparities in cancer care in the United States, we examined the impact of nonwhite race on operative outcomes after cancer surgery at American College of Surgeons National Surgical Quality Improvement Program hospitals (to be presented at the 2011 Southern Surgical Association Annual Meeting) [29]. This question is particularly important when the outcomes of racial minorities at quality-seeking hospitals, where cancer trials are typically conducted, remains unknown. In this study, nonwhites were more likely to have higher rates of co-morbidities ($P<.05$ for all). However, they had adverse adjusted short-term operative outcomes after cancer surgery that were comparable with those of white people, even after stratification by extent of surgical procedure. However, black, Hispanic, and American Indian/Alaskan Native patients were more likely to experience extended length of stay. These findings suggest that access to quality-driven hospitals may ameliorate racial disparities in cancer care and outcomes. Future policies should focus on expanding access to quality-driven surgical facilities as a step toward improving enrollment of these persons in cancer trials [29].

CONSIDERATIONS FOR VALID AND USEFUL CANCER TRIALS TO THE GENERAL SURGEON AND SURGICAL ONCOLOGIST IN THE REAL-WORLD

- Educating the public (as a stakeholder) on the importance of cancer clinical trials is an important task to engage and encourage more persons with cancer to enroll in cancer clinical trials. Surgeons need to take the lead on this task, because they represent the frontier to persons with early-stage solid organ malignant tumors.
- Community engagement to overcome issues such mistrust and abuse. Currently more than one-third of the US population is of a minority group. However, less than 1% of adult patients who have cancer enrolled in clinical trials are minorities. Several efforts are underway to increase minority recruitment and retention in clinical trials through developing networks of institutions and centers dedicated to minority health, establishing community-based participatory research and education programs to combat the underlying mistrust of the medical research community, and providing the environment for conducting clinical research for minority-related diseases.

- Streamlining the process of cancer clinical trials, especially when most trials have a long germination period from concept to completion. This lengthy process is further complicated by lack of completion of up to 40% of these trials; this was one of the main recommendations by the IOM on the status of cancer clinical trials in the United States.
- Education and engagement of more surgeons to be a crucial part of clinical trials. To date, surgery remains the most critical element of most solid malignant organ tumor treatments. In this regard, surgeons represent the gateway to both oncologic treatments and enrollment in investigational treatment protocols. To gain surgeon engagement in cancer clinical trials, strategies should mitigate key factors such as time demands, lack of support, infrastructure, patient and physician navigation systems, and realignment of incentives and compensations. Furthermore, surgeon-led organizations and NCI groups including the American College of Surgeons and American College of Surgeons Oncology Group can play a pivotal role in fulfilling these goals. These goals should also include creating a culture and an environment among current and future surgeons that will embrace cancer clinical trials.
- The American Society of Clinical Oncology recently published a blueprint of its vision to improve the treatment of cancer in 3 main domains: (1) establishing a new approach to therapeutic development, driven by a more thorough understanding of cancer biology; (2) designing smarter, faster clinical trials that are appropriate for the era of molecularly targeted therapies; and (3) harnessing information technology to seamlessly integrate clinical and translational research and patient care, ensuring that every patient's experience can inform research and improve care [30–33].
- Aggressive pursuit to include large health care systems, nonacademic centers, and Veterans Affairs, because these populations will add heterogeneity in terms of performance status, comorbidities, and race-based and age-based diversity (a trial's external validity to a surgeon's clinical practice).
- Design of diverse clinical trials that represent the cancer burden people carry in day-to-day clinical practice, including elders, ethnic/racial minorities, and those with comorbidities. Unless these persons with cancer are better represented in US cancer trials, surgeons will continue to question the applicability of these results to their practices.

SUMMARY

Cancer trials represent a rigorous and clear approach to testing whether an intervention or treatment will alter the outcomes of individuals with cancer in an experimental manner that is beyond the level of observational studies. As such, they remain useful and valid to the day-to-day practice of general surgeons and surgical oncologists. However, the shortcomings of current cancer clinical trials need to be recognized, especially when less than 1% of adults persons with cancer participate in cancer clinical trials, thus leaving the ability to generalize these trials to patients and their surgeons in the real-world setting an open question. Moving forward, physicians, payers, professional societies, advocates, the NCI, and other stakeholders need to develop broader cancer trials to benefit the millions of patients with cancer in the United States.

References

[1] A national cancer clinical trials system for the 21st century: reinvigorating the NCI cooperative group program. In: Nass SJ, Moses HL, Mendelsohn J, editors. Committee on Cancer Clinical Trials and the NCI Cooperative Group Program. Institute of Medicine. April, 2010.
[2] Brennan MF. Commentary: randomized controlled trials. Surg Oncol Clin North Am 2010;19(1):1–11.
[3] Rothenberger DA. Evidence-based practice requires evidence. Br J Surg 2004;91(11): 1387–8.
[4] "Comparative Effectiveness Research" workshop. Alliance Cooperative Meeting. Chicago (IL): Caner and Leukemia Group B; 2010.
[5] Elting LS, Cooksley C, Bekele BN, et al. Generalizability of cancer clinical trial results: prognostic differences between participants and nonparticipants. Cancer 2006;106(11): 2452–8.
[6] Stewart JH, Bertoni AG, Staten JL, et al. Participation in surgical oncology clinical trials: gender-, race/ethnicity-, and age-based disparities. Ann Surg Oncol 2007;14(12):3328–34.
[7] Hutchins LF, Unger JM, Crowley JJ, et al. Underrepresentation of patients 65 years of age or older in cancer-treatment trials. N Engl J Med 1999;341(27):2061–7.
[8] Murthy VH, Krumholz HM, Gross CP. Participation in cancer clinical trials: race-, sex-, and age-based disparities. JAMA 2004;291(22):2720–6.
[9] You YN, Ota D, Nelson H, et al. The American College of Surgeons Oncology Group. Surgery 2009;145(6):587–90.
[10] Luglio G, Nelson H. Laparoscopy for colon cancer: state of the art. Surg Oncol Clin North Am 2010;19:777–91.
[11] Dilts DM, Sandler AB. Invisible barriers to clinical trials: the impact of structural, infrastructural, and procedural barriers to opening oncology clinical trials. J Clin Oncol 2006;24: 4545–52.
[12] Pignatti F, Luria X, Abadie E, et al. Regulators, payers, and prescribers: can we fill the gaps? Lancet Oncol 2011;12(10):930–1.
[13] Rawlins MD, Chalkidou K. The opportunity cost of cancer care: a statement from NICE. Lancet Oncol 2011;12(10):931–2.
[14] Delivering affordable cancer care in high-income countries. The Lancet Oncology Commission. Lancet Oncol 2011;12:933–80.
[15] Siminoff LA, Zhang A, Colabianchi N, et al. Factors that predict the referral of breast cancer patients onto clinical trials by their surgeons and medical oncologists. J Clin Oncol 2000;18:1203–11.
[16] Martin RC 2nd, Polk HC Jr, Jaques DP. Does additional surgical training increase participation in randomized controlled trials? Am J Surg 2003;185:239–43.
[17] Jenkins V, Leach L, Fallowfield L, et al. Describing randomisation: patients' and the public's preferences compared with clinicians' practice. Br J Cancer 2002;87:854–8.
[18] Harrison JD, Solomon MJ, Young JM, et al. Surgical and oncology trials for rectal cancer: who will participate? Surgery 2007;142:94–101.
[19] Ford E, Jenkins V, Fallowfield L, et al. Clinicians' attitudes towards clinical trials of cancer therapy. Br J Cancer 2011;104:1535–43.
[20] Poonacha TK, Go RS. Level of scientific evidence underlying recommendations arising from the national comprehensive cancer network clinical practice guidelines. J Clin Oncol 2011;29:186–91.
[21] Begg CB, Engstrom PF. Eligibility and extrapolation in cancer clinical trials. J Clin Oncol 1987;5(6):962–8.
[22] Rusch VW. Surgeons: a future role in clinical trials? Oncologist 1997;2:v–vi.
[23] Lamont EB, Landrum MB, Keating NL, et al. Differences in clinical trial patient attributes and outcomes according to enrollment setting. J Clin Oncol 2010;28(2):215–21.
[24] Al-Refaie WB, Muluneh B, Zhong W, et al. Who receives their complex cancer surgery at low volume hospitals? J Am Coll Surg 2012;214(1):81–7.

[25] Al-Refaie WB, Vickers SM, Zhong W, et al. Cancer trials versus the real world. Ann Surg 2011;254(3):438–42.

[26] Dudeja V, Gay G, Habermann EB, et al. Do hospital attributes predict guideline-recommended gastric cancer care in the United States? Ann Surg Oncol 2012;19(2):365–72.

[27] Al-Refaie WB, Parsons HM, Henderson WG, et al. Results beyond 30-day operative mortality: colorectal cancer surgery in the oldest old. Ann Surg 2011;253(5):947–52.

[28] Dudeja V, Habermann EB, Zhong W, et al. Gastric cancer care in the elderly: insights into the generalizability of NCI-cancer trials. Ann Surg Oncol 2011;18(1):26–33.

[29] Al-Refaie W, Pisters PW, Rothenberger DA. Surgical oncology trials and surgeons in the real world! Ann Surg Oncol 2010;17(7):1727–8.

[30] Al-Refaie WB, Habermann E, Jensen EH, et al. Extremity soft tissue sarcoma care in the elderly: insights into the generalizability of NCI trials. Ann Surg Oncol 2010;17(7):1732–8.

[31] Al-Refaie W, Parsons HM, Henderson WG, et al. Major cancer surgery in the elderly: results from the American College of Surgeons National Surgical Quality Improvement Program. Ann Surg 2010;251(2):311–8.

[32] Al-Refaie W, Gay G, Virnig B, et al. Variations in gastric cancer care; a trend beyond racial disparities. Cancer 2010;116(2):465–75.

[33] Accelerating Progress against Cancer. ASCO's blueprint for transforming clinical and translational cancer research. American Society of Clinical Oncology; 2011.

The Current Management of Pancreatic Neuroendocrine Tumors

Trevor A. Ellison, MD, MBA, Barish H. Edil, MD*

Department of Surgery, The Johns Hopkins Hospital, 1550 Orleans Street, CRB II, Room 506, Baltimore, MD 21287, USA

Keywords
• Pancreas • Neuroendocrine tumor • PanNET • Hormones • Islet cell tumor
• Neuroendocrine neoplasm

Key Points
• A complete back ground of pancreatic neuroendocrine tumors. Including clinical presentation, evaluation and treatment.
• Pancreatic neuroendocrine tumors can be divided in functional and non functional tumors.
• New treatment chemotherapy regimens have entered the treatment paradigm.

INTRODUCTION

Pancreatic neuroendocrine tumors (PanNETs) are rare and heterogeneous. They constitute 3% to 5% of all pancreatic malignancies. Their incidence rate results in around 1000 new cases a year in the United States [1], with an associated prevalence of more than 100,000 individuals [2]. These tumors were first described by Nicholls [3] in 1902, and they are distinct from the more common pancreatic ductal adenocarcinoma (95% of pancreatic malignancies). PanNETs originate in the islet cells (ie, endocrine portion) of the pancreas rather than the exocrine pancreas and have a more indolent course with better overall survival (overall 5-year survival is about 42%) [1]. PanNETs present in 3 distinct fashions: as part of genetic syndromes, as functional tumors with dramatic clinical symptoms caused by overproduction of specific hormones and vasoactive peptides [4], and as nonfunctional tumors. Although they have a better prognosis than exocrine tumors, 50% to 60% of PanNETs, excluding insulinomas, have metastasized by the time of diagnosis [3], which can result in poor outcomes.

CLASSIFICATION

Gastrointestinal neuroendocrine tumors were first classified by an international body in 2000 when the World Health Organization (WHO) divided the

*Corresponding author. E-mail address: bedil1@jhmi.edu

0065-3411/12/$ – see front matter
doi:10.1016/j.yasu.2012.04.002

tumors into 5 general categories based on histologic differentiation: well-differentiated endocrine tumor, well-differentiated endocrine carcinoma, poorly differentiated endocrine/small cell carcinoma, mixed exocrine-endocrine tumor, and tumorlike lesion. This system proved to have prognostic efficacy as well as reproducibility [5]. The WHO also recommended that grade be measured by mitoses per 10 high-powered field or by Ki67 staining. The WHO subsequently published a classification specifically for PanNETs in 2004 and then a third classification system in 2010 for all gastroenteropancreatic neuroendocrine tumors.

The European Neuroendocrine Tumor Society (ENETS) issued a new staging and grading system in 2006 for foregut neuroendocrine tumors to further distinguish those tumors in the WHO classification system that had the same differentiation but different clinical behavior. The ENETS system was based on the tumor, node, metastasis (TNM) classification and they also suggested that grade be recorded. The ENETS system was proved in several series in providing stage separation [5].

It was not until 2010 that the American Joint Committee on Cancer (AJCC) in their seventh edition of the AJCC Cancer Staging Manual provided a staging system for PanNETs. The TNM staging system assigned to PanNETs was the same as used for exocrine pancreas cancer. The AJCC also suggested recording grade separately because of its prognostic influence on clinical behavior and survival outcome.

PRESENTATION AND DIAGNOSIS

PanNETs can be broadly divided into 3 distinct clinical presentations: syndromic, functional, and nonfunctional. The reason for this distinction is that the presentation, management, and prognosis vary between the 3 groups. Overall, nonfunctional Pan-NETs constitute most (85%) PanNETs, which is a change in trend from the past when functional PanNETs were most often recognized [4]. Functional PanNETs are typically detected because they present with sometimes severe clinical symptoms caused by hormone overproduction, whereas nonfunctional PanNETs usually present at later stages of the disease because of symptoms from space-occupying lesions or metastatic disease. However, recently, nonfunctional PanNETs are being discovered at earlier stages with the frequent use of computed tomography (CT) scans. CT scans are credited as the factor contributing to the more than 100% increase in the diagnosis of PanNET between the periods of 1977 to 1981 and 2002 to 2005 [6].

Syndromic PanNETs

PanNETs are associated with genetic syndromes in 5% to 25% of cases, with the most common syndrome being multiple endocrine neoplasia, type 1 (MEN-1) in which insulinomas and gastrinomas predominate [7]. It is important to recognize syndromic PanNETs for several reasons. First, recognizing these inherited, genetic syndromes allows for earlier surveillance of descendants. Second, these individuals are predisposed to multifocal pancreatic neoplasms and extrapancreatic neoplasm types so vigilance should be maintained for other organ systems. Third, the genetic defects in these syndromes can provide insight into the biologic pathways contributing to PanNETs. Fourth, recognizing a tumor related to a syndrome may alter management. For example resection of a gastrinoma in a patient with MEN-1/Zollinger-Ellison syndrome (ZES) rarely produces a cure so pancreatic surgery may not be considered the first-line option in these cases [3]. The following are some of the syndromes that include PanNETs.

MEN-I

These patients have an inherited mutation in the tumor suppressor gene, MEN1, located on chromosome 11q13. They have a defect in the menin protein and this predisposes them to parathyroid hyperplasia, pituitary tumors, and PanNETs. MEN-1 is most commonly associated with gastrinomas and these tumors occur in 20% to 30% of those with ZES and they tend to be more indolent and multifocal [3]. Although gastrinomas can occur in the pancreas, most are found in the submucosa of the duodenum, so careful inspection of the duodenum is required in any resection. With the multifocal character of syndromic patients, surgical cure of these PanNETs is less likely than for the sporadic form of PanNETs [1].

von Hippel-Lindau syndrome

These patient have an inherited mutation in the VHL gene located on chromosome 3p25, which predisposes them to PanNETs, pancreatic cysts, hemangioblastomas (retina, kidney, cerebellum, brain), renal cell carcinoma, and pheochromocytomas. Most of these individuals eventually develop pancreas tumors and these may be the first manifestations of this syndrome. Between 15% and 77% of patients have an associated pancreatic tumor including simple cysts (91%), serous cystadenomas(12%), and PanNETs (7%–12%). The PanNETs tend to be nonfunctional, asymptomatic, and multifocal [8].

Tuberous sclerosis complex

These patients have an inherited mutation in 1 of 2 genes (TSC1 on chromosome 9q34, which codes for the protein hamartin; or TSC2 on chromosome 16p13, which codes for the protein tuberin). These patients may show developmental delay, mental retardation, autism, brain lesions (subependymal giant cell astrocytomas, subependymal nodules, and cortical tubers), skin lesions (hypomelanotic macules and facial angiofibromas), angiomyolipomas of the kidneys, lymphangioleiomyomatosis of the lungs, rhabdomyomas of the heart, hamartomas of the eyes, and PanNETs. PanNETs are less common than the other manifestations.

Neurofibromatosis type I (von Recklinghausen disease)

These patients have an inherited mutation of the NF1 gene on chromosome 17q11, which codes for the protein neurofibromin. These patients develop skin lesions (café-au-lait spots), benign and malignant nervous system tumors (eg, neurofibromas and malignant peripheral nerve sheath tumors), Lisch nodules of the iris, and a small percentage develop PanNETs (somatostatinomas of the pancreas or duodenum).

Clinical genetic testing under the supervision of a trained genetic counselor is recommended for those with these syndromes.

Functional PanNETs

Functional PanNETs are typically distinguished by their dramatic clinical presentations secondary to the overproduction of specific pancreatic hormones. The clinical effects may be out of proportion to their size, which can make localization by conventional imaging techniques difficult. A list of the functional PanNETs with their associated presentation and diagnosis follows.

Insulinoma
Insulinomas are the most common functional PanNETs and are characteristically slow growing and benign (85%–90%). Ten percent may present as multiple tumors and 5% to 8% are associated with MEN-1 syndrome. Most tumors are intraparenchymal, with only 3% being ectopic (with the duodenal mucosa being the most common extrapancreatic location) [3]. When they are intrapancreatic, they are equally distributed throughout the pancreas, so blind resection is not warranted. If the tumor cannot be localized before surgery, 95% can be localized on surgical exploration with full pancreatic mobilization, palpation, and use of intraoperative ultrasound (IOUS) [3].

Presentation. These patients present clinically with the Whipple triad: fasting hypoglycemia (blood glucose <40 mg/dL), symptomatic hypoglycemia while fasting (tachycardia, palpitations, confusion, obtundation, seizures, changes in personality, coma, tremulousness, diaphoresis, fatigue, blurry vision, weakness), and relief of symptoms after administration of glucose.

Diagnosis. Diagnosis is confirmed by several biochemical tests in the clinical setting mentioned earlier. Biochemical abnormalities consist of documented fasting hypoglycemia (blood glucose <40 mg/dL) associated with an increased insulin level (blood insulin >5 mU/mL) and a fasting insulin/blood glucose ratio greater than 0.4. These biochemical determinations are best performed during a 72-hour monitored fast in the hospital, where blood glucose and insulin levels are drawn every 6 hours. At the time of hypoglycemic symptoms, blood glucose, insulin, proinsulin, and c-peptide are measured, after which intravenous glucose is administered and the fast terminated. Proinsulin and c-peptide levels should be increased in the case of insulinomas to rule out exogenous insulin administration.

Gastrinomas
Gastrinomas are the second most common functional PanNETs and they cause stomach and duodenal ulcers by releasing large amounts of gastrin. Drs Zollinger and Ellison first detailed a syndrome in 1955 in which they described 2 patients with severe peptic ulcer disease and PanNETs (ZES) [1]. Gastrinomas make up less than 1% of peptic ulcer disease [1], although they are present in 2% of individuals who have recurrent ulcers after ulcer surgery [4]. Gastrinomas have about a 50% malignant potential and up to 33% of those presenting with gastrinomas have liver metastases on diagnosis [1]. However, with increased CT scan screening, more gastrinomas are being picked up earlier without metastases so more are being found that are resectable [4]. Between 15% and 35% of gastrinomas are associated with MEN-1.

Presentation. Patients with gastrinomas present with unrelenting peptic ulcer disease, abdominal pain (90%), and diarrhea (50%) [4]. Ten percent of patients have diarrhea as their only symptom [4].

Diagnosis. There are several biochemical diagnostic tests for gastrinoma. The basal acid output (BAO)/maximal acid output (MAO) ratio greater than or equal to 0.6 is diagnostic, as is an overnight acid output greater than or equal to 100 mmol, BAO greater than or equal to 10 mmol/h, serum gastrin 10 times normal, or a positive secretin test. The secretin test (90% sensitive and specific) is performed to distinguish a gastrinoma from antral G-cell hyperplasia and other causes by rapidly injecting 1 unit of secretin per kilogram intravenously, and a 100% increase in gastrin within 10 minutes is considered positive for gastrinoma or, if a 2 unit per kilogram rapid intravenous (IV) infusion is given, then a 100% increase from the baseline gastrin level is considered positive for gastrinoma [1]. Proton pump inhibitors can mask the clinical manifestations of gastrinomas for extended periods of time, leading to more advanced disease by the time the gastrinoma is diagnosed. In addition, proton pump inhibitors have been implicated in false-positive secretin tests [9].

Glucagonoma
This is the third most common functional PanNET and 75% are malignant.

Presentation. Excess production of the hormone glucagon results in a clinical syndrome of a skin rash (necrolytic migratory erythema [NME]), venous thrombosis (which puts patients at high risk for pulmonary embolisms), and hyperglycemia. These 3 signs taken together are nearly diagnostic. Another classic constellation of symptoms is called the 4 Ds: dermatitis (NME), diabetes, deep venous thrombosis, and depression. Other symptoms may include stomatitis, weight loss, and anemia. NME is a severe dermatitis with highly pruritic, erythematous, scaly patches that migrate over the body in the perioral, intertriginous, and pretibial areas. The rash often precedes other symptoms by years and is the presenting feature in 70% of patients [3].

Diagnosis. Diagnosis can be made by skin biopsy of the NME rash as well as by increased fasting serum glucagon greater than 500 to 1000 pg/mL with low serum amino acids.

VIPoma
VIPoma (also known as the Verner-Morrison syndrome) is a rare tumor that may occur in the pancreas (usually the tail) or the duodenum. VIPomas are usually malignant and almost 50% present with metastases to the lymph nodes or liver.

Presentation. Patients with VIPomas present with the WDHA (watery diarrhea, hypokalemia, achlorhydria/hypochlorhydria) syndrome. The watery, secretory diarrhea is profuse and can be up to 5 to 10 L per day. The hypokalemia from fecal losses may be up to 400 mEq per day, leading to nausea, lethargy, and muscle weakness.

Diagnosis. The diagnosis is reached after other more common causes of diarrhea are ruled out. Fasting plasma vasoactive intestinal polypeptide levels are increased to more than 500 pg/mL and a minority of patients have increased levels of the peptide histidine-isoleucine (PHI) or prostaglandins.

Somatostatinoma
Somatostatinomas are the fifth most common functional PanNET and occur in fewer than 1 in 40 million people [4]. Most of these tumors are malignant and they are usually diagnosed as metastatic disease. They occur equally between the pancreas (usually the head of the pancreas) and duodenum (duodenal involvement is associated with von Recklinghausen disease).

Presentation. The clinical picture is that of diarrhea (caused by decreased pancreatic enzyme and bicarbonate secretion), steatorrhea, mild diabetes (caused by insulin inhibition), gallstones (caused by inhibition of cholecystokinin), and hypochlorhydria.

Diagnosis. These tumors are diagnosed by increased fasting serum somatostatin levels greater than 100 pg/mL in the clinical setting presented earlier.

Other rare functional PanNETs
There are other functional PanNETs that are exceedingly rare. They include tumors that secrete adrenocorticotropic hormone (ACTH) causing Cushing syndrome, parathyroid hormone–related protein (PTH-RP) causing hypercalcemia, serotonin causing flushing, neurotensin causing hypertension, and growth hormone–releasing factor causing acromegaly.

Nonfunctional PanNETs
Nonfunctional PanNETs are the most common type of PanNETs (85%) and they usually present with space-occupying symptoms such as abdominal pain, bowel obstruction, jaundice, and weight loss. Although they do not present with a clinical syndrome from hormone overproduction, these tumors may overproduce certain hormones that do not result in any clinical manifestations (eg, pancreatic polypeptide, neurotensin, α-subunit of human chorionic gonadotropin, neuron-specific enolase, and chromogranin A). These tumors have a more indolent course than pancreatic adenocarcinoma and also have a longer survival time, with overall 5-year survival in resected patients reaching 50% [4].

IMAGING
Currently, multidetector, thin-slice CT scan with contrast is the first-line imaging modality for localization and staging of all PanNETs. CT scans should be dual phase, allowing for both arterial and venous phases. PanNETs are solid masses on CT scan and they enhance on arterial phase owing to their vascularity (sensitivity can reach 82%) [7].

Magnetic resonance imaging (MRI) is useful if the tumor cannot be detected by the CT scan, because MRI may be marginally superior to CT scan in the localization of PanNETs. PanNETs on MRI reveal low signal density on T1-weighted images and high signal density on T2-weighted images [3]. Although gadolinium contrast used with MRI is more sensitive for detecting vascular lesions, MRI with gadolinium contrast may not be able to pick up tumors less than 1 cm, and their sensitivity for tumors between 1 and 2 cm may not be more than 50% [3].

Somatostatin receptor scintigraphy (SRS) is another imaging modality that is useful for tumors that express type 2 somatostatin receptors (which includes most PanNETs except for most insulinomas). Although it does not provide information on tumor size or resectability, it allows localization and evaluation of metastatic disease.

Endoscopic ultrasound (EUS) is a useful adjunct if the CT scan fails to identify a mass. EUS can detect lesions as small as 0.5 cm and has the added benefit of being able to obtain tissue via fine-needle aspiration [3]. EUS is best at localizing tumors in the head of the pancreas as opposed to more distal lesions, and EUS has a sensitivity of only 43% for detecting duodenal gastrinomas [3]. Traditional transabdominal ultrasound is not used routinely because it has a sensitivity of 9% to 64% for PanNETs [3].

IOUS is a tool for detecting small lesions not appreciated on conventional imaging or for planning the route of enucleation or resection. IOUS localizes 86% of insulinomas and, when combined with CT, it localizes 93% of insulinomas [3].

If CT, MRI, SRS, and EUS do not localize the PanNET, there are several invasive techniques to locate these lesions. First, selective arteriography consists of injecting contrast into different arteries that supply the pancreas and duodenum to see whether directed contrast will reveal their location. Second, for functional lesions, selective arterial stimulation with portal venous hormone sampling can be used. In this technique, a stimulation agent (eg, calcium gluconate in the case of insulinomas) is infused into the splenic, superior mesenteric, and gastroduodenal arteries, followed by sampling for the hormone in the hepatic vein. A positive localization test results when a 2-fold increase in hormone level after directed stimulation is detected in the hepatic vein (this has a 90% sensitivity for insulinomas) [3]. Third, percutaneous transhepatic portal venous sampling consists of taking venous samples from the splenic, superior mesenteric, and portal vein to localize the hormone-producing tumor.

Special considerations
Insulinomas
Insulinomas are usually diagnosed at a small size (<2 cm) so imaging can be challenging. If a contrast CT is unable to localize the lesion, then an MRI study can be ordered or the patient can undergo EUS. EUS has a sensitivity of 80% to 90%, although it is less sensitive for lesions in the tail of the pancreas [7], and the most effective imaging to localize an insulinomas is the combination of contrast CT and EUS [10]. Insulinomas appear sonolucent on EUS compared with the echoic pancreas and this modality has the advantage of providing a biopsy for tissue diagnosis. Even if a biochemically confirmed insulinoma cannot be localized by CT, MRI, or EUS, other localization modalities include selective angiography, selective arterial stimulation with portal venous hormone sampling, and percutaneous transhepatic portal venous sampling. These more invasive techniques are usually reserved for those lesions that are not detected by other imaging. Although SRS is commonly used for PanNET imaging, it is of little value with insulinomas

because most insulinomas fail to express type 2 somatostatin receptors. If all localization has failed, then exploratory laparotomy with IOUS is indicated because up to 93% of insulinomas can be localized in this manner [7]. IOUS with bimanual palpation has the advantage of being able to delineate the relationship between the lesion and vital structures in the pancreas so that a safe resection or enucleation can be planned. On the rare occasion when the insulinoma cannot be localized via exploratory laparotomy palpation with IOUS, then the patient should be closed and other localization modalities attempted; blind resection is not indicated because insulinomas are uniformly distributed throughout the pancreas.

Gastrinomas

Most tumors (85%) are found in the so-called gastrinoma triangle (the area bounded by the neck of the pancreas, the second and third portion of the duodenum, and the confluence of the cystic duct with the common bile duct), 40% are on the surface of the pancreas, 40% are extrapancreatic (including primary disease in the regional lymph nodes), and 15% are intrapancreatic [1].

It is important to evaluate the liver as well as the pancreas because most gastrinomas have metastasized by the time of presentation. If localization fails under other modalities, more invasive techniques (ie, selective angiography and percutaneous transhepatic portal venous sampling) can be undertaken. SRS is helpful in evaluating for distant metastases.

Glucagonomas and VIPomas

Glucagonomas and VIPomas tend to be large (5–10 cm and >3 cm, respectively) at presentation and so they are usually easily visible on pancreas protocol CT scan [7]. Most glucagonomas are in the body and tail of the pancreas. SRS is helpful in evaluating for distant metastases.

Nonfunctional PanNETs

Because of their insidious onset of symptoms, nonfunctional PanNETs usually present with large tumors that are easily localized with a contrast CT scan. These tumors are usually found in the head, neck, and uncinate process of the pancreas and, because up to 65% have metastasized at presentation, SRS is helpful in evaluating for distant metastases.

TREATMENT

There are 3 types of treatment of PanNETs: preoperative and postoperative treatment of any hormonal excess, surgery, and adjuvant therapy.

Current pharmaceutical treatment of hormonal excess is paramount in controlling symptoms in patients with functional tumors. Examples include diazoxide for insulinomas and proton pump inhibitors for gastrinomas. In addition to these tumor-specific pharmaceuticals, somatostatin analogues have played a role in all PanNETs. Somatostatin analogues have been proved to increase progression-free survival in metastatic disease for midgut neuroendocrine tumors [11] and, although they can stabilize disease (especially in tumors with high affinity to somatostatin receptors such as nonfunctional tumors, VIPomas, glucagonomas, and gastrinomas), they are unlikely to cause tumor regression [7].

Special considerations
Insulinomas
Preoperative control of hypoglycemic symptoms is warranted as part of the treatment of insulinomas. Management includes the institution of frequent small meals, including overnight snacks, and ensuring that any intravenous fluid is fortified with glucose [7]. In addition, 60% of those with insulinomas respond to diazoxide or a somatostatin analogue as a means to decrease their insulin secretion.

Gastrinomas
Gastric acid hypersecretion should be treated before surgery with a proton pump inhibitor.

Glucagonomas
Patients with glucagonomas are normally severely malnourished and their nutrition should be optimized with total parenteral nutrition (TPN) and insulin before any surgery. A somatostatin analogue has also proved effective in reducing glucagon levels and controlling hyperglycemia. In addition, correction of hypoaminoacidemia usually completely resolves the rash of NME.

VIPomas
It is important to correct fluid and electrolyte imbalances before surgery. The secretory diarrhea–induced dehydration and electrolyte imbalance of VIPomas is difficult to manage with IV fluids alone, so a somatostatin analogue can be used to rapidly control the diarrhea.

Surgery is the mainstay of all PanNET treatment and is the only curative modality. The most important prognostic factor on survival is whether the tumor can be surgically removed. Recent studies have suggested that surgical resection is underused, possibly because of the misconception that PanNETs are less malignant and the historical impression that pancreatic surgery is fraught with a high mortality. However, because all PanNETs have some malignant potential, pancreatic surgery has become safer in the past decades (especially in high-volume centers) and surgical intervention is the only possibility for cure, surgery should be offered to appropriate patients with PanNETs [7]. Plans for surgical intervention should always account for the risks or surgery, the extent of disease, and whether the patient is syndromic. For those who are eligible for resection at presentation for localized disease, surgical resection provides a 55% 5-year survival compared with the same patient without surgery, who has a 15% 5-year survival [1]. Even with unresectable (locally advanced or metastatic) disease, palliative surgery is appropriate for tumor debulking because of space-occupying or hormonal symptoms in all PanNETs as well as potentially offering increased survival. Because most PanNETs have metastasized by the time of diagnosis, special attention should be given to the liver, duodenum, small bowel, small bowel mesentery, peripancreatic lymph nodes, splenic hilum, and reproductive tract in women when operating on these tumors [4]. However, because of the indolent nature of PanNETs, slow-growing metastases may also be observed until palliation is required.

Enucleation is appropriate for small (usually <2 cm), benign tumors, as is the case for most insulinomas and some gastrinomas. At our institution, we have found laparoscopic surgery to be an option for PanNETs because we have achieved similar oncologic goals of negative margins and lymphadenectomy as with the traditional open technique with a lower complication rate, fewer wound complications, and less blood loss.

Special considerations

Insulinomas

Ninety percent of insulinomas are small, solitary tumors that are amenable to surgical resection and cure [4]. Because 90% of insulinomas are benign, enucleation is acceptable as long as the tumor is 2 to 3 mm removed from the pancreatic duct and surrounding vascular structures [3].

Gastrinomas

If gastrinomas are suspected to be benign and are in the pancreas, they can be removed by enucleation as long as they are small and not near ducts nor vessels. Liver transplantation for hepatic metastases has been used as an option in extreme cases. Resection in those with MEN-1/ZES rarely produces a cure [3].

Somatostatinomas

Even though most of these tumors are malignant and have metastasized by the time of diagnosis, precluding resection for cure, debulking of the primary and metastatic disease for symptomatic relief is appropriate. The gallbladder is always removed at the time of surgery because of concern for future stone development with increased somatostatin levels.

PanNETs do not respond strongly to systemic chemotherapy or radiation (radiation may offer a limited role in providing pain relief from bone metastases) because they are usually slow growing. Studies of chemotherapy show an objective response rate of 10% to 45%, with complete response being rare. In addition, chemotherapy regimens are associated with significant adverse events [12]. Targeted therapy for hepatic metastases for space-occupying or hormonal symptoms are also appropriate. As of May 2011, the US Food and Drug Administration (FDA) has approved 2 new targeted therapies for PanNETs.

Special considerations

Insulinomas

Chemotherapy agents used in insulinomas include streptozocin, dacarbazine (DTIC), doxorubicin, and 5-fluorouracil (5-FU; combination therapy provides the highest response rates) [4].

Gastrinomas
Liver transplant and interferon therapy have been used, although they have not shown reproducible survival improvements. Decreased survival is associated with bone or liver metastases or ectopic Cushing syndrome [1].

VIPomas
Although not prospectively studied, some VIPomas have been treated with a somatostatin analogue along with systemic chemotherapy (streptozocin) and interferon.

Nonfunctionals
Unresectable patients have shown partial response in some reports to combination chemotherapy (with the highest response rate being 69% in those receiving streptozocin and doxorubicin) [4].

Even though streptozocin has been one of the most studied chemotherapy regimens, it is toxic and therefore rarely used.

There follows a discussion of management approaches according to disease extent as adapted from the National Cancer Institute guidelines (last updated 11/10/2011 [1]).

Localized or locoregional disease
Surgery with intent to cure is the first-line therapy. Because there are no well-controlled trials for adjuvant therapy showing benefit, adjuvant therapy should still be considered investigational. Surgical approaches for this disease have not been well studied.

Metastatic disease
Most metastases are found in the liver and are caused by the slow-growing nature of PanNETs along with possible hormone overproduction, and cytoreductive surgery is appropriate as because it may be associated with long-term survival and relief from symptomatic hormone overproduction. Hepatic resection can include wedge resection or lobectomy, and reported 5-year survival of resected hepatic metastases has been 60% to 70% [7]. However, liver resection is not recommended for poorly differentiated tumors [7]. Although surgery is the standard approach to dealing with hepatic metastases, several other methods are used, including gel-foam embolization, transhepatic arterial chemoembolization (TACE), hepatic artery embolization with radioactive microspheres, percutaneous alcohol ablation, radiofrequency ablation, or cryoablation. There are currently no high-quality studies that compare the surgical approach with the alternatives, and even resection of all hepatic metastases is supported by only case studies.

Advanced and metastatic disease
Systemic therapy in this situation consists of somatostatin analogues for symptom relief in functional PanNETs, as well as cytotoxic regimens. It is unclear whether cytotoxic therapy improves overall survival but some regimens have been shown

to have antitumor effects as single agents or in combination. The most used and studied cytotoxic agents include streptozocin (reported response rates have been as high as 70%) [4], doxorubicin, 5-FU, temozolomide, dacarbazine, and chlorozotocin. However, these regimens result in significant toxicities. Case series have also reported that advanced progression of PanNETs has had favorable responses to several radiolabeled somatostatin analogues (eg, octreotide, octreotate, edotreotide, and lanreotide with attached radionuclides of 177lutrium, 90ytrium, or 111indium). Overall, there is a lack of evidence for these measures and there remains a need for randomized controlled trials. Most recently, in May of 2011, the FDA approved 2 new targeted therapies for PanNETs (a tyrosine kinase inhibitor, sunitinib, and a mammalian target of rapamycin [mTOR] inhibitor, everolimus). There are currently placebo-controlled trials including sunitinib and everolimus that have shown, in abstract form, that both agents increase progression-free survival, and sunitinib also increases overall survival [1,13,14]. This finding is particularly interesting because, at Johns Hopkins, we recently found mTOR pathway genes, in addition to other novel cancer pathways, to be frequently altered in PanNETs [15].

Progressive or recurrent disease
There are no established guidelines for this type of disease and options have included reoperation (including debulking for symptom relief from space-occupying or hormonal effects) and systemic chemotherapy as described for advanced and metastatic disease. Therapy should be based on the individual's characteristics, site of recurrence, and prior therapy. One series reporting reoperation noted a 10-year survival of 72% [7].

SURVEILLANCE AND PROGNOSIS
PanNETs have an indolent course compared with pancreatic adenocarcinoma and therefore have a longer overall survival (50%–70%) [4]. However, prognosis is generally difficult to predict because the natural history of PanNETs is largely unknown. Five-year overall survival can range from 97% in benign insulinomas to 30% in metastatic nonfunctional tumors [11]. Therefore, all PanNETs should not be categorized together and they should be differentiated by the categories described earlier (ie, syndromic, functional, and nonfunctional). Because most PanNETs are nonfunctional and have a late presentation, about 65% of PanNETs are unresectable or metastatic (mostly to the regional lymph nodes and liver) on presentation [6].

After surgical resection, a surveillance program should be instituted to follow for recurrence and should be tailored to the patient and type of PanNET removed. This program typically involves some type of cross-sectional imaging and the following of tumor markers such as chromogranin A [16,17].

LATEST UPDATES
For most patients who are not eligible for surgery, many combinations of adjuvant therapy have been tried; however, this tumor is resistant to chemotherapy

and radiation. Before 2011, streptozocin was the only approved agent for unresectable disease. This agent was originally approved in 1984 and subsequent research has shed doubt on the efficacy of streptozocin [6]. The outlook for metastatic disease has been constant for several decades, with median survival time being 24 months and 5-year overall survival from 30% to 40% [6]. Because of its rarity, PanNETs have not been rigorously researched [2].

In May of 2011, the FDA approved both sunitinib and everolimus for the treatment of unresectable PanNETs. Sunitinib (Sutent; Pfizer, New York, NY, USA) is an oral multikinase inhibitor that inhibits vascular endothelial growth factor (VEGF) receptors and platelet-derived growth factor (PDGF) receptors, thereby affecting tumor angiogenesis and proliferation. Sunitinib provided increased progression-free survival as well as overall survival in a phase III, multicenter, double-blind, randomized, placebo-controlled trial [12]. Everolimus (Afinitor; Novartis Pharmaceuticals Co., East Hanover, NJ, USA) is an mTOR inhibitor and inhibits tumor angiogenesis, proliferation, and growth. Everolimus also has been shown in studies to increase progression-free survival by about 65% compared with placebo in unresectable patients (this effect is independent of somatostatin analogue or chemotherapy use) [11].

There are several ongoing clinical trials of the effectiveness of medical management of PanNETs. These trials include combination therapies (eg, everolimus with a somatostatin analogue, multikinase inhibitor with a monoclonal antibody to VEGF), radiolabeled somatostatin analogues, oral alkylating agents, and radioembolization for hepatic metastases. Other trials studying the treatment of hepatic metastases via surgical resection, TACE, or both, and early results suggest that, used in combination, they are more efficacious than resection alone or TACE alone, although this was not a specific study of PanNETs [18,19].

The National Cancer Institute convened a NET Task Force within the GI (gastrointestinal) Steering Committee to plan for clinical trials based on unmet needs while developing appropriate study end points, standardizing trial inclusion criteria, and establishing future goals for the PanNET studies [2]. Guidelines were established, including separating PanNETs from other GI NETs in trials, separating out poorly differentiated tumors when studying low-grade tumors, avoiding somatostatin analogue washout periods when possible when studying control of hormonal syndromes, including quality-of-life endpoints in clinical trials, and establishing progression-free survival as a feasible and relevant primary endpoint because of the long survival after progression of disease [2].

SUMMARY

PanNETs constitute a rare and heterogeneous group of pancreatic neoplasms whose overall prognosis is better than the more common pancreatic adenocarcinoma. Although surgery is the only treatment that provides a cure, many adjuvant therapies have been explored with some new, exciting, targeted therapies just approved for PanNETs. With growing interest in this type of neoplasm, an increasing number of clinical trials and natural history studies should shed light on the best management for these patients.

References

[1] NCI at NIH. Pancreatic neuroendocrine tumors (islet cell tumors) treatment (PDQ ®). Available at: http://www.cancer.gov/cancertopics/pdq/treatment/isletcell/HealthProfessional. Accessed April 2, 2012.

[2] Kulke MH, Siu LL, Tepper JE, et al. Future directions in the treatment of neuroendocrine tumors: consensus report of the national cancer institute neuroendocrine tumor clinical trials planning meeting. J Clin Oncol 2011;29(7):934–43.

[3] O'Grady HL, Conlon KC. Pancreatic neuroendocrine tumours. Eur J Surg Oncol 2008;34: 324–32.

[4] Johns Hopkins Medicine, The Sol Goldman Pancreatic Cancer Research Center. Islet cell tumors of the pancreas/endocrine neoplasms of the pancreas. Available at: http://pathology.jhu.edu/pc/TreatmentEndocrine.php?area=tr#causes. Accessed April 2, 2012.

[5] Rindi G. The ENETS guidelines: the new TNM classification system. Tumori 2010;96(5): 806–9.

[6] Oberstein PE, Saif MW. Novel agents in the treatment of unresectable neuroendocrine tumors. JOP 2011;12(4):358–61.

[7] Morrow EH, Norton JA. Management of pancreatic islet cell tumors excluding gastrinoma. In: Cameron JL, Cameron AM, editors. Current surgical therapy. 10th edition. Philadelphia: Elsevier Saunders; 2011. p. 456–60.

[8] Taouli B, Ghouadni M, Corréas JM, et al. Spectrum of abdominal imaging findings in von Hippel-Lindau disease. Am J Roentgenol 2003;181(4):1049–54.

[9] Goldman JA, Blanton WP, Hay DW, et al. False-positive secretin stimulation test for gastrinoma associated with the use of proton pump inhibitor therapy. Clin Gastroenterol Hepatol 2009;7(5):600–2.

[10] Gouya H, Vignaux O, Augui J, et al. CT, endoscopic sonography, and a combined protocol for preoperative evaluation of pancreatic insulinomas. Am J Roentgenol 2003;181(4): 987–92.

[11] Saif MW. Pancreatic neoplasm in 2011: an update. JOP 2011;12(4):316–21.

[12] Jensen RT, Fave GD. Promising advances in the treatment of malignant pancreatic endocrine tumors. N Engl J Med 2011;364(6):564–5.

[13] Raymond E, Dahan L, Raoul J-L, et al. Sunitinib malate for the treatment of pancreatic neuroendocrine tumors. N Engl J Med 2011;364(6):501–13.

[14] Yao JC, Shah MH, Ito T, et al. Everolimus for advanced pancreatic neuroendocrine tumors. N Engl J Med 2011;364(6):514–23.

[15] Jiao Y, Shi C, Edil BH, et al. DAXX/ATRX, MEN1, and mTOR pathway genes are frequently altered in pancreatic neuroendocrine tumors. Science 2011;331(6021):1199–203.

[16] Seregni E, Ferrari L, Bajetta E, et al. Clinical significance of blood chromogranin A measurement in neuroendocrine tumours. Ann Oncol 2001;12(Suppl 2):S69–72.

[17] Tomassetti P, Migliori M, Simoni P, et al. Diagnostic value of plasma chromogranin A in neuroendocrine tumors. Eur J Gastroenterol Hepatol 2001;13(1):55–8.

[18] Dimou AT, Syrigos KN, Saif MW. Neuroendocrine tumors of the pancreas: what's new. JOP 2010;11(2):135–8.

[19] Celinski SA, Nguyen KT, Steel JL, et al. Multimodality management of neuroendocrine tumors metastatic to the liver. 2010 Gastrointestinal Cancers Symposium. Pittsburgh (PA): UPMC Neuroendocrine Cancer Treatment Center; 2010.

INDEX

A

Abdominal aortic aneurysms, medical screening for, 102
  multivariate risk score, 106
  repair of, readmission rates following, 166–167
  ruptured, 101–102
  screening for, **101–109**
    new directions in, 105–107
    screening recommendations in, 105
    screening techniques for, 102–104
    screening trials in, 104–105

Abdominal surgery, readmission rates for, **155–170**

Adenoma, parathyroid. See *Hyperparathyroidism, primary.*

American College of Surgeons Oncology Group trials, 7–8, 11, 12, 13

Aneurysms, abdominal aortic. See *Abdominal aortic aneurysms.*

Axial imaging, in primary hyperparathyroidism, 177

Axilla, clinically negative, surgical approaches for, 4
  clinically positive, surgical approaches for, 3
  management of, in breast cancer, 3

Axillary node dissection, for breast cancer, evolution of, 1–3
  who should have or not have, **1–18**
  versus sentinel lymph node biopsy, 11–14

B

Bariatric operations, readmission rates following, 160–162

Breast, regional lymph nodes of, 2

Breast cancer, axillary surgery for, evolution of, 1–3
  lymph node biopsy in. See *Lymph node biopsy.*
  management of axilla in, 3

who should have or not have axillary node dissection with, **1–18**

C

Cancer, hereditary, identification of, 140
  predisposition syndromes, 138

Cancer clinical trials, and importance to all stakeholders, 269–270
  are they valid and useful for general surgeon and surgical oncologist ?, **269–281**
  enhancing applicability of, to real-world settings, 275–278
  participation in, 273–274
  valid and useful, considerations for, for general surgeon, 278–279
  versus real-world, in United States, 274
  why are they unique to persons with cancer ?, 270–271
  wide-scale dissemination and adoption of, 271–273

Cancer patient, genetic counselors as surgical ally in optimal care of, **137–153**

Candida, peristomal, 30

Capillary leak syndrome, trauma-induced, **237–253**
  abdominal compartment syndrome in, 242–243
  catabolism in, 241–242
  description of, 237
  diagnosis of, 238–239
  direct tissue injury in, 242
  epidemiology of, 238
  etiology of, 239–242
  fluid administration in, 240–241
  goal-directed resuscitation in, 246
  hemostatic resuscitation and, 245–246
  inflammation in, 240
  lung injury in, 243–244
  neurologic injury in, 244
  organ-specific effects of, 242–244
  pathophysiology of, 239–242
  postcapillary hypertension in, 242

0065-3411/12/$ – see front matter
Doi:10.1016/S0065-3411(12)00029-2

Moving?

Make sure your subscription moves with you!

To notify us of your new address, find your **Clinics Account Number** (located on your mailing label above your name), and contact customer service at:

Email: journalscustomerservice-usa@elsevier.com

800-654-2452 (subscribers in the U.S. & Canada)
314-447-8871 (subscribers outside of the U.S. & Canada)

Fax number: 314-447-8029

Elsevier Health Sciences Division
Subscription Customer Service
3251 Riverport Lane
Maryland Heights, MO 63043

*To ensure uninterrupted delivery of your subscription, please notify us at least 4 weeks in advance of move.